# The Legacy of Milton H. Erickson:

## Selected Papers of Stephen Gilligan

## *Other Works by Stephen Gilligan*

*Therapeutic Trances: The Cooperation Principle in Ericksonian Hypnotherapy*. New York: Brunner/Mazel, 1987.

*The Courage to Love: Principles and Practices of Self-Relations Psychotherapy*. New York: Norton, 1997.

### Edited Books

*Brief Therapy: Myths, Methods, Metaphors*. Edited by J. Zeig and S. Gilligan. New York: Brunner/Mazel, 1988.

*Therapeutic Conversations*. Edited by S. Gilligan and R. Price. New York: Norton, 1993.

For further information about books, tapes, and workshops by Stephen Gilligan, visit the website at: www.StephenGilligan.com.

# The Legacy of Milton H. Erickson:

## Selected Papers of Stephen Gilligan

*edited by*

Stephen Gilligan, Ph.D.

Zeig, Tucker, & Theisen, Inc.
Phoenix, Arizona

**Library of Congress Cataloging-in-Publication Data**

The legacy of Milton H. Erickson : selected papers of Stephen Gilligan / edited by Stephen Gilligan

p. cm.

Includes bibliographical references and index.

ISBN 1-891944-90-8 (alk. paper)

1. Hypnotism — Therapeutic use. 2. Erickson, Milton H. I. Erickson, Milton H. II. Gilligan, Stephen G., 1954–

RC495.L44 2002
615.89'162—dc21 2002035828



Published by

ZEIG, TUCKER & THEISEN, INC.
3614 North 24th Street
Phoenix, AZ 85016

Manufactured in the United States of America

10 9 8 7 6 5 4 3 2 1

**TO ZOE:**

May you find happiness

in this life.

Your dad loves you very much.

# Contents

## Contents

# *Foreword*

I first met Stephen Gilligan some twenty-five years ago when we were students at the University of California at Santa Cruz. At that time (in the mid-1970s) we were embarking on a remarkable journey that would be central to our later professional lives. We were both members of the original group of students who studied with Richard Bandler and John Grinder at the foundation of the field of NLP (Neuro-Linguistic Programming).

Bandler and Grinder were at the crest of the wave that was transforming psychology and our understanding of human thought and behavior — a revolution fueled by people such as Noam Chomsky, Gregory Bateson, Fritz Perls, Virginia Satir, and Milton Erickson. Bandler and Grinder had just begun their attempt to unravel some of the mysteries of Ericksonian hypnosis, identifying many of the key verbal patterns and non-verbal skills that Erickson applied in his remarkable psychiatric work. Bandler and Grinder would refine their ideas and try out their techniques by working with a group of devoted college students (whom they sometimes humorously referred to as cadets of their "Academy of Space").

Even though I joined the group relatively early on, Stephen already had the reputation as the "star student," rivaling Bandler and Grinder in skill, creativity and cleverness. I felt a deep connection with Stephen, perhaps because we shared an Irish heritage and Catholic upbringing in the San Francisco Bay area during the 1960s. Further, in addition to Grinder, Bandler, and Erickson, we were students of Gregory Bateson, and shared an admiration for Bateson's wisdom and integrity. I looked up to Stephen, admiring his commitment, complexity and depth, and have, to this day, found myself impressed over and over again with Stephen's brilliance.

# FOREWORD

Our paths diverged for some years beginning in the later 1970s. Stephen chose to focus on hypnosis and to attain a Ph.D. at prestigious Stanford University, while I concentrated on NLP. Stephen went on to become a leading teacher of Ericksonian hypnosis and psychotherapy all and change. Stephen shows clearly that Erickson functioned more from principles than technique, and emphasizes the deeper, generative nature of Erickson's work. Drawing also from his extensive experience with aikido and the martial arts, Stephen paints a rich portrait of Erickson's methods.

In recent years I have had the privilege of working together with Stephen again in a number of capacities. I have found Stephen's work in self-relations, sponsorship and relational archetypes some of the most personally stimulating and fertile developments in psychology and self-development in the last decade. The seminars that we have presented together, *Love in the Face of Violence* and *Skills of Sponsorship*, have been some of the most personally rewarding and transformational of my teaching career. And, as with Erickson, I have come to admire Stephen's heart as much as his mind.

Readers will find Stephen's writing style to be clear, sincere, insightful and pragmatic; it is also enriched by a good balance of self-revelation and humor (what Stephen refers to as his "Irish twinkle"). Furthermore, Stephen has an impressive ability to identify and formulate fundamental principles that can be applied in many different situations. Readers will walk away with both a deeper understanding of and a deeper appreciation for Erickson's work.

Robert Dilts
Santa Cruz, California
January, 2000

# *Introduction*

I first met Milton Erickson 27 years ago. I was a 19-year old college kid desperately trying to find his way in the world. I had always been interested in psychology, but felt deadened by the pathology-oriented emphasis of most clinical approaches. Erickson's creative, life-affirming approach resonated deep within me, and his human presence touched me profoundly. My soul caught fire, and its flame still burns to this day (despite my frequent inattention to it). For this I am forever grateful to Dr. Erickson and the legacy that he left.

This book contains many of the chapters and articles I have written about that legacy. I have arranged them more or less chronologically, so the reader might see a certain progression that has occurred over the years. For example, one can see a gradual shift from a technical, more hierarchical position to a more relational one. Also, the therapeutic use of altered states generally broadens from an emphasis on hypnotic trance in the early chapters to include additional body-mind healing states in later chapters.

Even with these changes, however, certain ideas remain constant. The most basic one is the principle of utilization, which I believe is Erickson's great contribution to psychotherapy. Erickson brilliantly showed how the person's problem or symptoms could be accepted and used as the basis for creative solutions. A second basic idea has to do with the profound intelligence of the unconscious, primarily when it is incorporated into a human relationship that includes cognitive cooperation skills. A third idea has to do with the creative relationship between therapist and client that can supersede the capacities of therapist or client alone.

In reading back through some of the chapters, I more than occasionally was embarrassed by the wordiness and inaccessibiity of some of the writing, especially the earlier pieces. I hope the reader will kindly bear with me through some of this earlier writing, if only to realize that even the most heady of writers can gradually evolve.

Jeff Zeig once commented that while there have been a number of extraordinary psychotherapists, few could match Milton Erickson's record of inspiring a younger generation of clinicians to teach and carry on his work. So much has been written by a diverse number of students. My own work is but a single example of how one could continue Erickson's legacy.

In this regard, I will conclude with a brief story. Near the end of the five years I studied with Milton Erickson, I asked him how I could pay him back for all of the generosity and help he gave me. He replied, in his kind, mischievous way, "Whatever you have found useful to you during this time, you can repay me by passing it on to others!" This book is an attempt to do just that: pass on the extraordinary legacy left by an extraordinary human being. Whatever you find here that is useful to you, keep passing it to others!

Stephen Gilligan, Ph.D.
March, 2002

# Part I:

# Theoretical Views

## Chapter 1

# ERICKSONIAN APPROACHES TO CLINICAL HYPNOSIS[1]

I would like to discuss in this paper what I consider to be some essential aspects of an Ericksonian approach to hypnosis and hypnotherapy. I want to first contrast briefly the Ericksonian view of the hypnotic relationship to other more traditional views, and then to identify what I consider to be the general principles of communication in the Ericksonian approach and their application to the specific situation of hypnotic inductions. Finally, I want to comment about the need for integrity in applying these principles and techniques. Each of these topics is a major one, and in a short discussion I can convey only a general sense of their significance. Therefore, my remarks will be highly selective and necessarily incomplete. A more comprehensive treatment of these issues can be found in *Therapeutic Trances: The Cooperation Principle in Ericksonian Hypnotherapy*.

## THE HYPNOTIC RELATIONSHIP

The first issue is the nature of the hypnotic relationship. Below I list the three main views of the hypnotic relationship: (1) the authoritarian approach; (2) the standardized approach; and (3) the utilization approach.

The *authoritarian approach* emphasizes the power of the hypnotist. This approach, spawned by Mesmer and others, is still explicitly exploited by stage

---

[1] This essay appeared previously in Jeffrey K. Zeig. 1982. *Ericksonian approaches to hypnosis and psychotherapy*. New York: Brunner/Mazel.

hypnotists and is consequently often the conceptualization held by the uninformed layperson. Even many trained clinicians implicitly adhere to this view, which in its extreme form involves some powerful and charismatic operator (usually a male) exercising some strange power over some hapless and weak-willed subject (often a female). In essence, the operator gets the subject to do something he or she wouldn't ordinarily do (e.g., bark like a dog or stop smoking). This approach generally assumes that the unconscious is some passive receptacle into which suggestions are "placed" or some fertile ground which the hypnotist "digs into" so that he can "plant" suggestions. Frankly, I don't think the unconscious should be treated like a piece of dirt. For this and other reasons — such as the fact that direct suggestions generally don't work very well, and people often don't like to be told authoritatively what to do — this approach has rather limited value.

Many people have realized these limitations and subsequently developed what might be called the *standardized approach*. This conceptualization, adhered to by many experimentalists, is in part a reaction to the misplaced emphasis of the authoritarian approach on the power of the hypnotist. The standardized approach generally assumes that hypnotic responsiveness is determined by some inherent trait or ability of the subject. The hypnotist really isn't important — the subject is either hypnotizable or he isn't. This view further assumes that you can assess a person's "susceptibility" to trance by presenting 10 or 20 minutes of standardized and repetitive suggestions and then administering some quick behavioral tests, such as hand immobility or heaviness. If the subject passes most of these tests, he is considered a good hypnotic subject; otherwise, too bad. I might note that the hypnotist is considered so unimportant in this approach that suggestions are sometimes put on tape. So, if you're a busy person, you can put the tape on, go out and drink coffee for 10 or 20 minutes, and then come back and administer the tests.

There is nothing inherently wrong with this approach, especially in a research setting, where sometimes it is necessary. However, it doesn't work very well for a lot of subjects, especially those in clinical situations. The standardized approach interprets the large percentage of unresponsive subjects as evidence that some people are just not susceptible to the phenomenon of trance. I think their unresponsiveness is more a reflection of the limitations of the approach. The standardized inductions are usually poor in quality and essentially tell the subject to relax about 40 or 50 times. The standardized form demands that the subject attempt to fit his experience into some predetermined structure; it cannot handle or utilize any difficulties a subject might be having, such as a nagging internal dialogue.

Another problem in the standardized approach is that trance is defined in terms of the number of behavioral items passed on a test. I think this is like defining love in terms of the number of kisses emitted by a person or saying that I can't dance because I don't know the fox trot. I think this approach misses a major point about trance: *It is a subjective internal experience whose behavioral manifestations will vary across individuals.*

This point is central to the Ericksonian approach, which I put under the heading of being the *utilization approach.* In contrast to the authoritarian and standardized approaches, it stresses the *interactional* nature of the hypnotic relationship. Neither hypnotist nor subject is of prime importance; what is of major importance is the *interaction* between the two. The hypnotic endeavor is a *cooperative* effort in which responsibility is mutually assumed. The hypnotist's task is to guide and supervise the subject; the subject's task is to decide if, how, and when to respond to the hypnotist's communications.

The utilization approach also assumes that each person is unique in terms of the strategies used to create his or her own experience and that, consequently, the hypnotist's effectiveness depends upon how well he is able to adapt his strategies to those of a given subject. Thus, standardized communications are not used. The approach further assumes that unconscious processes can operate in an intelligent, autonomous, and creative fashion, and that people have stored in their unconscious all the resources necessary to transform their experience. This is what trance is all about: It is an opportunity for the subject to set aside his identification with any limiting conscious processes and shift into a context (i.e., trance) where he/she can access and utilize unconscious resources for therapeutic gain.

## PRINCIPLES OF ERICKSONIAN COMMUNICATION

The question thus becomes: How does the hypnotist facilitate hypnotic processes in the subject? Instead of standardized techniques, he has to use general principles to guide his efforts. I consider the most important of these principles to be: (1) accept and utilize the client's reality; (2) pace and lead the subject's behavior; and (3) interpret "resistance" as lack of pacing.

The first principle — accept and utilize — was stressed again and again by Erickson and is the essential theme of Erickson and Rossi's *Hypnotherapy*

(1979). Briefly stated, *accepting* means assuming and communicating to the subject that "What you're doing at this point in time is exactly what I'd like you to be doing. It's fine; it's perfect." *Utilizing* means assuming and communicating the attitude that "What you're doing right now is exactly that which will allow you to do X." The process of accepting and utilizing is one of communicating that what the subject is doing is fine *and* it will allow him/her to do something else (e.g., experience trance).

Bandler and Grinder (1975) discussed these principles in the more process-oriented terms of *pacing and leading the subject's behavior.* Pacing communications essentially feed back the subject's experience; they add nothing new. Their major intent is to enhance the rapport between hypnotist and subject. This enables the subject to be more trustful and cooperative and the hypnotist to be more understanding. Once rapport has been developed, the hypnotist can *lead* by introducing behaviors that are different from, but consistent with, the subject's present state and slightly closer to the desired state (e.g., trance).

According to these principles of Ericksonian communication, the effective hypnotic communicator assumes all experience is valid and utilizable and then behaviorally paces and leads toward the desired state. He freely admits that he does not know exactly which path will lead to the desired state and really does not know which techniques will work best. But he does know that he can "get in tune with" the subject, thereby establishing a rhythmic, continuous feedback loop in which one closely observes, accepts, and utilizes the subject's ongoing response. In this sort of interaction, the trek toward the desired state unfolds in a nonlinear, spiral-like fashion.

Within this feedback loop of interaction, the principles of pacing and leading can be applied in many different ways and at many different levels. One of the simplest forms of pacing and leading involves direct verbal description of the subject's ongoing behavior. This is often a good way to start a hypnotic induction. For example, you, as hypnotist, might note to a subject:

1. You're sitting there, (*pacing statement*)
2. You're looking at me, (*pacing statement*)
3. You're breathing in and out, (*pacing statement*)
4. Eyes blinking up and then down, (*pacing statement*)
5. And as you shift in your chair, (*pacing statement*)
6. You can also begin to shift into a state of comfortable relaxation. (*leading statement*)

The first five clauses are all pacing statements; they simply describe the undeniable reality of the subject's observable behaviors. The final clause, however, uses pacing to introduce a leading statement (develop relaxation).

Of course, just any leading statement will not do. Sometimes you will lead too quickly or inappropriately. But that's fine; you simply observe how the subject responds and pace and utilize that. If he/she follows, fine, that becomes your new state to pace; if not, fine, simply pace what he/she is doing. This whole interaction is one of pacing and leading, pacing and leading, again and again and again and again.

Pacing and leading can be done nonverbally, too. For instance, if you wanted to calm down an excited client, you could begin to mirror or reflect back his nonverbal excitedness by speaking in the same breathless, high-pitched and frantic way. After a while you could begin to lead by slowing down just a bit and relaxing just a bit more. If you lead too quickly and the subject continues in his frenetic rhythm, that's fine; you can shift back into the quick pace once again, talking about how fast things can really get and then again begin to gradually slow down. You can continue this process until the subject reaches the desired state.

Another way to nonverbally pace and lead is to synchronize one of your behavioral parameters — such as the tonal inflections in your voice — to a different behavioral parameter of the subject — say his breathing rate — so that every time he breathes out, your tonal inflection goes down. You might nod your head subtly every time the subject blinks his eyes and then begin to nod occasionally when the subject is not blinking. This leading can be gradually increased to the point that you can elicit eyelid flutters from the subject, a response that can easily be utilized to develop a trance. This technique, which I call *cross-behavioral pacing and leading*, is usually quite effective. It is indirect and thus bypasses the subject's conscious processes.

Pacing and leading can be more complex and sophisticated. For example, a co-therapist and I worked with a psychotic who terrorized the psychiatrists on his ward with gross hallucinations of dead babies, hot dogs coming out of his ears, and other bizarre images. When we first interviewed him, he looked wildly about and asked us if we saw the hallucinations. We agreed with him in a matter-of-fact fashion and then looked crazily into space before asking him if he saw *our* hallucinations. Of course, this was all done quite elaborately and dramatically. He was understandably stunned by our response. He tried to counter with more hallucinations, which we again accepted and then led by introducing more of our own. After a while we disappointedly confessed that we had asked to see him because we were interested in becoming better hallucinators and had been told that he was an expert. However, we pointed out, there had obviously been a mistake; after all, we had 10 good hallucinations, while he only had three mediocre ones. Besides, we continued, the guy on the next ward had half a dozen hallucinations of a much better variety.

Needless to say, this produced a state of confusion in the patient, which we used by offering to teach him to be a better hallucinator. He agreed, so over the next several months we showed him how to generate other hallucinations, how to hallucinate in a relaxed fashion, and how to have comforting hallucinations. We gradually led from scary and uncontrolled hallucinative processes, to more relaxed and valuable sorts of hallucinations, and then to dropping hallucinations altogether.

Another client of mine was a successful corporate president who suffered from intense internal conflicts. As part of the therapeutic strategy I hypnotized him and had him visualize himself at a "board meeting" where all of the different "parts" of himself were present. He was directed to use his position as "chairman" to solve the various disagreements between the "board members." This was done over several sessions and produced favorable results.

The point to be drawn from these examples is that you take what the person gives you and use it. That becomes your strategy. One of the profound consequences of this way of thinking and acting is that there really is no such thing as "resistance" in a utilization approach. *Everything the person is doing is exactly what you would like him to be doing.* Your task is to generate communications that use ongoing experiences. When you are not fully using them, the subject will tell you, usually indirectly and nonverbally. You will find yourself accusing the person of being "resistant" or branding him/her as "nonsusceptible." You are reacting to communications from the subject that are saying, "What you're doing is not pacing me at this time. You're not using some behavior or experience of mine." Neither the hypnotist nor the subject is a "bad person" or "wrong" or "sick" or "crazy." "Resistance" is just a message that you need to synchronize yourself with the subject again. I think this is a radical concept that is incredibly useful to the clinician.

## THE PROCESS OF INDUCTION

How do these utilization principles apply to the specific situation of inductions? The main strategies or principles that the Ericksonian hypnotist uses to induce trance are: (1) secure and maintain the subject's attentional absorption; (2) access and develop unconscious processes (associational strategies); and (3) pace and distract conscious processes (dissociational strategies).

The first thing you want to do in an induction is to secure the subject's attention and then maintain that absorption. To do this, you use nonverbal processes in certain ways: (1) stay externally oriented; (2) remain flexible; (3) communicate meaningfully; and (4) be confident.

The first — staying externally oriented — is critical, because your major task as a hypnotist is to use the subject's ongoing processes. It is therefore rather important that you remain aware of what the subject is doing all the time. To best do this, you might develop what Bandler and Grinder call an *up-time state*, which I call an *externally-oriented trance*. In this state the hypnotist breathes comfortably and focuses fully and continually on the subject. He gets into a rhythmic feedback loop where he feels strong contact with the subject. In this state the hypnotist's behavior is not mediated by conscious processes; rather, he allows himself to drop into trance and let his unconscious respond. Stated another way, the sole contents of the hypnotist's consciousness are the subject's behavior, rather than the internal imagery that normally pervades thinking processes. It is as if the notion of mind extends beyond the normal boundaries of the body to include the subject. This is not a state of total empathy; it is a paradoxical state in which the hypnotist simultaneously experiences complete rapport with the subject *and* an observational detachment from the interaction. This process enhances both the hypnotist's and subject's feelings of rapport. It also helps both participants to develop focused but effortless styles of processing. Furthermore, it helps the hypnotist to detect subtle aspects of the subject's experience.

Now all of this may sound a bit strange, but I train my students to develop and use this style of processing while operating as hypnotists. Most of them find it easy to develop and almost all of them claim that it markedly enhances their effectiveness as hypnotists. It is a process not unlike those used by great entertainers and athletes. These master practitioners spend endless hours using conscious, analytical processes to develop and refine their skills, but they "stop thinking" and let their unconscious do it for them when it comes time for the actual performance. An effective Ericksonian hypnotherapist thinks long and hard before and after a clinical session, but while actually interacting with a client, he lets his unconscious use the products of those contemplations.

I learned of this process from Erickson, who used it rather often. For example, during the early part of my training with him I watched him do a marvelous piece of work with a patient. Assuming that his sophisticated strategies had to be generated from complex conscious cognitions, I was determined to identify the exact thought processes he used. After the patient left, I poised pencil on paper and resolutely began to interrogate him.

"Milton, do you make a lot of pictures?"

"No," he slowly but firmly stated.

"No pictures," I muttered, crossing that category out on my sheet. "OK. Do you have a lot of internal dialogue in that situation?"

"No," he again convincingly replied.

"OK. No internal dialogue. Let me write that down here. OK. Well, do you have kinesthetic sensations? You know, feelings in the body, that sort of thing."

"No."

I was beginning to grow both suspicious and confused. "Let's see. No pictures, no internal dialogue, no kinesthetic sensation. Well, Milton, I don't understand. How do you know what to do?"

"I don't know. I don't know what I'm going to do, I don't know what I'm going to say. All I know is that I trust my unconscious to shelve into my conscious that which is appropriate. And I don't know how they're going to respond. All I know is that *they will respond.* I don't know why. I don't know when. All I know is that they'll respond in an appropriate fashion, in a way which best suits them as an individual. And so I become intrigued with wondering exactly *how* their unconscious will choose to respond. And so I comfortably await their response, knowing that when it occurs, I can accept and utilize it."

He paused, his eyes twinkling. "Now I know that sounds ridiculous. *But it works*!!"

And after my initial confusion, I checked it out and found that indeed it did work.

The second process involves *remaining flexible* when you're in this externally-oriented trance state. If a technique doesn't work, fine, use another one. If a communication does not seem appropriate, fine, shift to a different one. *There are really no mistakes you can make in well-intentioned hypnotic communication.* There are only outcomes, and every outcome is useful. You offer behavioral communications and then observe and use the responses. To do this, you must really stay in tune with the subject, not trying to fit him/her into any rigid, preformed category.

Another interaction I had with Erickson illustrates the importance of this point. It was one of the most important learning experiences in my life. After years of diligently studying his approach, I felt I had a fairly good grasp of his sophisticated strategies, yet clearly sensed that I was lacking something. My work was not as effective as I knew it could be, but I was unclear about how I was limiting myself. Finally, on the last day of a week-long visit with Erickson, I respectfully requested some guidance in the matter. Instead of launching one of his lengthy and indirect answers, he stated in a simple but intensely meaningful fashion, "You've got a tendency to overcompartmentalize your experience, and it gets in the way of your unconscious." He then immediately ended the session.

As I walked out with a colleague, I confessed my disappointment about not being given any useful feedback, but sympathetically suggested that it was because Erickson was getting old, and besides, he never did have a good conscious understanding of what he did. In other words, I "compartmentalized" his response! Several months later, at the end of a similar training session, I again advanced the question, to which he replied a bit more sternly, "You've got a tendency to overcompartmentalize your experience, and it gets in the way of your unconscious!" My disappointment was even more marked this time, for Erickson was clearly getting a bit senile; he didn't even remember what he had told me before.

Four months later, my despair deepened when a third phrasing of the question was met with the same response. Why was Milton being so uninformative? Why couldn't he remember what he had told me before? Did he give such unhelpful advice on such matters to all his students? If so, what happened to his emphasis on unique solutions for each person? I gave the question one more try several months later, to which he replied: "You've got a tendency to overcompartmentalize your experience, and it gets in the way of your unconscious!" FLASH!! Four times and eight months later, I was startled with the blinding (or rather unblinking) insight: *I had a tendency to overcompartmentalize my experience, and did it ever get in the way of my unconscious*!! When I finally looked at Erickson, his eyes were twinkling. "That's right," he said softly.

My realization really unfolded and developed over the next months. It became all too clear that most of my time as a hypnotist was spent in internal dialogue, trying to classify the subject's behavior and then come up with some sophisticated response. The more I indulged in these conceptual evaluations, the less I attended to what the subject was actually experiencing and doing. In addition, I was forced to "objectify" the subject into this or that class, thereby limiting the degree of possible rapport. As I relinquished the need for such "compartmentalizations," my appreciation of the uniqueness of each individual grew. Most importantly, my communications became more fitting and my work more effective.

Of course, I sometimes find myself mired again in this evaluative mode. But when I do, I think back to Erickson's simple but persistent suggestion. It is difficult to resist such a suggestion.

The final two points are that you must communicate in a meaningful and confident fashion to the subject. This process was a major part of what Erickson emphasized in his writings. Your nonverbal delivery must unequivocally communicate to the subject that what you're saying is important and that he/she can respond to it. In many respects your nonverbal communication is more important than your verbalizations. If what you're saying *seems* meaningful and important, the person will feel compelled to respond.

Once the subject is attentive, you use rapport to develop unconscious processes; that is, you want to develop hypnotic experiences in the subject. You can accomplish this in a number of ways. A nice technique to begin an induction is with questions that access trance-relevant experiences from the person's memory. For instance, you might ask general questions:

- Do you remember what you felt like during your last trance?
- What did it feel like when you were in the deepest trance you've ever been in?

Or, if the subject has no previous trance experience:

- Can you imagine and begin to describe to me what it would be like for you to begin to develop a trance?
- Do you remember a time when you felt very relaxed?

Or, if you wish to develop a particular trance phenomenon, such as age regression, you might ask more specific questions:

- Did you have a nickname as a child?
- Did you have a favorite game as a youngster?
- Did you have an imaginary playmate as a child?

There are countless numbers of these questions, which essentially ask the subject to revivify some naturalistic experience relevant to trance processes. It is important to realize that the subject's response to such inquiries will depend in large part on *how* they are delivered. Generally speaking, the subject will access and become absorbed in the revivified experiences to the extent that the hypnotist asks the question(s) in a meaningful, compelling, and expectant fashion.

The subject's responses can then be developed, either through further questions or through other, more elaborate techniques. Many of these techniques are well known already, so I will not say much about them except that most traditional techniques are suitable, as long as you adapt them to the particular subject. For example, you might use progressive relaxation techniques with kinesthetically-oriented subjects, or guided imagery methods with visually-oriented persons. With a person whose conscious processes (e.g., internal dialogue) interfere with the development of trance, you might tell metaphorical stories. Such stories, which were a trademark of Erickson's work, have content that is dissimilar to the subject's experience or problems, but specify processes or themes that are quite similar to those salient in the subject's experience. So you talk about other people going into a trance, or interactions with other clients, or even personal experiences. The subject is consciously distracted because he/she thinks, "Gee, that's not about me," and yet unconsciously identifies with the story and thus gains access to the experiences suggested by it.

This last point leads to the third induction principle, that of pacing and distracting the conscious processes. Distraction or confusion techniques are useful because accessing techniques alone will generally be effective only to the extent that the subject allows them to be. That is, the subject not only must be willing to participate, but must also be *able* to let unconscious experiences develop. Many subjects have difficulty doing this. Specifically, their conscious processes interfere by continually questioning, analyzing, or trying to help with the development of the hypnotic experience. To the extent that such conscious participation occurs, the hypnotist needs to employ techniques and strategies that depotentiate such interference.

There are many ways in which this can be done. For example, the hypnotist can use techniques that totally occupy the subject's internal processes with tasks irrelevant to the trance development. One such technique involves instructing the subject to count backwards (silently) from a thousand to one, by three's. While the subject does this, the hypnotist goes on with his induction patter. If the subject seems to be able to do this without any problem, you can use an overloading technique such as having him verbalize the letters of the alphabet in a forward fashion while visualizing them backward. The subject begins by verbalizing an "a" to himself, and at the same visualizing the letter "z"; the letter "b" is then verbalized while "y" is visualized; and so on. If you try this yourself, you quickly will realize how overloading and disorienting it can be. Meanwhile back at the unconscious, the hypnotist is using accessing techniques for the development of trance.

In addition to distraction techniques, Erickson developed a large body of confusion techniques. Briefly stated, underlying the use of confusion techniques are the following assumptions: (1) there are many automatic and predictable patterns in a person's behavioral processes; (2) the unexpected discontinuation of any of these patterns will create an uncertainty state dominated by undifferentiated arousal (e.g., confusion); (3) the arousal will increase unless the person can cognitively attribute it to something; (4) most people strongly dislike uncertainty states and are motivated to avoid them; (5) consequently, most people will grab onto the first thing that enters their consciousness that reduces the uncertainty.

Based on these assumptions, most confusion techniques involve the following five steps:

1. *Identify* a dominant pattern in the subject's behavior.
2. *Pace* the pattern for awhile.
3. *Interrupt* or *overload* the pattern in a way which confuses the subject.
4. *Amplify* the confusion a bit.
5. *Use* the confusion by introducing a simple leading statement (e.g., "drop into trance").

These principles can be understood through a few examples. My first experience of involuntarily dropping into trance illustrates how relatively simple interruption techniques are easily effected. I was sitting in Erickson's office. As I intently listened to him tell a number of metaphorical stories, I was strongly dominated by the cognitive pattern of analyzing and then "compartmentalizing" every statement he made in terms of what it "really" meant. I was therefore startled when all of a sudden he intently looked at my hand, pointed to it, and said in the most surprised and incredulous fashion, "Isn't that your left hand *not* lifting? . . . Yet? . . . Now?" My recollection of the experience is still rather hazy. All I remember is seeing the room swimming about and feeling my hand beginning to involuntarily float upwards. I found myself looking right into Erickson's eyes as he said, "That's right, close your eyes and drop into trance *nowww*!!!" Believe me, I did so at once. He then added, "And let your unconscious do the work for you." I did that also. The most effective confusion techniques are those that use the very pattern that is keeping the person out of trance — in this case, my "compartmentalization" processes — as the basis for the induction. Again, whatever the person is doing is exactly that which will allow him to experience trance.

Other confusion techniques involve *overloading* the subject's conscious processes. For example, a double induction is a process in which two hypnotists perform simultaneous inductions on one subject. The hypnotists play off each other, both verbally and nonverbally. After a while, most subjects find it nearly impossible to continue to pay full attention to all they are experiencing. Some simply give up and retreat into trance; others become so disoriented that simply instructing them to "let go fully and simply drop all the way into trance" is usually quite effective. Many clinicians tell me that they like this double induction technique, but they can't use it because they work alone. There is no need for despair. A modified procedure is to instruct the subject to pay close attention to a taped induction. While the tape is playing, you do a "live" induction in the other ear.

Confusional overload can also be accomplished by telling stories involving spatial and/or temporal disorientation. One story I have found to be particularly effective involves an automobile trip in which the driver is unclear about the exact sequence of directional turns. An abbreviated example of this technique, which I call the *autohypnosis directional maneuver*, is as follows:

(After about 15 minutes of general inductional communications)

> And there are so many directions you can follow when you allow your unconscious to do it for you . . . just as there are many different directions you can follow physically . . . I'll give you an example. . . . Some summers ago, I was traveling all alone on the highway in my car, just paying close attention to the sound of the engine, and knowing that slowly but surely I was heading into another state. And in that state there was a particular destination I was headed for, a particular person I wished to see, a particular experience I was looking forward to in that other state. . . . However, while I knew the general set of directions regarding how to get to where I wanted to go, I could not for the life of me remember the proper order in which those turns occurred. I did know that from where I was *there* then, I thought to myself, I don't want to be *here now*; I want to be *there now*, and all I can remember is that to get *there now*, or at least soon from *now* from *here*, I take a com-

> bination of three *right* turns and three *left* turns . . . but I don't know quite which is the *right* series of *rights* and *lefts* . . . but I do want to get *there* and I am *here now*, and so I said, all *right, pay attention very closely* (embedded suggestion to subject), because we've got to make it *right* or we'll be *left* behind. . . . And *then* I said, all *right*, let's begin. . . . I'll take a *right here* (I think that's *right*), and *then* a *left* and *now* I'm *left* with two *lefts* and two *rights*. So all *right*, I'll take another *left*, which means I'm now *left* with a *left* and a *right* and a *right*. *If* I take a *right*, I'll be *left* with a *right* and a *left*, but if I take a *left*, I'll be *left* with a *right* and another *right*. . . . But I don't think that is *right*, so I'll take a *right* first, and *then a left*, and *now* I'm *left* with a *right*, and so I take the *right*, and . . . dead end. It's the *wrong* way. And so now I've got to go back to the starting point, so as not to get completely *left* behind . . . so I begin to backtrack and *now* take three *rights* and three *lefts* again, except that each turn is *now* the opposite from the other direction . . . *Everything is reversed*. . . . Now which was *then* a *right* is *now* a *left* . . . and that which was *left then* is *now a right* . . . so for every *right then* it is *right now* to take a *left* . . . and for every *left then* it is *right now* to take a *right*, and *now* I'm back at the beginning, ready to begin again . . . and so I begin. . . .

You can then repeat the story with a different sequence of directions and continue until the subject looks completely confused, at which point you can offer trance suggestions within the story. For example, to continue from above:

> And after a while I became so tired, so confused, that I didn't know and didn't care where to turn next. . . . I couldn't tell a *right* from a *left*, nor a *left* from a *left*. . . . I couldn't figure out whether taking a *left* was *right*, or whether taking a *right* was *right*. So I pulled off to the side of the road, turned off the engine, and sat there with my eyes closed, and said to myself, "*To hell with trying to figure it out. Stop all this activity and just relax into a trance!!*" (This statement is uttered in a slower, softer, but more intense and emphatic fashion.) And I did. (The hypnotist now shifts to a more relaxed, almost relieved tone.) . . . And I was able to *just allow that trance to develop*. . . . There was the recognition that there is no need to pay attention to anything except the need to attend to one's own internal needs . . . and what a nice thing to know that you can simply let *your unconscious do the work for you*.

All of these statements are valid and consistent with each other. Also, the effectiveness of the story depends in large part on the hypnotist's nonverbal communications. As with any Ericksonian technique, the hypnotist needs to capture and maintain the subject's conscious attention and must therefore speak meaningfully, impressively, and congruently. In addition, because the intent is to create and then use informational overload, the hypnotist begins with a relatively quick tempo, increases and intensifies it even more when the subject starts to get confused, but then dramatically reduces it (to a slower, softer voice) right at the point of utilization. Finally, it is quite useful to employ special tonal markings to subtly emphasize both (a) the directional and ambiguous terms (e.g., right/left), and (b) the several embedded suggestions regarding paying attention and dropping into trance. When these and other nonverbal techniques are judiciously applied, the story will usually work quite well as an induction device.

One final technique for depotentiating conscious processes is boredom. As Erickson used to say, "I've got an unconscious mind, and they've got an unconscious mind. Therefore, as long as we're in the room together, sooner or later they'll go into trance. And if nothing else works, I'll bore them into trance. It might take them five minutes, 10 minutes, 30 minutes, one hour, several hours, or many hours. That's fine; I can wait." And, boy, could he ever wait. You might tell two or three hours of metaphorical stories, gradually wearing down the person to the point that he/she is unable or unwilling to offer any conscious resistances to shifting into trance. In fact, many people retreat into trance to get away from all those boring stories.

To summarize, induction is a process in which the hypnotist uses his body as a musical instrument, tuning it to get into rhythm with the "behavioral dance" of the subject. The hypnotist works to secure and hold the subject's attentional processes, thereby making it possible to access unconscious processes to develop hypnotic experiences. To the extent that the subject's conscious processes interfere with this development, the hypnotist uses distraction, confusion, and boredom techniques. In short, the most effective induction strategy is one that maximally uses the subject's ongoing experience as the basis for trance development.

## THE INTEGRITY OF THE HYPNOTIST

Before closing, I'd like to comment briefly on the issue of integrity. Simply put, the principles, strategies, and techniques of the Ericksonian approach are incredibly powerful tools. And while tools are value-free, *their capacity to enhance or create is equivalent to their potential to oppress or destroy*. I think that one need only look at similarities in the communication patterns of great humanitarians like Christ and great oppressors like Hitler to realize this. The important point here is that the effect of a tool on the quality of human experience depends on its user. Consequently, the integrity of the hypnotist is a major issue.

Incidentally, I don't think you can ignore this issue, even if you try. As Bateson, Haley, and others have pointed out, you cannot *not* affect another person's behavior. In this sense, all behavior is manipulation. What the Ericksonian approach does is make explicit a lot of the ways in which we are constantly influencing each other. By becoming aware of such patterns, you can use them systematically; that is, you can align your behavior with your intent, thereby making you a powerful communicator. What becomes critical, then, is getting clear about your intent.

*This is not a trivial matter to be sidestepped or disregarded.* In training mental health professionals, I have noticed that failing to come to grips with it creates many problems. Some trainees have difficulty acknowledging that they can and do powerfully influence human behavior and thus find themselves unable to use Ericksonian techniques in any powerfully effective fashion. Other trainees are initially overpowered by an insecure need to prove themselves and consequently wield techniques in a domineering and insensitive fashion. Both types of students are controlled by their ability to manipulate, the former by attempting to dissociate from it, the latter by using it irresponsibly. In both cases, the true power to enhance experience is stifled.

Once a person becomes aware of the intent and effect of his behavior, he can use communication in a powerful manner. Here the issue of integrity becomes particularly important. By integrity I mean the degree to which the hypnotist is able to *refrain* from imposing his own solutions and beliefs on the subject, to *refrain* from having to prove his own worth at the subject's expense, and instead fully to *support* the person in his/her quest for change.

The hypnotist's integrity has many practical consequences. Lacking integrity, even the highly skilled hypnotherapist will find that his clients can develop hypnotic phenomena but *not* hypnotherapeutic changes; or they will become impressed with his abilities but *not* their own; or they will try to take on his beliefs and lifestyle, rather than developing their own. In short, the hypnotist lacking integrity will be in no position to really help the client.

Conversely, the hypnotist operating with integrity can easily secure rapport with the client. By trusting the hypnotist, the client begins to trust himself more. He consequently becomes more willing to examine his shortcomings and more able to develop new ways of being. He also becomes more willing, both in trance and waking states, to comply with directives, no matter how strange or bizarre they may seem. This is important to the Ericksonian practitioner, who uses many unorthodox strategies.

In fact, I firmly believe that the most powerful aspect of Erickson's communication was his integrity. Before training with him, I would read about all these wild things he did with his patients and I could never quite figure out how he could get these people to cooperate with him. After watching him in action, it became crystal clear that he had an unwavering intention to fully respect and support his patients and students. He wasn't out to manipulate or control for his own personal gains. Consequently, people would really let go and fully cooperate with him.

In conclusion, this whole issue of integrity needs to be thought about long, hard, and often. You must dearly decide whether you wish to support or oppress others. Of course, the second choice cannot always be implemented. Most hypnotic subjects will quickly learn to distrust and hence not cooperate with a nonsupportive hypnotist. Choosing to *support* the subject is a lot easier, since there really can be no "resistance" when one is totally aligned with another individual. Besides, it's a far more personally satisfying and professionally effective position. Simply stated, the more integrity you develop, the more fun and success you are likely to experience, and I think that's what "it" is all about.

# Chapter 2

# SYMPTOM PHENOMENA AS TRANCE PHENOMENA[1]

The major thesis of this chapter is that inherent in symptom phenomena are naturalistic versions of classical hypnotic phenomena. The interactional sequence leading to symptomatic expressions is viewed as a hypnotic induction, and the resulting symptom phenomena are acknowledged as hypnotic trance phenomena. This view allows therapists to accept symptoms as legitimate hypnotic expressions already being practiced by the client, and thus to work to transform such admittedly self-devaluing acts into self-valuing, flexible solutions.

The approach taken here is based on the utilization principle pioneered by Milton Erickson. Erickson (1948, 1952, 1959, 1965) advocated accepting and amplifying the client's processes as the means for therapeutic changes. His special emphasis on the relevance of hypnosis in this regard continues to be developed by his students, and one of the major contributions of Ericksonian psychotherapy has been to elucidate the relationship between hypnotic processes and symptomatic processes.

## SIMILARITIES OF SYMPTOM PHENOMENA AND HYPNOTIC PHENOMENA

A central assumption is that a person expressing a symptom is a person im-

[1] This essay appeared previously in Jeffrey K. Zeig and Stephen R. Lankton (Eds.). 1988. *Developing Ericksonian therapy: State of the art.* New York: Brunner/Mazel.

mersed in a naturalistic, albeit self-devaluing, trance. The therapist's task is to join the hypnotic processes inherent in the problematic expression and to cooperate in ways that allow their transformation into self-valuing solutions. To effectively do this, the therapist must be clear about the elements shared by symptomatic trances and therapeutic trances. Following are the eight shared characteristics we will explore in this section:

1. Paradoxical injunctions
2. Both/and logic
3. Ideodynamicism
4. Intensified experiential involvement
5. Sustained attention
6. Temporal variability
7. Somatic changes
8. Other phenomenological alterations

### *Paradoxical Injunctions*

Induction of trance, like all communications, emerges within a relationship context. It is therefore important to consider the transactional patterns that give rise to this experiential state, one of which is the paradoxical injunction, wherein two seemingly contradictory directives are presented simultaneously. For example:

1. Hear what I say/Don't pay attention to me.
2. I want you to go into trance/I want you to stay out of trance.
3. I want you to let that hand lift/I don't want you to lift that hand.

Figure 2.1 illustrates the general form of this pattern, which is assumed here as fundamental to the development of trance states. The figure also indicates how the resulting trances may be generative or symptomatic, depending on the relationship context.

The idea that paradoxical injunctions create altered states is rooted in the Bateson group's formulation of the double bind hypothesis (Bateson, Jackson, Haley, & Weakland, 1956; Haley, 1963). In studying schizophrenics within a family systems context, the Bateson group observed that their altered states developed in response to contradictory parental "suggestions." For example, a parent may repeatedly communicate messages of this sort:

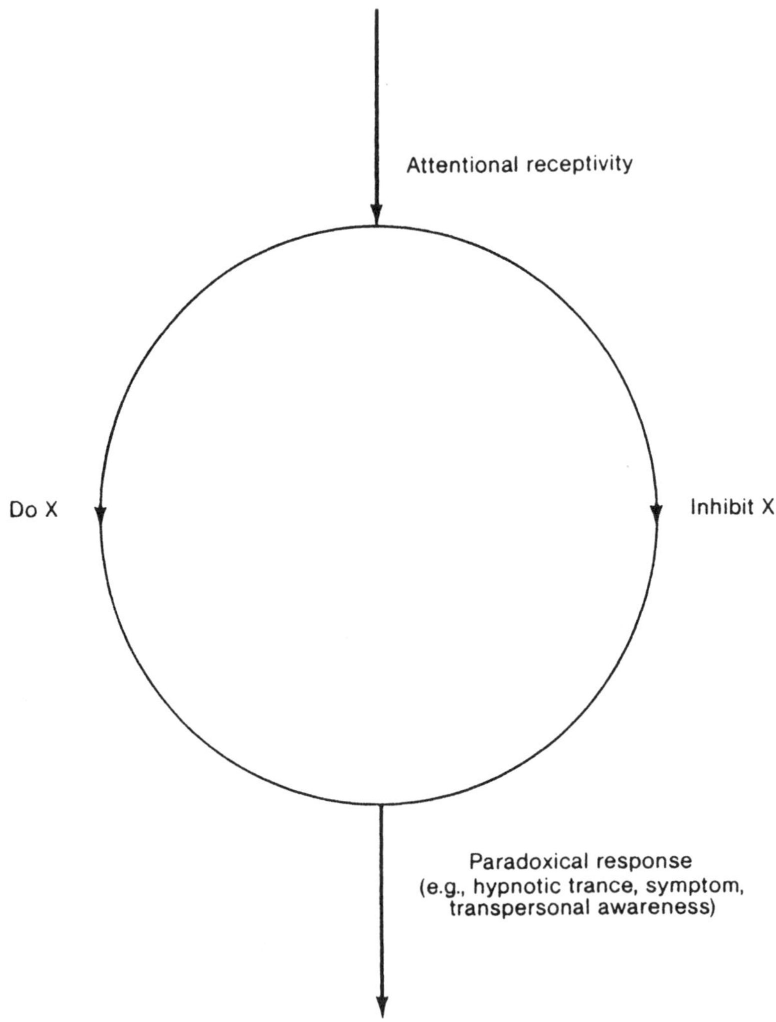


Figure 2.1.
The generation of altered states from paradoxical injunctions.

1. This is funny/This is not funny.
2. Listen to me/Disregard what I say.
3. Love me/Don't express your love.

These contradictory messages are typically delivered simultaneously, though usually in different channels (e.g., verbal and nonverbal).[2] Bateson et al. (1956) proposed that the repeated offering of such statements stimulates (schizophrenic) altered states in a person who is unable to leave the context, comment on the communications, or respond to just one or the other side of the message.

Haley (1963) extended this hypothesis by applying it to the contexts of hypnosis and psychotherapy. He noted that a person expressing symptoms is a person giving paradoxical directives. For example:

1. I am communicating this (symptom)/It is not me who is communicating this (symptom).
2. I want to change/I don't want to change.
3. Come closer/Stay away.

Haley further observed that psychotherapists would typically use their own paradoxical injunctions when communicating with clients. For example:

1. Follow my directives/I am non-directive.
2. I cannot help you/I can help you help yourself.
3. Our relationship is personal/Our relationship is impersonal.

Haley (1963) suggested that such therapeutic paradoxes were effective precisely because they mapped into the contradictions inherent in a person's symptomatic behavior. Thus, psychotherapists may be successful to the extent that they execute judo-like counter-inductions to the "hypnotic inductions" of clients (cf. Watts, 1961).

Erickson and Rossi (1975) elaborated these ideas further in the context of

---

[2] Double binds may be distinguished from paradoxes in that the former involves messages at different logical levels, whereas paradoxes contain messages at the same logical level. While Bateson and his group made much of this distinction (e.g., see Haley, 1955, 1963), I do not think it so important for practical concerns.

hypnotherapy. They discussed techniques of therapeutic double bind wherein naturalistic hypnosis could be utilized via paradoxical communications such as:

1. I want you to respond (unconsciously)/I don't want you to respond (consciously).
2. You can be all alone in trance/You can be alone with me in trance.
3. You can remember to forget OR forget to remember.

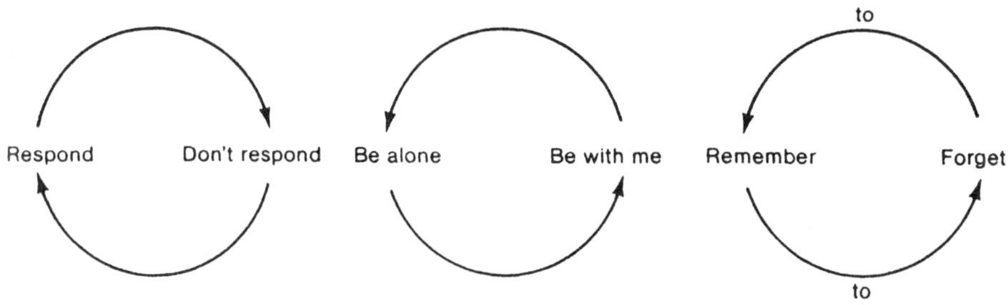


Figure 2.2.
Examples of paradoxical injunctions.

As Figure 2.2 illustrates, each of these examples involves asking the subject to respond simultaneously to both sides of a complementarity. In contrast to the paradoxical injunctions underlying symptomatic communication, such "suggestions" also convey an underlying support for the individual. But in common with symptomatic communications, the respondent is expected to remain in the context, to respond to both sides simultaneously, and to not comment on (e.g., try to explain or talk about) the paradox. To reiterate, it is this formula which seems to be dramatically effective in inducing altered states of consciousness characterized by the emergence of trance phenomena, whether they be symptomatic or therapeutic in nature.

Paradoxical injunctions are inherent in most of the techniques developed by Erickson. Metaphorical stories include the paradox of "This story is not about you/This story is about you." Symptom prescription and "encouraging resistance" techniques instruct the person to change by not changing. Dissociation involves asking the person to respond spontaneously (i.e., unconsciously), but to deliberately not respond (consciously). In these and other techniques, paradoxical directives depotentiate the linear orientation of the conscious mind and amplify the circular and systemic orientation of the unconscious mind, thereby giving rise to trance and its symptoms. Haley (1963) proposed that the effectiveness of such techniques may arise primarily from their ability to join and recontextualize the paradoxical injunctions inherent in the client's symptomatic "trance."

Paradoxical messages occur in many contexts. Bateson (1954) and Haley (1955) have described their relevance to play, humor, fantasy, and dreaming. Watts (1961) and Rossi and Jichaku (1984) elaborated on their use in transpersonal contexts such as Zen Buddhism. Since this communicational form is prevalent in various contexts but produces extended trances in only some, it should be appreciated as a necessary but not sufficient condition for trance development. Other factors must also be present for a sustained trance to occur.

### *Both/and Logic*

A corollary to the communication of paradoxical directives is the experience of both/and logic in entranced individuals. Both/and logics allow for something (X) and its opposite (X') to simultaneously be true, in contrast to the more traditional either/or logic which postulates that if X is true, its opposite (X') is not. This experience of "trance logic" (Orne, 1959) was beautifully illustrated in hypnosis experiments described by Beahrs (1982). Subjects actually hypnotized ("reals") and subjects merely pretending to be hypnotized ("simulators") were both given suggestions to not see ("negatively hallucinate") an individual actually standing in the room. Another person was then placed directly in front of this individual, and subjects were asked to walk a direct path to the other person. The experimental question was thus one of how subjects would respond to the individual standing in their path, since they were asked to not perceive him. As expected, simulating subjects did what they thought a negatively hallucinating person would do: They bumped into the individual standing in their path. However, subjects actually experiencing trance responded quite differently: They walked around the individual they were told to negatively hallucinate.

In extensive post-test interviews, a fascinating story emerged. When asked if they "saw" the person standing in their path, hypnotized subjects insisted they did not. When asked why they forged a circuitous path, they claimed not wanting to bump into the person standing there whom they did not see! In short, entranced subjects entertained two experiential states without contradiction: They did not "see" the person AND they did see the person. Thus, the experience of trance seems to allow for an organizational state wherein opposing states or values can co-exist simultaneously.

We can see from these data a natural function of trance: It allows individuals an opportunity to experience both sides of a relationship simultaneously. The relationship can be distinguished in many ways: subject/object, observer/observed, self/other, conscious/unconscious, and so forth. This capacity for the experience of both/and logic may contribute to problems in a variety of ways.

For example, problems often develop and persevere when a person dissociates from (e.g., denies) a relationship at a conscious level even while identifying with it deeply at an unconscious level. A person may claim to not want to eat (smoke, drink, take drugs, etc.) even while vigorously engaging in a systematic abuse of that activity. A marital relationship might be painfully balanced by the simultaneous feelings of love and hate, approach and avoidance. In these and other problems, individuals may be observed to express both sides of a relationship simultaneously. As they do so, other characteristics of trance discussed below also show up.

Both/and logics may also play a central role in solutions. For example, a pregnant mother being trained in hypnotic pain control for natural childbirth was told she could experience herself "apart from while a part of" her body when needles were inserted into her arms and hands. She later reported having felt a curious sensation at the insertion sites while simultaneously wondering (in a detached and comfortable state) whether this was what "they normally referred to as pain."

With another client, a change in a behavioral pattern of overeating was achieved by hypnotically training the woman to experience a "phantom body" that could step outside of her physical body and binge when needed "even while her unconscious could take care of all the REST needed." (This "phantom body" technique has been used successfully in a variety of cases involving addictions.)

Finally, significant therapeutic progress was made with a couple via "mutual hypnosis" exercises wherein partners learn to develop a "together yet apart" trance state. The both/and logic of trance may allow for creative interaction between normally conflicting parts.

### *Ideodynamicism*

Self-expression in trance states is felt to occur independently of normal conscious mediation. Feelings, thoughts, behaviors, etc., just seem to happen, without planning or effort. In hypnotic terminology, this phenomenon is called *ideodynamicism* ("ideas" into "dynamics" without conscious interference), which may involve ideo-motor, ideo-sensory, ideo-cognitive, ideo-affective, ideo-perceptual, or ideo-imaginal expressions. As Bernheim (1895) noted, ideodynamicism is intensified by trance.

Ideodynamicism is a primary feature of symptomatic trances. Problem descriptions invariably contain some references to being "out of control," in terms of interpersonal (e.g., behaviors) or intrapersonal (e.g., cognitions) communication. While traditional therapy typically attempts to bring these "out of control" processes under the dominance of the conscious mind, the approach in Ericksonian therapy is often different. Such expressions are acknowledged as legitimate processes, however they occur in self-devaluing or socially unacceptable fashions. Thus, therapeutic efforts are focused on recontextualizing or reframing such processes in ways that allow change. For example, a client complained of recurrent internal dialogue that "suggested" imminent failure. After his attention was suitably absorbed, intense and repetitive use of the "failure" theme was used as the basis for hypnotherapeutic communications:

> Now, John, I'm going to ask you to do some things here which I am confident you will succeed in failing to fully do even now. Now what do I mean by that? Simply this: You're thinking a lot about failure. You're thinking about failing at work. You're thinking about failing at home. You can think about failing to fully respond here in the office. So what I will not fail to continue to remind you to do is to wonder and wander unconsciously in terms of how much you can enjoy that failure as you hear now my words. I want to suggest that your hand will fail to lift up. I want to suggest that your eyelids will fail to blink or not blink. I want to suggest that you may fail to not wonder about how you will continue to wonder. I want you to fail to fully relax only part ways. . . .

Hypnotic elaboration on this "failure" theme served to absorb attention, elicit a therapeutic trance, and develop a variety of therapeutic trance phenomena.

This utilization approach to "out of control" processes in Ericksonian therapy stems from its hypnotic roots. The hypnotic subject is encouraged to "just let things happen." This may involve a hand lifting without a sense of conscious volition; a memory being recalled in a surprising way; a feeling of not being able to move; or a sense of thoughts "thinking themselves." In short, the hypnotist encourages the development of self-expressions independent from the control of the conscious mind. It is thus a natural step to appreciate symptoms as spontaneous ideodynamic processes that may be accepted and utilized as legitimate hypnotic phenomena.

In utilizing ideodynamic phenomena, it is important to recognize that they may be attributed to a variety of sources, including the devil, the unconscious, the deceased, or family members. Actually, all such ideodynamic processes are naturalistic expressions for which a person is responsible (i.e., has the ability to respond to). Thus, naming the source (e.g., "the unconscious") is relevant only to securing a person's cooperation in participating in the process of accepting experience.

### *Intensified Experiential Involvement*

As discussed earlier, trance amplifies experiential involvement. Ordinary psychological processes are intensified to the extent of seeming phenomenologically different. Remembering becomes hypermnesia; forgetting can be experienced as amnesia. Memory deepens to regression, future projection to age progression. Detachment evolves into dissociation, attachment into full identification. These amplified phenomena are present in both therapeutic and symptomatic trance processes; as such, they may be experienced as self-valuing (e.g., revivifying a happy childhood event) or self-devaluing (e.g., internal dialogue intensifying into haunting voices). Trance augments the basic processes by which experience is generated.

Amplified expression in trance means deeper immersion in the experience. Just as would happen if the radio you were listening to were turned up or the colors you were watching grew more intense, the sense of involvement increases as trance augments whatever "shows up" in experience. At the same time, attention diminishes to stimuli outside the psychological field of the trance. Thus, if you were to go into trance with a friend in a crowded room, you might grow oblivious to all the neighboring stimuli. Or if you were to develop a symptomatic trance around a sense of anxiety in your chest, awareness of the environment (including the rest of your body) might fade away.

Trance increases absorption in stimuli inside the established psychological field and decreases it in stimuli outside of the field. In self-valuing states, this is quite an asset: Artists may become totally immersed in their artistic works; therapy clients can experience full absorption in a feeling of self-acceptance; thinkers may develop complete involvement in letting thoughts unfold. But in self-devaluing states, this same skill becomes a liability: A person victimized by incest remains deeply withdrawn into the horror of the experience; a couple in an argument can literally see nothing but each partner's cues indicating mistrust. Flexibility and other skills must be available if increased experiential absorption in trance is to be advantageous.

Part of the reason that experiential absorption is deepened in trance is that critical processes are dampened. Awareness becomes less laden with analytical processes and more filled with "concrete" phenomenological experience. As with any development, this may help or hinder, depending on the relationship context. On the one hand, less critical processes allow more creative and spontaneous processes to unfold; on the other hand, a person stuck in a symptomatic trance may require critical faculties to recognize what is happening. As we shall see, it is therefore important to develop trances that have error-correcting capacities within them.

### *Sustained Attention*

In addition to deeper experiential absorption, trance enables more sustained attentional orientation to a given idea or experience. This is in contrast to a normal waking state, where attention usually shifts across different facets of the environment. The ability to focus attention in trance was noted by James Braid in the 18th century, who replaced his original term of monoideism ("single idea" state) with the term hypnosis ("sleep" state). It was also noted by Bernheim in the 1890s, who described psychological problems in terms of "idea fixations" and proposes the use of repetitively suggesting other ideas via hypnosis.

These "idea fixations" distinguish both symptomatic and therapeutic trance states. In symptomatic trances, individuals organize their experience around some recurrent stimulus. Possibilities include the voice of a parent, a feeling in the part of the body, and the expression of some ritualized behavior (e.g., handwashing, smoking). This same sustained attention to a stimulus characterizes therapeutic trances. Here the focus may be on the hypnotist's voice, a thumbtack on the wall, a mantra, or a rhythmic dance. Thus, the sustained absorption of trance may make for ruts or grooves, depending on the relationship context.

### *Temporal Variability*

As trance intensifies experiential involvement and sustains attentional focus, a person's sense of time changes. In particular, the linear sense of time as having beginning and end (thereby creating "past," "present," and "future") often disappears, giving way in trance to a "timeless" quality. This development makes sense when we think of psychological time as a construct of analytical thinking, useful for organizing goal-oriented actions and sequencing events (cf. Ornstein, 1969). As analytical thinking dissipates in trance, individuals are less inclined to process experience in sequential terms, and the ability to accurately estimate the temporal duration of the experience is thus reduced. This seems to be true for both hypnotic trances (Schwartz, 1978) and symptomatic trances (Melges, 1982).

One consequence of the disruption in temporal sequencing is that individuals are less able to distinguish the order in which events transpired (Evans & Kihlstrom, 1973). Alternatively stated, individuals in trance are more able to "jumble" the order of a sequence, thereby freeing behavior from a rigid linear chain of events. Since this rigidity seems to distinguish problem sequences, where A automatically triggers B which automatically triggers C, trance can thus facilitate the use of "scramble techniques" (Lankton & Lankton, 1983) and other interventions designed to alter invariant sequences (see Haley, 1976).

Another consequence of "timelessness" is difficulty in distinguishing a past and future from the present (Melges, 1982). Thus, individuals in trance are less inclined to represent a "future" distinction from "now" (Zimbardo, Maslach, & Marshall, 1972). This state enables more aliveness, creativity, and spontaneity in the present.

At the same time, timelessness in a symptomatic trance may be quite problematic. Individuals engulfed in a "depressive trance" have extreme difficulty in sensing the possibility of a future different from their present state. Likewise, couples engaged in an altered state sequence of arguing have little access to other "times" that may provide resources for the present challenge.

The temporal variability of trance can be used for therapeutic advantage. For example, a client may be trained to experience a minute as an hour, or an hour like a minute. Thus, a few moments of relaxation in between labor contractions or before a public performance may provide a person with "all the time in the world" to retrieve and integrate needed resources. Alternatively, several hours of pain (e.g., following a surgery) might be psychologically felt as involving only minutes of clock time. As Cooper and Erickson (1959) and Masters and Houston (1972) have elaborated, time distortion can facilitate development in many areas.

### *Somatic Changes*

Any significant shift in psychological experience will be accompanied by a shift in somatic experience. It is therefore not surprising that a variety of bodily changes are felt in the course of trance experiences. A person may feel relaxed and drowsy (the body becoming heavy and warm), or perhaps alert and immobilized (cataleptic). As such changes develop, a person may feel greater association with and/or greater dissociation from the body; for example, a person may feel oriented within the body or observing it from a distance. Either way, there will generally be less of a sense of active control over the movements or experiences of the body; expression will be felt as being initiated from some other source (e.g., "the unconscious," an enemy, the hypnotist).

These alterations will be accompanied by shifts in the person's patterning of physical expressions. As trance develops, changes may be observed in behavioral patterns of breathing, movement, eye focus, talking, pulse rate, and so forth. (Erickson, Rossi, & Rossi, 1976; Gilligan, 1987). Observation of such cues thus reveals the onset of trance. As we will see, the behavioral patterns involved in therapeutic trances are clearly distinguishable from those accompanying symptomatic trances.

The variability of somatic experience during trance can be therapeutically utilized. For example, an obese client desiring weight loss reported in trance that her body felt like an expanding round balloon. Over time, elaborate suggestions to experience the "balloon body" expand and contract gently, along with specific breathing suggestions, enabled the gradual shrinking of the body image, which correlated with weight loss.[3] Thus, the therapist may utilize

[3] It may be assumed that people regulate their body weight partly by unconscious body

spontaneous bodily changes in trance as naturalistic "techniques" useful in establishing desired changes.

### *Other Phenomenological Alterations*

In addition to the changes thus far discussed, other phenomenological alterations occur in trance. For the open-eyed person, vision may become blurry, light patterns may change, a face may distort or turn into that of another person (familiar or unfamiliar). When eyes are closed, unusual images may develop: geometric patterns, void-like spaces, archetypal characters, or dream-like figures.

As with all trance characteristics, such phenomenological alterations may be symptomatic or therapeutic. For example, a client described a recurrent symptomatic trance in which she felt imprisoned by a circular brick wall that rose high to the sky, leaving her with a painful sense of disconnection. A similar "hallucinated wall" technique was spontaneously developed by a hypnotized psychotherapy client interested in developing ways to experience safety and solitude. Thus, any of the many unusual phenomenological developments that occur in trance may be exhilarating and satisfying or frightening and debilitating, depending on context.

## CONTEXT DIFFERENCES: SYMPTOMATIC TRANCES VS. THERAPEUTIC TRANCES

As we have seen, symptom phenomena and hypnotic phenomena share numerous characteristics. Both are developed from paradoxical injunctions and involve paradoxical (both/and) experience; both feature the principle of ideodynamicism, whereby expressions (thoughts, behaviors, feelings, etc.) develop outside of conscious control; and both involve intensified experiential absorption, sustained attention, temporal alterations, somatic changes, and other phenomenological shifts. In short, a person expressing a symptom is a person in trance.

In this view, the variable of therapeutic interest is the relationship context

images that serve as "homeostats" (Pribram, 1971). Thus, modification of this fixed image facilitates modification of the actual physical body (Achterberg, 1985).

in which trance processes occur. The following are seven context variables that will be discussed:

1. Self-valuation process
2. Level of trust
3. Biological context
4. Content variability
5. Frame variability
6. Context sensitivity
7. Relationship style: cooperation vs. competition

### *Self-Valuation*

In any experience, two levels of participation may be distinguished. The first is phenomenological — the expressions that actually appear in the experience. The second is psychological — how a person chooses to relate to the experience. For example, a client complained that when she closed her eyes to relax, a pair of disembodied eyes would be staring at her intensely. Coincidentally, a therapy trainee reported a similar image of disembodied eyes appearing during a group trance some months later. The client felt afraid and attempted in various ways to negate the experience, while the trainee felt comfortable and chose to welcome the unusual development. Thus, different relationships were established toward the same trance phenomenon.

As might be expected, the experience was a problem for the client and a solution for the trainee. The claim here is that the "difference making the difference" was the valuation process. Whether aware of it or not, every person "votes" on each life experience: This vote is to either value or devalue the experience, thereby establishing it as either ally or enemy, resource or deficit. A self-valuing vote enables a therapeutic trance, while a self-devaluing vote makes for a symptomatic trance. Thus, a major task for the therapist is to validate symptom phenomena, thereby paving the way for a translation of problems into solutions.

This valuation process underlies the cornerstone principle of utilization in Ericksonian psychotherapy. This principle, which advocates accepting and using whatever a person is doing as the basis for change, seems to have emerged from Erickson's personal challenges with polio, dyslexia, tone deafness, and color blindness, phenomena normally devalued as major deficits (Erickson & Rossi, 1977). As Erickson demonstrated with himself and others, such "problems" can be appreciated as opportunities for unique learning and self-development.

This appreciation does not require trying to frame an experience as "good" or "pleasant," since many experiences are naturally unpleasant. Rather, it involves viewing each experience that arises as a viable human expression that can be integrated into the overall fabric of a person's developmental tapestry. To develop such an appreciation, the therapist often needs to "deframe" perceptual orientation, such that a phenomenon can be observed independently of its ascribed value (Gilligan, 1987). A therapist can recognize this neutral state by an ability to equally generate ways in which the phenomenon could be socially desirable or undesirable. For example, the process of withdrawing may be a problem or a solution, depending on the context.

Once the therapist is able to value the client's expression, various methods can be used to promote the client's doing the same. One technique is to simply feed back in a self-valuing way those aspects of a symptomatic experience in which a person is especially absorbed. For example, a client began to recount multiple childhood experiences of sexual and physical abuse. As she became increasingly upset and self-absorbed, I tried to reassure her. After about 30 minutes, I finally "heard" her repeated chants about feeling "crazy" and thus immediately proclaimed in an intense fashion, "You are crazy!" The woman's demeanor became centered and focused, and asked, "Do you really think so?" Maintaining the same intensity and sincerity, I continued to validate that her experience was indeed "crazy," while periodically wondering how this craziness was going to be approached in a way that would allow new choices. Thus, joining and valuing the person's dominant experience of feeling "crazy" was a first step in the therapeutic task of transforming her relationship to it.

A similar technique is symptom prescription, which in its simplest form directs a person to continue to do what they are doing (Erickson, 1965). Thus, a depressed person might be asked to practice his depression. In traditional therapy, this strategy may seem unusual or paradoxical. It is straightforward and common sense within the Ericksonian approach. The assumption is that joining an ongoing process allows one to gradually modify that process. Symptom prescription enables the client to shift from a self-valuing strategy of attempted negation to a self-valuing process of choosing (and thereby accepting) the recurrent process.

Another way to value symptomatic experience is to re-language and develop it as a hypnotic skill. For example, a person complaining of overeating reported experiencing a burning sensation in her stomach shortly before binging. I accepted and defined this phenomenon as the spontaneous development of hypnotic sensations, then worked with the woman to "allow the unconscious" to amplify this trance phenomenon in ways that led to different responses.

The above methods assume that the way a person relates to a phenomenon determines its value and the response to it. Such methods seek to translate problems into solutions by changing the way a person "votes" on the experience. When the relationship is shifted from self-devaluation to self-valuation, a symptomatic trance can be translated into a therapeutic trance.

## *Level of Trust*

Another major difference between symptomatic and therapeutic trances is the level of trust. A person immersed in a problematic trance experiences little in self and others, while someone engaged in a solution-oriented trance experiences enhanced trust. Trust is crucial to the quality of a trance, since without it a person will be unable to "let go" and allow unconscious expression. An untrusting individual will "fight" the trance experience, which can distort it and make it painful. Thus, the therapist interested in joining and working with symptomatic expressions must first secure the person's trust.

For example, an incest survivor requested hypnosis in hopes of "reconnecting with feelings," but warned of a strong need to establish boundaries. Accordingly, I emphasized the need for safety and trust as paramount to the process, then asked her to reflect on what might allow her to satisfy that need. After some contemplation, she reported with mild embarrassment a recurrent sense of needing to be all alone in the room. Contemplating this "hypnotic koan" of how to stay in the room while leaving it, I imagined myself sitting in the doorway to the office, with nothing but my feet visible to the client. I did a brief hypnotic induction in this unusual position, and the client felt tremendously relieved that her considerations were being respected while her needs were met. Further work gradually decreased the physical distance, so by the end of several sessions she felt comfortable with me in close physical proximity, though it was important for her to keep her eyes open during this time.

With the client who had reported disembodied eyes staring at her, the following communications helped to develop trust:

> Now Joan, you are experiencing a lot of different things, some of which you are concerned about. Your conscious mind is participating

> in various ways, and so is your unconscious. And your unconscious is expressing a lot of different things, all the way from the way you're breathing, the way you're feeling, and other ways you can learn naturally to allow changes to occur comfortably. And so what I'd like you to do is simply look at me here, because it's important to know safely that you can feel grounded and secure as your unconscious begins to communicate. Because even while you look at me here, no matter what I say or don't say, your unconscious can feel safe and secure in the knowledge that you can continue to sit there comfortably and let your unconscious operate according to your needs as an individual. . . . And you have plenty of needs as an individual. . . . You have a need for safety . . . you have a need to operate at the rate which is appropriate to you . . . you have a need and a right to experience comfort in your breathing . . . you have a need to experience security . . . you have a need to be able to know that you can withdraw and stay here simultaneously . . . you have a need to know that even as you look at me and my eyes remain here with you, other meaningful changes can happen in accord with the needs of the entire self . . . my face may begin to change, and you have a need and a right to know that you can continue with that security even as the eyes remain and the identity and the relationship and the feeling and the sense of the ability of the eyes to transform as you develop that integration at your rate. . . .

Delivered in a soft yet absorbing manner, these communications served to experientially secure Joan's attention in a way that allowed rapport to develop. This context of trust was then used to elicit and recontextualize the trance phenomena of the disembodied eyes.

Trust is essential to transform a symptomatic trance into one that is therapeutic. The therapist seeks to find those conditions that will enable clients to realize that it is safe for them to explore their experience.

### *Biological Context*

One of the most striking differences between symptomatic and therapeutic trances is in physical patterning. In symptomatic trances, individuals are typically distinguished by arrhythmic and nonfluid motor patterns, chronic muscular contractions (especially in the neck and stomach), irregular and shallow breathing patterns, and overall tension (i.e., physical holding patterns). In contrast, individuals in therapeutic trances tend to exhibit a greater sense of grace and rhythm in movements, balanced muscular tonicity, deeper and more rhythmic breathing patterns, general flexibility, and relaxed eye movements.

As the most rudimentary experimentation or observation will show, these different ways of organizing biological experience dramatically influence the perceived value of a psychological experience. A person with disrupted rhythms, poor breathing patterns, and chronic muscular tension will be hard pressed to accept and interact with hypnotic experience. On the other hand, an individual with balanced rhythms, breathing patterns, and muscle tonicity is generally willing and able to integrate experiences of all sorts. In short, the biological patterning of the self may determine whether a psychological event is experienced as a problem or a solution.

One of the most critical tasks of the therapist is thus to develop and maintain balanced biological states. This is especially important at the outset of hypnotic exploration. Since it involves transactions at a primary (nonverbal) level, the therapist should begin by ensuring a balanced, centered state within him or herself. As I have described in detail (1987), this orientation is then extended to include the client. Only when attention has been experientially absorbed in a fashion that allows rhythms to be synchronized does the therapist proceed with hypnotic directives.

Once hypnotic explorations are underway, the therapist continues to monitor nonverbal patterning. Changes in expression (rhythm, breathing, muscle tone, posture, etc.) signal changes in psychological orientation, thereby suggesting modifications in therapeutic communications. Specific interventions are needed if any changes involve sustained holding patterns (e.g., in breathing or muscles) or arrhythmic expressions, since this indicates a fundamental shift in biological context (from self-valuing to self-devaluing). For example, a man complaining of recurrent nightmares was directed to (hypnotically) redream the nightmare with a new ending. Halfway through the dream the man's nonverbal patterning abruptly shifted: His face paled, breathing stopped, muscles contracted (especially in his throat), and posture stiffened. The following direct suggestions were immediately given:

> That's right . . . and there is that experience again . . . So I want you to breathe deeply and automatically now, Bob . . . breathe and let the tensions move through you . . . breathe and let the fears dissipate . . . breathe and allow that new dream to complete itself . . . and you don't know and I don't know how your unconscious will and is now going

> to dream a different dream from here on in ... but I do know that it is important that you breathe, Bob, as you develop that new relationship ... that's it ... breathe ... and as you do, feel free to hear my voice in the background as much as is needed to recognize that you can feel safe here and now and there and then and here and now, a part of and apart from ... and all the while, breathing, Bob, as you hear my voice and let your muscles relax and really enjoy that surprise of watching and feeling those integrations developing even more now ... you can feel it, Bob ... breathe ... that's it ... you can feel it ... breathe ... that's it ... you can watch and feel those integrations ... that's it ... that's it ... that's it. ...

While these hypnotic directives were being given, Bob appeared to move through an array of intense emotional experiences, including anger, fear, sadness, and (finally) relief. From a pragmatic perspective, these emotional processes were of little concern to me; of primary importance was the biological context in which they developed. As with most clients, Bob had developed a way of intensely rigidifying his nonverbal patterning during the experience, thereby ensuring an unpleasant experience and undesirable outcome. With hypnotic "coaching" regarding new biological patterns (especially breathing), a new response developed. He dreamed a different ending to the dream, and experienced no further nightmares.

Sometimes additional interventions are needed to balance nonverbal patterns. With one mesomorphic client, who upon entering trance would develop intense muscular contractions, I did a great deal of hypnotic work while relaxing and supporting his neck muscles with my hands. With another client, a woman who complained of intense jealousy of her husband, I interrupted the extreme "tunnel vision" involved in the jealousy pattern by having her go into trance by looking at her husband while simultaneously seeing her own hands in peripheral vision. This strategy redistributed her attention in a way that disabled the focal intensity while enabling her to connect with her own body. With many other clients, I have found it useful to have them hold my hand and/or keep their eyes open while in trance. These are some of the different ways in which the therapist can satisfy the major responsibility of ensuring that hypnotic explorations occur within self-valuing biological contexts.

### *Content Variability*

For a process to remain generative, its content must periodically change. Conversely, for a process to remain problematic, some of its aspects must be invariant. Thus, while the content of a person's therapeutic trances varies over time, an individual's symptomatic trances feature the same focal content again and again. Consider the general hypnotic process of ideosensory phenomena. It might appear recurrently in a symptomatic trance as a migraine headache or a burning in the stomach. Regardless of the selected content, it would tend to repeat itself across successive symptomatic trances. In contrast, an individual experiencing a series of therapeutic trances might develop warmth in the hands during one trance, a tingling in the chest in the next trance, and heaviness in the feet in another trance. In short, a general skill or process will tend to be expressed in different times, depending on the situation.[4]

Looked at in this way, a major role assumed by the hypnotherapist is that of variety generator. The dictum in this regard is, "Where singular fixity was, flexible variability shall be." To function as a variety generator, the therapist identifies repetitive content in a person's symptomatic trance. For example, a depressed man complained of an overwhelming "feeling of emptiness" in his chest. A series of therapeutic trances were used to vary the content of this trance phenomenon, such that successive experiences included a vision of emptiness, a picture of emptiness, a symbol of emptiness, a feeling of emptiness in the stomach, a feeling of emptiness in the head, a feeling of emptiness in the feet while noting a "full symbol" develop in the head, a comfortable feeling of full emptiness, a suggestive vision of empty fullness, and "a surprising dream integrating fullness and emptiness in regard to the whole body of experiential learnings." By using multiple trials to generate a variety of possible modifications of the focal content of the symptom, new possibilities emerged. A symptom can only be maintained when certain parameters (what, where, when, with whom, how, what called, attributions) are fixed in content. When the content is varied, the process begins to shift and changes can be made.

---

[4] In this sense, a person in symptomatic trance is engaging in idolatry ("an idea frozen into a specific image"). Just as God is not the statue on the dashboard, an idea is not the content used to represent it in a given situation. When content is invariant, this distinction is forgotten.

## *Frame Variability*

Individuals usually operate in relationship with (1) goals or intentions and (2) reference structures or frames for achieving those goals. This means that (1) the contents of consciousness are usually represented within a matrix or network of other associations; and (2) the person views this frame from a certain perspective (e.g., goal orientation). These frames serve as filters for experience, ensuring selective orientation and biased interpretations. Far from being undesirable, frames are essential for achieving specific goals. However, frames must be altered in accord with changing values and situations, so a person must periodically set aside frames to allow new structures to develop.[5]

If this is not done deliberately, it will happen "spontaneously." For example, symptomatic trances may develop when the conscious mind is no longer able to handle a situation with its activated frames, thereby prompting the unconscious mind to become dominant (via spontaneous trance development) as a means to generate new possibilities.

How a person responds to this deframing process can determine whether a trance is symptomatic or therapeutic. In general, a person in a symptomatic trance maintains rigidity in regard to psychological frames, while a person in a therapeutic trance is highly flexible. Frame invariance thus makes for a self-devaluing trance, while frame variability enables a self-valuing trance.

Frame variability is relevant in at least three ways. First, the person in a symptomatic trance tends to repeatedly view a psychological event from the same perspective. For example, a man in therapy attributed his troubles to his alcoholic father's abuse of him as a child. He recalled such abusive events often, each time viewing them from the same self-defeating, depression-induction perspective. In contrast to this fixed position, a person in therapeutic trance is capable of relating to an event from multiple perspectives. Thus, the above client was guided in therapeutic trance to successfully examine a key

---

[5] Historically, such frame transformations have occurred at developmental transitions such as initiation into adulthood, marriage, war, death, etc. In the present view, it is not coincidental that hypnotic processes usually played a central role in marking these shifts. With the modern (Western) emphasis on individual development, it seems that frame transformation occurs more often and at different times for different people, thereby requiring additional ritualistic contexts wherein individuals can "deframe to reframe" (i.e., develop a trance to allow new structures to emerge). Psychotherapy seems to have arisen as the social institution for guiding persons through the altered states inherent in such transformations.

abusive event from the perspectives of the young boy, the father 20 years later, the mother, a kindly and wise stranger, and the boy as an old man.

In a different set of trances, a series of emotional states (sadness, then anger, then contentment) was developed before having the man again access the key experience. This variability in perspective freed him from responding to the event as the "cause" of his unhappiness, and new ways of being became available.

Second, symptomatic trances typically involve rigid attachment to a frame. In contrast, a person in a therapeutic trance is more able and willing to deframe experience. A person in therapeutic trance can experience this deframing experience in such a way that thoughts, feelings, and other associations drift in and out of awareness even as attention absorbs in a single distinction. The person hallucinating within a fixed frame can be guided to experience hallucinations within a drift of changing frames while grounded in relationship to the therapist, with the result that the fixed frame (and hence invariant meaning) normally binding the hallucination is deframed. This allows new possibilities to develop, since a distinction has no value independent from a frame of reference. Thus, the therapist first deframes a distinction, then uses the therapy context to promote new frames that reflect the present needs and values of the person.

A third distinction regarding the operation of frames in trances concerns their relationship to intentions or goals. Symptomatic trances usually involve a condensation (or enmeshment) of intentions and frames, whereas therapeutic trances enable intentions to operate independently from frames. For example, typically the desire for safety in a symptomatic trance automatically activates the same frame or program used previously to achieve safety (e.g., withdrawal, substance abuse, violence).

In contrast, the person in therapeutic trance may contemplate a goal without committing to a specific structure for achieving it. This allows multiple possibilities to be examined, and only those most appropriate for the present situation to be actualized. Thus, a client needing security (or any other outcome) may take time in therapeutic trance to "allow the unconscious" to serve up a variety of possible ways to achieve the goal according to the present needs. By "deframing" goals from structures, the intentions or motivations underlying problem processes can be acknowledged and satisfied in self-valuing fashions.

To summarize, therapeutic trance allows a much greater flexibility in relationship to psychological frames. In contrast to symptomatic trances, therapeutic trances enable variability in terms of: (1) the perspective from which an event is viewed; (2) the unbinding (or deframing) of a distinction from a matrix of other associations; and (3) the independence of an intention from a frame to satisfy that intention. The therapist can translate problems into solutions by introducing variability in these framing parameters.

### *Context Sensitivity*

The experience of trance has traditionally been associated with increased suggestibility. This is misleading to the extent that it depicts the hypnotized person as somehow gullible. However, trance does influence sensitivity to new relationships in the social or environmental fields. Interestingly, it seems that context sensitivity is enhanced by therapeutic trance. That is, individuals in therapeutic trances are open to new possibilities and generally willing and able to experiment with new ways of being. In contrast, persons in symptomatic trances tend to close down to new possibilities while trying to avoid potentially threatening changes.

Since context sensitivity is essential for adaptive behavior, the therapist works to transform the insensitivity of symptomatic trances into the sensitivity of therapeutic trances. Given that a person will generally be closed to "outside" influences around the symptom area, this is accomplished by joining a person's verbal and nonverbal patterns to first get "inside" the system. Once pattern matching has allowed the therapist to join a system, gradual pattern modification enables the experiential changes necessary for renewed context sensitivity.

### *Relationship Style: Cooperation vs. Competition*

Trance allows both sides of a relationship to be experienced simultaneously. This can be a problem or a solution, as it requires an appreciation of differences as well as the realization of "common-unities." For example, a husband and wife (or two different "parts" of an individual) are "a part of yet apart from" each other, and thus must discover how to acknowledge not only both "sides" but "the middle third" as well. The quality of experience in this paradoxical "both/and" relationship depends partly on the relationship style used to guide transactions. In this regard, symptomatic trances tend to be dominated by competitive relationships while therapeutic trances are distinguished by cooperational strategies. Suppose a person has both an urge to smoke and an injunction to not smoke. That person can develop a symptomatic trance by attempting to have one side (e.g., not smoke) dominate the other side (smoke). Since negation is impossible at a primary level (e.g., "don't think of blue"), the competitive style produces at best a splitting of the self into a conscious and unconscious experience. If the situation continues, a symptom usually projects out of the struggle of these opposing injunctions (e.g., an identified patient emerges from the conflict between parents).

The therapist is thus faced with the task of transforming competitive "win-lose" relationships into cooperative "win-win" relationships. The challenge is to solve the "hypnotic koan" (see Gilligan, 1987) of "How can X and X' be equally acknowledged?" While a straightforward answer or an immediate integration is usually not forthcoming, a therapeutic trance will allow a cooperational context wherein "opposites" or "enemies" can find common ground and generate solutions. Thus, the "smoker/non-smoker" relationship can be contemplated in trance as a "hypnotic koan": How can you satisfy the smoker's needs and the non-smoker's needs? When this question was posed in therapeutic trance recently to a man struggling with this complementarity, he responded with a variety of experiential processes. Later inquiry revealed that the koan triggered an experience of (hallucinated) mist and fog enshrouding the man. From a distant observer position he realized after awhile that both "sides" really needed to be "lost in the clouds" now and again during the day. In other words, his unconscious developed a symbolic solution (withdrawing into a cloudy daydream) that satisfied both sides of himself. Thus, a cooperative relationship in therapeutic relationship allowed a "win-lose" relationship to be translated into a "win-win" creative solution.

## SUMMARY

We have proceeded from the naturalistic view that trance is a cross-contextual process by which unconscious processes are amplified. As we have seen, this process features paradoxical injunctions and paradoxical experience, ideodynamic expression, intensified experiential absorption, sustained attention, temporal alterations, somatic changes, and other phenomenological shifts. Trance may or may not be useful, depending on contextual factors such as self-valuation, trust, biological patterning, content and frame variability, context sensitivity, and relationship style. In other words, the relationship context provides the value for any experience; the therapist's task is to recontextualize symptoms so that solutions emerge. As Erickson (1948, 1952, 1959, 1965) emphasized, there are many ways to accomplish this task. The success of any method generally derives from its capacity to join and empower the client's reality. Modification and even outright rejection of a method will sometimes be necessary, depending on the unique needs and patterns of the individual client. Whatever the case, the main idea to remember is that solutions are inherent in the client's ongoing processes, not in the therapist's cleverness.

## Chapter 3

# GENERATIVE AUTONOMY: PRINCIPLES FOR AN ERICKSONIAN HYPNOTHERAPY[1]

I do not know much about gods; but I think that the river
Is a strong brown god — sullen, untamed, and intractable,
Patient to some degree, at first recognised as a frontier;
Useful, untrustworthy, as a conveyor of commerce;
Then only a problem confronting the builder of bridges.
The problem once solved, the brown god is almost forgotten
By the dwellers in cities — ever, however, implacable.
Keeping his seasons and rages, destroyer, reminder
Of what men choose to forget. Unhonored, unpropitiated
By worshippers of the machine, but waiting, watching and waiting.
His rhythm was present in the nursery bedroom,
In the rank ailanthus of the April dooryard,
In the smell of grapes of the autumn table,
And the evening circle in winter gaslight.
The river is within us, the sea is all about us.

— From *Four Quartets*, by T. S. Eliot

[1] This essay appeared previously in Jeffrey K. Zeig. 1985. *Ericksonian psychotherapy, Vol. I: Structures*. New York: Brunner/Mazel.

## INTRODUCTION

I think the "strong brown god" flowed through Milton Erickson. He moved with the life rhythms that most of us have forgotten, but from which we can never escape. His words and his expressions washed away the dust of our everyday living and freed many feet entrenched in the dried mud of frozen positions. Like water, Erickson adapted his form of expression to the ruts, grooves, and patterns of the everchanging, unfolding terrain.

Sadly, Milton Erickson is no longer with us. Yet he was around long enough to inspire many people to realize that the river is within each of us and that the sea *does* surround us all. What do we do with this realization? We can sink or swim; we can dam or build bridges that lead us to forget; we can continue to explore these waters on our own.

Generations pass and pass on their "living ideas" to the next generation. Now that a new season is upon us, how shall we as a "common-unity" of individuals inspired by Milton Erickson respond? Milton Erickson was one of a kind, especially in his special ability to experientially convey that *each of us is one of a kind*, though we all share a deep common-unity. Thus, a shared set of values, ideas, and principles will be expressed in different ways by different individuals.

Realizing this "autonomy in common-unity" was easier when Erickson was the unitary *embodiment* of "Ericksonian approaches." Now, I believe the challenge is to cooperate, rather than compete — to further develop some extraordinary ideas.

This chapter is offered as a possible contribution to the process.[2] It presents the view that the "reality" we experience is self-generated by processes circular (and thus usually unconscious) in nature. A further assumption is that these self-reflexive processes can culminate in either expanding circles of autonomy or "vicious" circles (cycles) of unchanging patterns, depending on whether experience is valued or devalued.

The problem procesess also are seen to be the solution processes; this is the fundamental Ericksonian principles of utilization. Thus, the structure of therapy is determined by the structure of the client's "reality," not by some *a priori*

[2] Among those to whom I owe debts of intellectual and personal gratitude are Milton Erickson, Gregory Bateson, T. S. Eliot, Gordon Bower, Buckminster Fuller, John Lilly, G. Spenser Brown, and Francisco Varela. I also deeply acknowledge Denise Ross, who inspired and supported my explorations with her irreplaceable love and partnership.

frame held by the therapist. The hypnotherapist joins a client's "circle" of recursive looping to expand a self-devaluing "intrapersonal trance" to a self-valuing "interpersonal trance" state. Hypnotherapeutic skills of (1) context valuing; (2) balancing complementary relationships; and (3) generating multiple associative pathways are utilized to "re-source" a client's "circle of autonomy." This "circle" accesses the "generative unconscious" which is a source of transformational change.

To develop these themes, the first section overviews key ideas regarding how a reality comes into being via acts of distinction. The second section applies these ideas to seven representative areas of Ericksonian hypnotherapy: (1) problems as double binds; (2) the hypnotherapy relationship; (3) the hypnotherapist's personal absorption in the hypnotic interaction; (4) generating interpersonal trance loops; (5) the circular structure of ideas in the hypnotic loop; (6) "circuit breaking" loops as diagnostic cues; and (7) a general hypnotherapy procedure for reuniting organizational structures within their circle of autonomy.

## DRAWING DISTINCTIONS

A major tenet of this chapter is that we actively participate in generating our experience. The Ericksonian therapist thus seeks to identify *how* a client is generating painful realities, and then utilizes these very processes to enable their transformation. This approach assumes that no "objective reality" exists independent of observers, and that all experience and behavior emerges from, and indicates values of, relationships. Accordingly, self-referential paradoxes are unavoidable, i.e., all relationships are circular in nature. This applies not only to a client's interactions in "problem" situations, but to the therapist's interactions with clients. All expressions — interpersonal experience, diagnoses, techniques, etc. — simultaneously indicate the "reality" of *both* "subject" *and* "object" (and thus are neither "subjective" nor "objective").

In this "both/and" view, the therapist is a "cooperator" in an *interpersonal* relationship, *not* a "programmmer" or impersonal (i.e., depersonalized) operator. This relationship, like any other, can be either a "vicious cycle" in which the client's experience continues to be devalued or a "common-unity context" enabling autonomous and self-valuing change processes.

In this view, the distinctions one makes are fundamental to the reality one experiences. This section briefly overviews key ideas underlying this orientation.

*Distinctions as Purposive Acts*

Any reality is the result of self-generated distinctions. This view is expressed most cogently by the work of G. Spencer Brown (1979), who observed:

> A universe comes into being when a space is severed or taken apart. The skin of a living organism cuts off an outside from an inside. So does the circumference of a circle in a plane. By tracing the way we represent such a severance, we can begin to reconstruct, with an accuracy and coverage that appear almost uncanny, the basic forms underlying linguistic, mathematical, physical, and biological science, and can begin to see how the familiar laws of our own experience follow inexorably from the original act of severance. The act is itself already remembered, even if unconsciously, as our first attempt to distinguish different things in a world where, in the first place, the boundaries can be drawn anywhere we please. At this stage the universe cannot be distinguished from how we act upon it, and the world may seem like shifting sand beneath out feet. (p. xxix)

Thus, a reality — individual or collective — arises and is maintained by self-distinguished relationships. A primary distinction is an act or injunction that crosses the boundary of a unified space and cleaves it into "inner" and "outer" states, thereby calling into existence a complementary correlation within a common-unity space.[3]

---

[3] As will be elaborated throughout the paper, the view is not one of causality but rather "co-relation"; that is, a phenomenological reality "e-merges" to express relationship values. We can choose how to cooperate with these self-distinguished relationships (and thereby determine the quality of our experience), but we can never unilaterally control them, because all relationships have the paradoxical quality of being "a part of and apart from" the observer-participant.

This view differs radically ("from the root or center") from the rational ("ratio-making" or "dividing") doctrine which most of us have learned to accept without question. It does not reject the "either/or" logic of the rational approach, but emphasizes it within the deeper and more inclusive context of "both/and" logic. A major foundation for this new epistemology is modern physics (e.g., see Zukav, 1979). In this regard, it is ironic that psychology developed its structural foundations according to those of 19th-century physics, but has virtually ignored the revolutionary developments in physics in this century that have shown these foundations to be markedly inadequate.

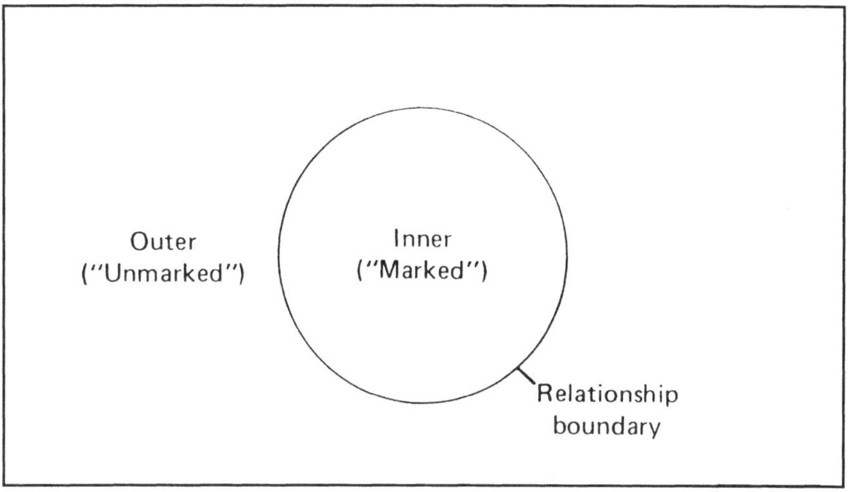


Figure 3.1.
The act of distinction.

As can be seen in the simple illustration of Figure 3.1, distinction is a form of closure, an act of generating boundaries. A distinction is a correlation, a distinguished relationship, an indication of "this and not that."

A distinction expresses the values and intentions of the distinguisher, indicating a "difference which make a difference" (Bateson, 1979). As Brown (1979, p. 1) notes, "There can be no distinction without motive, and there can be no motive unless contents are seen to differ in value."

Thus, one side of a distinction is "marked" (i.e., exhibited, emphasized, "pointed to," identified) as having some particular value; the other is "unmarked" (i.e., inhibited). The marked state is a figure within the "ground" or "field" of the unmarked state. Both states are united in a deeper common-unity, although this is not evident phenomenologically ("in appearances").

Thus, every distinction contains: (1) a marked state; (2) a complementary unmarked state; (3) a correlational boundary (i.e., a mutually specifying relationship); and (4) a deeper common-unity. Also, every distinction is self-referential; i.e., it refers back to its maker.

In this regard, the most primitive distinction we make is the self-definition of our respective identities as autonomous (self-regulating) persons within a "common-unity." This self-identity is fundamental to our existence, serving as the constant context filter which generates (i.e., determines) what we experience (and don't experience), what we do (and don't do), what we value (and don't value), etc.

Precisely because it is a primitive distinction (i.e., a fundamental *context*), self-identity is not directly observable. It can, however, be inferred from invariances and regularities in its structural interactions (behavioral, cognitive, imaginal, etc.). Some parameters we will consider in this regard include: (1) where the primary boundaries are drawn (e.g., individual, family, group); (2) the criteria of a distinction (e.g., What outside state(s) mutually define the distinguished boundaries? How are the complementary states seen to differ in content and value? Are these differences valued or devalued?); (3) the flexibility (or rigidity) of relationship boundaries (e.g., Do they contract and expand rhythmically according to organismic needs?); and (4) any devaluing and dissociated "loops" (i.e., recurrent patterns of self-devaluation).

### *Depths of Self-Distinctions*

An individual operates in domains of experience in patterned fashions. These patterns are essential for stability and for growth but, like all artifacts, they have equal potential to limit or liberate. To appreciate how they are used in Self-expression, four levels of Self-distinction may he distinguished: (1) Self-common-unity as the life essence; (2) Self-autonomy as organizational unity; (3) Self as complementary correlator; and (4) Self as varying correlations of interactional content.

The illustration shown in Figure 3.2 may be considered from an inner-outer or outer-inner viewpoint. That is, movement can and does occur in both directions: outwards (towards more awareness) and inwards (awareness and more reference). From this view, an experiential reality is a phenomenological "standing wave" or "interference pattern" generated from the interaction of outward- and inward-directed signals.

#### **Level 1. Self as common-unity (Self as field).**

This primary distinction may he considered as the source of generativity referred to by Erickson (1980b, p. 345) as "that vital sense of the beingness of the self (that) is often overlooked." It is usually overlooked precisely because it is not phenomenologically apparent. In fact, it cannot be represented in any way other than metaphor. It is the unnameable, the Tao, the essence of

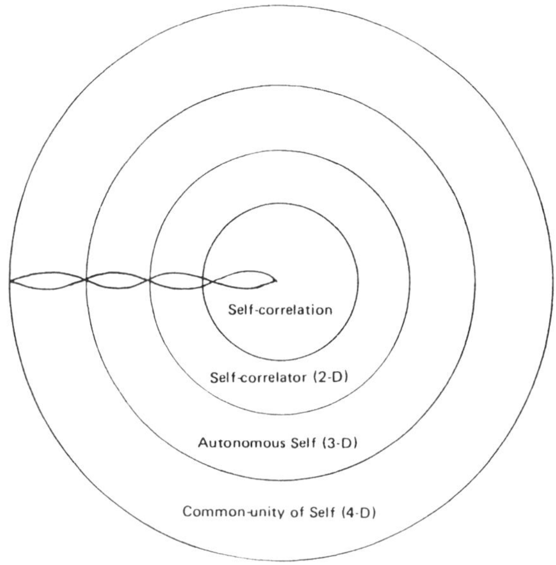


Figure 3.2.
Depths of self-distinction: One possible set of boundaries.

essence of common-unity, the Deep Self, the collective unconscious. It is, to use the words of T. S. Eliot (1963), "a condition of complete simplicity costing not less than everything."

We might imagine the Deep Self as a four-dimensional hypersphere enfolded in the topological form of a torus. The torus ("Möbius sphere" or "doughnut sphere") has been used by Einstein and Eddington as a model of the universe (Davis & Hersh, 1981: Young, 1972; Zukav, 1979). Among its fascinating properties is that every point in the sphere is a center point, being described by the same Fourier transform mathematics used to generate holograms (Davis & Hersh, 1981). Thus, the whole is contained in each of the points (as in holograms). In this view, each person is a unique representation of the same "seed."

A dynamic representation of the torus is a tornado, whose complementary actions are illustrated in Figure 3.3.

**Level 2. Self as organizational autonomy (Self as being).**

This next level is the spherical domain of phenomenological experience and of systemic organization. It is the domain of the "personal unconscious"

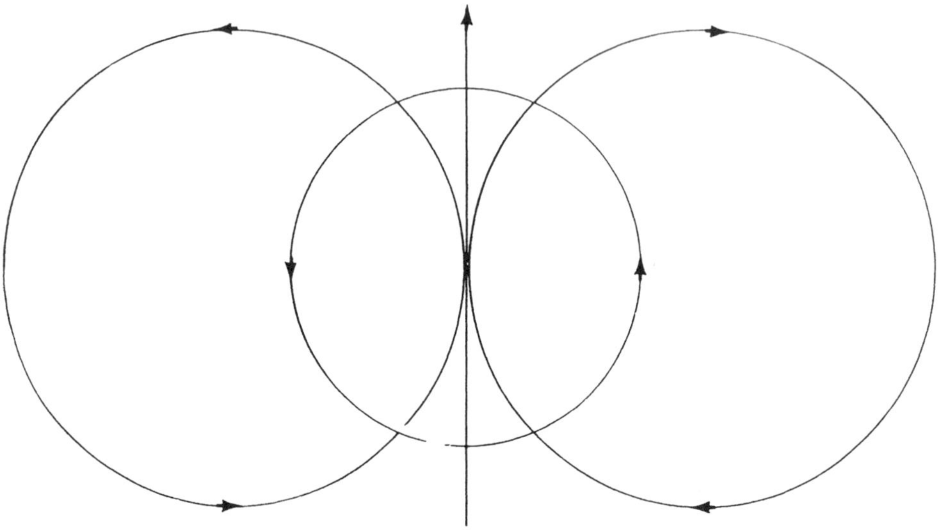

Figure 3.3.
Separate motions of the torus vortex.

that distinguishes "self" (as individual, family, culture, etc.) from "other." Critical at this level is the notion of autonomy ("self-regulation"). Autonomy reflects the wonder of a unique life (within the common-unity of Life), a distinct form within (the universe of) Form. Autonomy does not separate but distinguishes a being as "a part of and apart from" the common-unity. This complementary relationship implies complementary goals: (a) preserve the circle of organizational identity; and (b) regenerate and expand autonomy (i.e., grow).

The concept of autonomy is central in Ericksonian therapy. Erickson (1952) distinguished the "core personality" of the patient from the expressed personality patterns, and suggested that even though the client was unaware of this "core," it was that which the therapist needed to align with and stimulate for therapeutic change.

A system's sphere of autonomy is the organizational identity through which it can interact with integrity ("wholeness") in the common-unity. The sphere of autonomy expands through developmental cycles ("circles") of transformation which expand its domain. A transformational cycle is like a quantum (whole unit) leap to a next wave orbit; learnings from previous cycles remain along with fundamental relationships, but their values and expressions are modified by the additional "response-abilities," capacities, and challenges of the next autonomous context.

For example, one's parents will always be one's parents and the biological and social patterns inherited from them are non-negatable; but growth in autonomy achieves increased response-ability for individual (individuating) modifications of these patterns, thereby enabling (though not assuring) the continued growth of individual and common-unity.

**Level 3. Self as complementary correlator (Self as mind).**

To express autonomy within common-unity, a system requires relationship ("correlational") structures. Thus, this two-dimensional level is the domain of the "conscious mind," the correlator and intentional actor, the symbolic ("re-presenting") self. It might be represented topologically as "hemispheres," triangles, or circles. It is the domain of roles, sensory-motor cybernetic loops, goal-achieving programs, analysis, rationality ("ratio-making"). Distinctions may be organized at this level in terms of triadic unities such as those shown in Figure 3.4.

**Level 4. Self as correlational content (Self as symbol).**

From the correlation of complementary structures, the content of experience emerges. The transitory content of experience (behavior, thoughts, feelings, images, cognitions, etc.) "e-merges" from relationship. The content is the form resulting from ongoing interference patterns (e.g., correlations).

## *Concluding Notes*

To conclude this overview of the centrality of distinction in generating experience, a few additional points might be made.

**1. We cannot NOT participate!**

We can never operate "outside" of the universe. We actively participate in constructing our reality. No observation (description, relationship, perception, etc.) occurs independently from the actions (i.e., distinctions) of an observer. *Reality* is not "out there" in an "object" sense; "reality" is the constellation of experiential correlations expressing distinctions that *we* draw (mostly unconsciously). Thus, we are responsible for (and thus able to respond to) our experience.

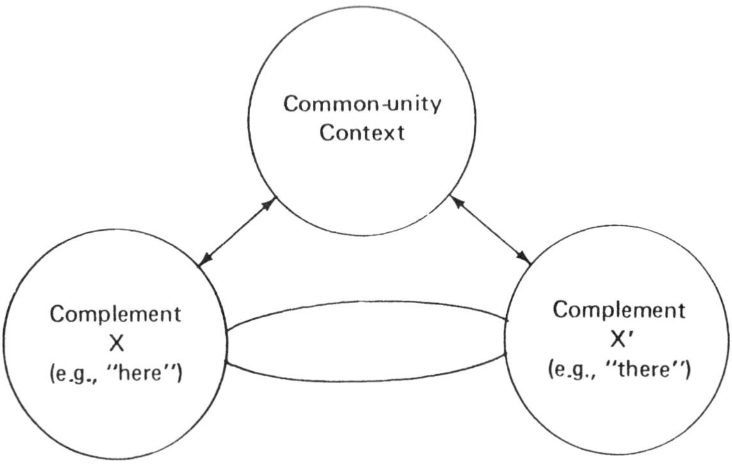


Figure 3.4.
The triadic unity of complements in common-unity.

**2. The principles of unity, complementarity, and multiplicity are extremely generative for Ericksonian hypnotherapy.**

Organizational unity is assumed to underlie all correlations and distinctions. Unity forms a common-unity context in which all complementary structures interact — e.g., "inner/outer," "observer/observed," "friend/enemy," "sound/silence," "self/other," "thinker/thought," etc. This common-unity is often not realized. Complements become framed in an either/or relationship of opposition ("standing in the way of ") or dissociation, thereby prompting attempts to develop (or identify with) one complement and control ("defeat," "overcome," "get rid of," etc.) the other. Since complements are inseparable (though distinguishable) and negation is impossible, such control strategies usually create increasingly "vicious" cycles (i.e., circles) of dissociational functioning. As we will see, a major therapeutic value of trance is its "both/and" quality ("a part of and apart from," as in "my hand is lifting but I'm not lifting it") which allows integration of common-unity complements.

**3. Distinctions are arbitrary, but their consequences are not.**

The integrity ("wholeness") of our distinctions is reflected in the consequences of our actions. Any representation (e.g., image, theory, description, interpretation) is a biased "suggestion" regarding what to observe and where to observe it from. A representation is a time-frozen, fixed-position "pointer" to a pattern which it is not. Thus, multiple instances of complementary ("double") descriptions are generally needed.

**4. We are the territory, but only perceive the maps.**

Korzybski's (1933) dictum that the map is not the territory is often used to claim that we don't have direct access to "the world of experience." This proposal does not jibe well with the view that we create our world of experience. While our phenomenological experience is limited to three-dimensional transformations, our Self is undeniably part of the unitary, four-dimensional universe. We can only talk about or conceptualize maps, but primary knowing (such as in deep trance) can be made of the territory from which such maps are derived. Stated in another way, we can know the territory but not know we know the territory.

**5. A distinction may be called ("indicated" or "named") in many ways: commands, instructions, names, descriptions, expressions, etc.**

This indication may be recalled also in many ways: posthypnotic cues, images, internal dialogue, posture, names. Calls may differ in appearance, but are identical in indicating the underlying motive and marked value of a distinction. This equivalency allows condensation or reducibility of a number of calls to the value of the primary distinction. The value of a call made again (and again, however many times one wishes) is thus simply the value of one call (Brown, 1979).

This equivalency of different names of a distinction may help or hamper change. For example, individuals seeking therapy are typically dominated by "re-calls" of some self-devaluing state. That is, they repeatedly call forth some undesirable and threatening state which they (erroneously) perceive as being "caused" by "non-self" actions — i.e., by uncontrollable "outside" influences such as harassing thoughts, "the past," family members or other persons, etc. In such cases, individuals are generally not aware that the problem states are self-generated, for straightforward reasons to be addressed later.

A somewhat less obvious example concerns the theoretical frames of the therapist. A therapist using models specifying *a priori* content values (e.g., diagnostic categories) will generally perceive only the values and distinctions projected by that model (e.g., Rosenhan, 1984). Many argue that no viable alternatives exist, that some biased structure is needed. Erickson demonstrated otherwise in his emphasis on creating a "new theory" for every client. He emphasized the need for the therapist to "degenerate" his or her description frames and tune to (and utilize) those unavoidably expressed by the client. Tuning to how the client recalls an undesirable state, the hypnotherapist can then apply the Ericksonian cornerstone principle of utilization by acting in accord with the client's distinctions. This synchronization makes the "external" experience of the client equivalent in value to his or her "internal" experience. This enhances trust and cooperation, allowing for the dissipation of rigid frameworks and the autonomous development of generative trance processes.

With these distinctions in mind, let us turn to consideration of their clinical applications.

## GENERATIVE AUTONOMY IN THE HYPNOTHERAPEUTIC RELATIONSHIP

To give a flavor of how ideas of generative autonomy can be applied in Ericksonian hypnotherapy, seven representative topics are overviewed in this section: (1) problems as double binds; (2) the hypnotherapy relationship; (3) the hypnotherapist's personal absorption in the hypnotic interaction; (4) generating interpersonal trance loops; (5) the circular structuring of ideas in the hypnotic loop; (6) "circuit-breaking" loops as diagnostic cues; and (7) a general hypnotherapy procedure for reuniting organizational structures within their circle of autonomy.

### *Problems as Double Binds*

Autonomy ("self-regulation") is essential to the existence of any organizational unity, and therefore will always be the dominant intention underlying expressions. Autonomy does not separate but distinguishes a being as "a part of and apart from" the community. This complementary relationship implies complementary goals: (1) preserve the circle of organizational identity; and (2) regenerate and expand autonomy (i.e., grow). When these complementary goals are not achieved, contradictory expressions and recurrent problems are the result.

In other words, problems develop when a correlational complement is devalued, forbidden, dissociated, etc. The result is that the system is split into oppositional camps, with the autonomy of the common-unity thus lost to both complements. To understand how this might occur, imagine a person cycling through dynamic complement loops within the circle of autonomy. At some point in this sequence, the person might interrupt participation in the dynamic loop. Rest might be needed, or threat to the integrity of the circle of autonomy may be encountered. In the latter case, the immediate priority of the system will be to desist from complementary interaction, "freeze" the circular loop in its present state (i.e., time-bind it, as in making an image), and withdraw into the circle of autonomy to protect and be protected.

This withdrawal is natural, common, and essential, and will be evidenced by autonomic "fight or flee" cues such as restriction of breathing and motoric movements in general, disruption of natural rhythm in expression, increased tension, etc. These responses are necessary and vital messages reminding the person that as a precious and unique autonomous being, he or she is vulnerable (i.e., sensitive, alive) and therefore needs to balance contact and withdrawal in common-unity interactions.

The defensive state of tension, conscious monitoring, and physical rigidity will *not* dissipate until it is acknowledged and valued. While such a state is active, the person cannot participate directly (i.e., spontaneously) in the Natural domain; his or her actions will be regulated by computations made in the Imaginal and Symbolic domains. If this restriction persists, the tension ("holding pattern") will become "condensed" into symbolic and imaginal (i.e., time-frozen) distinctions, thereby giving rise to derived (mis)identification states such as "ego," "anxiety," and "conscious mind." The circle of autonomy will become dissociated from the dynamic expressions of its complements, though the underlying common-unity will always remain. (An individual is "indivisible," regardless of his or her experience or conceptions. Thus, you can't go anywhere without "your" Self or can't "find" your Self anywhere but where it always is — right where you are.)

At some point, however, the person will need to reconnect with and complete the *relationship* in the dynamic loop from which he or she "exited." (The alternative is to have the dissociated structure dominate your experience with absolute, life-denying certainty.) Reuniting Self with self-distinction (e.g., organizational identity) requires a sense of security and autonomy; *a person will never attempt to recross "time-frozen" boundaries if their integrity is in jeopardy.* The needed security can often be gained from a rest period or a recentering (e.g., trance), but sometimes one must develop greater integrity (i.e., increased autonomy) before reuniting the severed states. An example of this is traumatic incidents (e.g., rape or war victims), where the violation of integrity that prompted the dissociative withdrawal is so severe ("severing") that reuniting Self and expressions is often only possible after autonomous growth has been achieved.

It is important to realize that dissociation is not from a place or thing or object, but from an *experiential correlation* (i.e., a relationship pattern). These correlations are not time/space structures but patterns or forms of severing a unified space (Brown, 1979). (As T. S. Eliot [1963] remarked, "History is a pattern of timeless moments.") Paradoxically, dissociation affirms association at a deeper level. (As Freud noted about repression, the denial always affirms.) One cannot negate or escape self-correlations, because they never "go" anywhere; they are "time-frozen" states which can be transformed only by reentry and revaluation.

In this view, there is no "past" to "go back into"; problems are expressions of self-devaluing, time-frozen (i.e.. nonrhythmic) oscillation patterns that are "a part of and apart from" a person's organizational identity. These time-frozen patterns act as screens to separate a person from others. Because all transactions will be conducted through these screens, problems are always in the "present tense," staring a person right in the face (so to speak). The transitory content of the problem — e.g., where it first started — is quite irrelevant. The "pattern which disconnects" — to subvert Bateson's (1979) distinction — is "the thing."

In life, the patterns which connect are always deeper (and thus less apparent) than those which disconnect. Thus, while a person may be dissociated at functional levels, he or she is always unitary ("indivisible") at the deeper (autonomy in common-unity) level of Self. Consequently, *a person's "unconscious" autonomy will always be generating that which is needed for integration and growth.*

In other words, solutions are always present, awaiting discovery. They will become apparent (i.e., phenomenologically realized) only when dissociated experience (i.e., devalued relationships) is valued; they become more obscure when experience is devalued, as when a person identifies with one complement and attempts to dissociate from the other. In this sense, the solution is always contained in the problem, while the attempted solution contains (i.e., constrains) the problem from resolution.

This paradoxical relationship will be evidenced by a person "spinning" reiteratively through the same problem loop sequence — i.e., through structural invariance in interaction processes. In hypnotherapy, trance is used as an opportunity to allow a person to stop "spinning his wheels," and return to the

Self center in the circle of autonomy in order to rebalance the system and allow generative autonomy to develop new expressions more suitable for the present needs.

Problems become chronic when a person (mis)identifies with one complement (X or X') and disidentifies with the other complement. Such a Self-(mis)identification initiates a vicious cycle of devaluation which cannot be changed through any consciously attempted solutions. (Mis)identifying with one complement, a person (mis)perceives the other complement as a threat to his or her identity and therefore devalues it as the "opposition" (i.e., the position of acting against). This self-generated devaluation is misattributed to the "reality" of the "world out there," thereby again severing "inner" and "outer" (self/other) complements. Severation becomes perseveration, and the individual becomes "locked" in the "cells" of his or her time-frozen pattern, barred from spontaneously participating or directly experiencing the natural domain.

Thus develops a reiterative cycle of self-defeating, dysfunctional dissociation. The paradoxical complements of self-expression become devalued, and a both/and complementarity degenerates into a neither/nor "no win" situation masquerading as "either/or" logic with "we shall conquer" rationality ("ratio" meaning dividing X/X'). Instead of the two hands of indivisible common-unity self-referentially drawing each other (as in the famous Escher prints), they viciously attack each other, oblivious of their interdependence.

This situation is never self-reflectively (i.e., "consciously") apparent, precisely because of the (mis)identification with the complements. Not only will the person be oblivious to their essential contributions in generating and maintaining a recurrent ("re-circling") problem, investigation will reveal that what the person thinks he or she is expressing in a problem situation is exactly the opposite of the actual expressions.

The more the person tries to overcome the problem, the more he or she creates and strengthens it. Oppositional splits between complements deepen and mutual devaluation increases, thereby intensifying the dissociation from the common-unity circle of autonomy which is the sole source of generativity for any integral solution.

In other words, individuals become increasingly dissociated from their "unconscious mind" and more and more (mis)identified with the regulation of the "conscious mind." The generative autonomy they desperately seek is the generative autonomy they continually deny. This double bind creates "symptoms" which ingeniously express the nature of the devalued unconscious autonomy characterizing the system. This is the position the person is typically inhabiting when entering the therapy office. Let us move to examine some ways in which this state of affairs might be utilized and transformed.

### *The Paradoxical Nature of the Hypnotherapy Relationship*

First and foremost, hypnotherapy is a cooperative correlation between autonomous individuals in a common-unity context. Therapist and client are equals at the most fundamental level; both are unique, incomparable individuals sharing a common ground of being. Realization of this fact is the basis for generative autonomy. The client is first and foremost a person to be valued and respected, not a depersonalized category or object to be manipulated.

Within this context of mutual autonomy, the therapist assumes the problem is also the solution. (This is the basis of Erickson's utilization principle.) The therapist experientially joins the client's system to expand its intrapersonal loops to an interpersonal circle. As a complementary co-operator both "inside" and "outside" the system, the therapist stimulates transformation by valuing its context, balancing its complements, and eliciting new modes of expression.

The therapist becomes "a part of" the system by *absorbing* the client's patterns, but operates "apart from" the devaluing correlations which disallow generative autonomy. This paradoxical "both/and" process is best accomplished through hypnotic processes, because a distinguishing characteristic of trance is this experience of operating as "a part of yet apart from" (e.g., Erickson & Rossi, 1981; Gilligan, 1987).

To the extent that the therapist matches client patterns while protecting client autonomy, therapeutic communications are "irresistible." The form (i.e., patterns) of the client's "inner" and "outer" world becomes indistinguishable, thereby voiding the "wall" between these states. *Trance emerges spontaneously as a result.* Thus, trance isn't induced by one person "doing something" to another (e.g., "putting them under"); it unfolds from experiential co-operation.

*This trance is interpersonal in nature.* The client feels "a part of but apart from" both his or her experience and from the hypnotherapist. It is a paradoxical "trinity" relationship in which therapist, client, and the therapist/client relationship are autonomous systems co-operating in common-unity.[4]

---

[4] It might be noted that this same "trinity" obtains in other mutually valuing relationships of intimacy. There is "me" plus "you" plus "us"; 1 + 1 = 3. The illusions of control or separateness dissipate in such interactions, making possible the generative autonomy of creative expression.

This experiential relationship may be viewed as a mutual trance developed from a mutual induction. The client serves up the structural induction (i.e., the patterns of his or her "reality"); the therapist counters with the context induction which values the presented patterns. The therapist does not identify with the binds or devaluing processes of the client's induction, but rather remains centered in an autonomous, externally directed state of experiential absorption in which his or her primary commitment is to protect and support the client's autonomy. (This relationship is not unlike the nondominating supervision an adult provides a child playing in a playground.) The therapist does not directly challenge the problem "trance" but rather develops complementary relationships, and diversifies the ways in which it is expressed.

### *The Hypnotherapist's Personal Absorption in Hypnotic Processes*

Many difficulties arise from the time-frozen view that a therapist can or should be impersonally involved with clients. Many therapists believe that "one cannot not communicate" (Watzlawick, Beavin, & Jackson, 1967), but ignore or deny that an important correlate is "one cannot not experience." Consequently, false dichotomies between "objective" behavioral observations and "subjective" feeling processes are often constructed. This forces a "choice" between whether the therapist should deny feelings or indulgently focus on them. Both roads empty into the same ditch: feelings becoming dissociated and condensed with images and cognitions into "e-motions" ("away from motion"). To reiterate, feelings express ongoing correlations in physical domains (rhythm, resonance, shifts), while emotions are condensed feeling/cognition/image units symbolizing personal values (Gilligan, 1982; Gilligan & Bower, 1984). In other words, feelings are properties of natural *environment*, while emotions express values of constructed *systems*.

Feelings are essential to establishing any rhythmic and continuous expression. They are a major channel for tuning and remaining sensitive to the client's processes, and are fundamental to effective hypnotic communications and therapeutic observations. Feelings are analogical (continuous), not digital (discrete) communications. Thus, prolonged *discussion* of feeling often leads to a reified conceptual exchange where attempts are made to be "warm, empathetic and genuine." Thus, the hypnotherapist doesn't really talk about or categorize the content of feelings too much, but rather feels them like a continuous vibration (as in listening/feeling music) to modulate experiential involvement.

The hypnotherapist invites personal involvement in trance processes through experiential feelings. In this regard, I find the following principle tremendously valuable as an ethical and practical guide:

*Do not ask, direct, or expect the client to do or experience anything hypnotically until you (the hypnotherapist) have experientially demonstrated to yourself and to the client your own willingness and ability to do the same.*

In other words, respond to your own suggestions before asking the client to do so. Generate the general state within yourself, and then invite the client to participate in it in their own fashion. As Erickson noted:

> It is your attitude toward the patient that determines the results you achieve. . . . Whenever you want any hypnotic results with your patients, you had better mean what you say. All you need to do (in order to convince yourself) is to look back through your own personal history as a functioning human being. Look back to when you've had an anesthesia, when you've had analgesia. Recognize that you've had amnesia . . . on innumerable occasions. You really don't differ from other, normal human beings. Your total experience should teach that you are not asking anything of your patients that is beyond their abilities. When you give a suggestion to a patient, you'd better keep in mind, "I *know* this patient can develop an analgesia — I *know* this patient can develop an anesthesia — I *know* this patient can develop amnesia." (In Rossi, Ryan, & Sharp, 1983, p. 125)

### *Generating the Interpersonal Trance Loop*

To generate an "interpersonal trance" with a client, the therapist must first "degenerate" his or her frames of correlation (i.e., "conscious mind"). Having emptied his or her own "tea cup," the therapist can absorb the client's "cup of tea." This is achieved by developing a trance-like state characterized by enhanced sensory awareness, balanced tonicity, experiential absorption, rhythmic continuity, effortlessness, nonlinear thinking, and complete orientation to the client. Erickson commented on the therapeutic value of operating from such a state (Erickson & Rossi, 1977):

> If I have any doubts about my capacity to see the important things I go into a trance. When there is a crucial issue with a patient and I don't want to miss any of the clues I go into a trance. . . . I start keeping close track of every movement, sign, or behavioral manifestation that could be important. And as I began speaking to you just now my vi-

> sion becomes tunnel-like and I saw only you and your chair. It happened automatically, that terrible intensity, as I was looking at you. The word "terrible" is wrong; it's pleasurable. (p. 42)

I suggest that these "working trances" may be essential to understanding and practicing Ericksonian hypnotherapy. Their paradoxes and complementarities — and especially their emphasis on a generative "unconscious mind" — seem to lie outside the boundaries (i.e., limitations) of a "normal" waking state.

*Generating and utilizing this "both/and" state of generative autonomy is a clinical skill that needs to be learned and refined.* The autonomy of both therapist and client needs to be maintained while the deeper common-unity between the two is realized. This generally requires a warm-up period in which participants "feel each other out." The connection will unfold differently on each occasion.

There are many ways this process might be developed. I will note here in a general way some aspects of what I commonly experience in this regard. I usually begin by engaging the client in addressing general, open-ended issues. I'll initiate a transition process by fixating "over there" on the client. This allows me to enter trance while fully absorbed in the client's processes, not my own. Eyes may be softened or diverted if the connection between participants seems too intense for either participant, but the maintenance of an absorbed gaze is one of the quickest ways to develop trance in both self and other. (People need to shift their eyes to stay in an analytical state!) Tunnel vision usually develops within several minutes, and things get a little hazy momentarily as this dissociative state develops. I find it essential to remain fixated externally on the subject while also monitoring my physical comfort (e.g., breathing, distributed tension) during this time of boundary remarking.

Posture, muscle tension, breathing, and physical distance are all important factors. I find it important to adjust to a balanced symmetry in postural orientation (with slight forward tilting), with both feet flat on the floor. I begin to "suspend" my rhythms and "feel out" for the underlying rhythm of the client. (Breathing, pulse rate, and motor movements can be used as indicators, but these are not sufficient.) Everybody has a unique rhythm! At some point, a very distinct sense of a flowing feeling loop begins to develop.[5] Both parties

[5] For reviews of the extensive research on rhythmic synchronization ("entrainment"), see Leonard (1978) and Hall (1983).

usually soften, and I usually shift to an innocuous topic to allow time to adjust to this interpersonal trance. Muscle tonus takes on the balanced tonicity characteristic of ideodynamic (i.e., generative autonomy) expression (Erickson & Rossi, 1981), and an effortless sense of interpersonal connection develops.

While hypnotically synchronizing with a person, I find it essential to periodically veer away from attending to any specific aspect of the client's communications (especially their verbalizations), and work instead to develop a state of equi-potential attentional distribution, such that no "figures" exist (i.e., stand out) from the perceptual "ground." In this unusual attentional state, sensory modalities begin to merge together and perceptual blurring often occurs temporarily. It is at this point that synchronized hypnotic responses with the client develop, along with a heightened sense of autonomy (in both parties typically). This correlation is partly the result of the therapist having developed the trance by absorbing the client's patterns. To reiterate, such "interpersonal trances" can be developed only at a rate and pace suitable to both parties. If either party pulls away at any point, this indicates the need to slow down and perhaps take a break.

As the "interpersonal trance" loop unfolds, the therapist will often discover various images, feelings, or minute details (e.g., a particular emphasis given to a word) "popping out" into awareness. That is, attention is drawn to some idiosyncratic pattern. These are often spontaneous unconscious indicators of "where the action is." Thus, the hypnotherapist might puzzle over the possible significance of such cues even while continuing the general loop of the interpersonal trance.

These descriptions may seem rather bizarre, or too complex, or otherwise disconcerting to the reader. Again, it should be noted that the processes of hypnotherapy are naturalistic and therefore represented in other situational interactions as well. The "far-out" experiences one can have in reading science fiction, watching an engaging drama, listening to favorite music, playing competitive sports, making love, or daydreaming may be relevant reference structures. A major difference may be that the processes just described involve personal and professional responsibilities with another person. I believe that the exceedingly complex task of hypnotherapy requires both systematic, sincere and careful planning and creative, nonlinear, and hypnotic interaction. To master this complementary balance, rigorous training is required.

## *The Balance Principle in Hypnotic Communications*

The principle can be stated as follows: *Generative autonomy is generated, maintained, and expanded by a co-operative expression of complementary forms.*

The balance principle assumes that the mutually inclusive logic of "both/and" is a deeper and more generative relationship structure than the mutually exclusive logic of "either/or." "Either/or" relationships represent symmetrical complements (X, X') as {X and not X'}, and are therefore useful in indicating preference, bias, sequence, intention, and so on. If the complements are expressed in a *rhythmic* and balanced (i.e., oscillating) fashion over time, such biasing is valuable. If an imbalance develops, the autonomy of the system will be threatened and behavior will become rigid and defensive.

The balance principle assumes that *generative autonomy* is expressed by "both/and" relationships. For example, the miracle of life emerges from the complementarity of biological complements. A key requirement for generativity is that the autonomous context of Self common-unity is valued (and not "e-valued"). This circle of autonomy always exists. It isn't created from a Hegelian "synthesis" of thesis and antithesis; it is the unitary common-unity context from which complements are distinguished.

However, generative autonomy is actualized only through a "both/and" relationship of interacting complements. An example is the "runner's high" achieved in jogging. Here the runner goes through a series of cycles (right foot/left foot, inhale/exhale, etc.) until at some indeterminate point an altered state of effortless expression may develop.

Another example is learning to walk. Milton Erickson described this process in recollecting how as an adolescent crippled by polio he learned to walk again:

> I learned to stand up by watching baby sister learn to stand up: use two hands for a base, uncross your legs, use the knees for a wide base, and then put more pressure on one arm and hand to get up. Sway back and forth to get balance. Practice knee bends and keep balance. Move head after the body balances. Move hand and shoulder after the body balances. Put one foot in front of the other with balance. Fall. Try again. (Ross, Ryan, & Sharp, 1983, pp. 13–14)

This beautiful description can be applied to virtually any learning process. A final example of the balance principle is in the process of hypnotic induction. One of the dynamic complements characterizing trance development is holding on and letting go. For example, you may begin to relax some, then orient externally a bit, wander a little more into trance before wondering. "Is it happening? Will it happen? Can it happen?" You might then discover yourself letting go a little bit more, holding on for security, and so on. At some point, "it" happens: you discover yourself experiencing the effortlessness, the autonomy, the hypnotic quality of trance.

In applying the balance principle in hypnotherapy, it is useful to keep in mind Erickson's description of hypnosis as a process of communicating ideas in an experiential fashion. To develop generative autonomy, these ideas may be expressed in a number of different complementary structures. One simple yet effective structure involves triplet statements indicating complements in autonomy. For example:

> I don't know and you don't know exactly how you'll go into trance, but what a nice thing to know that (your unconscious knows) how and when to respond in a manner appropriate for you as an individual.
>
> You can consciously wonder about trance and experientially wander into trance, and autonomously operate in co-operative security as you do so.
>
> Now you should hold on to your need for security and only let go now of any unnecessary tension. holding on to doubts and letting go of any need to actively attend here, all the while discovering a secure balance of unconscious development.
>
> And you have had some past experiences you didn't like, and there are some potential future experiences you'd like to develop, and here we are in the gifts and presents of the present presence of undeniable actuality of unconscious expression.

A related loop structure is the following six-statement sequence:

1. A *general statement* of a universal skill, experience, response, etc.
2. A *general statement* indicating that (1) can occur in many ways.
3. A *specific possibility* x (of how "it" might occur).
4. A *specific possibility* y.

5. A *specific possibility* z.
6. A *general statement* concluding that subject will respond in some way.

For example:

1. Everybody has the ability to experience absorption.
2. And we all can develop absorption in different ways, at different rates, at different times. . . .
3. Some people become absorbed in feelings of security.
4. Some people become absorbed listening to a voice.
5. Some people become absorbed by allowing themselves to visually become immersed.
6. So I don't know how exactly which way you will discover that security of internal absorption developing. . . .

This structure can be modified by adding complements to each specific possibility [(x, x'), (y, y'), (z, z')]:

1. We all experience many different kinds of sensations. . . .
2. And those sensations develop in so many different ways. . . .
3. So I don't know whether your hand will get *cool* or *warm*.
4. Or whether your *left* or *right* earlobe will feel that lack of sensation.
5. Or whether your shoulders will feel *light* or *heavy*. . . .
6. But I do know that you really can enjoy those autonomous developments and then some.

These simple examples indicate how various idea loops might be used to experientially develop autonomous unity, complementary balance, and multiple possibilities.

The simplicity of such "chunking structures" makes them extremely valuable tools for unfolding a trance process in a systematic yet unpredictable fashion. To appreciate this fact, an excellent training exercise is to write out (and/or tape) inductions consisting solely of such structures. This will demonstrate how such forms can provide structure and assure complementary balance for both hypnotherapist and client, thereby enabling the hypnotherapist to generate a circular flow of hypnotic communications.

These simple patterns are especially useful in the absorption and orientation of attentional processes. Thus they can be utilized to develop experiential absorption, disperse focus, displace symptoms, distract analysis, destabilize rigid patterns, and develop generative autonomy (i.e., therapeutic dissociation) in hypnotic explorations. They can enhance receptivity (by reducing dominant conscious loops); enable suggestions to be seeded; and encourage trust, spontaneity, and self-appreciation.

Virtually any distinction — i.e., therapeutic idea — can be looped in such structures, and multiple distinctions — e.g., regarding unconscious generativity, the client's ongoing patterns, client resources, client problems — can be interwoven to form new tapestries of expressions. This "weaving" style reflects, I believe, Erickson's emphasis on therapeutic hypnosis as the communication of *simple ideas* in experientially absorbing fashions. (In addressing problems, a degeneration of the problem description into many simple components is first required.)

It should be recognized that the balance principle applies in many other ways. For example, complementary styles of communication should be balanced within and across hypnotherapy sessions. Examples of complementary styles include:

associational/dissociational
direct/indirect
general/specific
serious/humorous
pacing/leading
agreeing/disagreeing
cryptic/straightforward
predictable/unpredictable
focusing/distracting
permissive/directive
global/detailed
self-referential/other-referential

Thus, the Ericksonian hypnotherapist will complement indirect methods with direct approaches, a humorous style with a serious side, pacing with leading, etc. The particular complements used should reflect what is natural for the hypnotherapist and what is appropriate for the client. I usually spend time identifying the cognitive style a client is most dependent upon (e.g., global). After some rapport has been achieved, I then take on the complementary style (e.g., detailed). By oscillating rhythmically between these complements during hypnotherapeutic interaction. the client is led away from rigid identification with any one way of being and toward a balanced and generative expression of complementary styles.

## *Diagnostic Cues: Exits from the Circle of Autonomy*

Problems may be viewed as time-frozen double binds reflecting self-devaluing acts of e-valuation ("value pushed away") of a complementary co-relation. The intra- or inter-personal "co-relators" consequently shift from mutually inclusive double binds to mutually exclusive double binds caught in a "vicious cycle" of painful violence. Thus, a major diagnostic task in therapy is to identify "split" correlational complements. This requires orientation to, and interaction with, the unique processes of each client. The hypnotherapist "deframes" by setting aside personal and theoretical biases, experientially "tunes" to the client's self-essence (via processes described above), and through circular and complementary probing identifies where and how the client dissociates.

A major assumption here is that form-specified diagnostic categories are unnecessary and probably counterproductive, because the client's experience is already formed in a unique yet discernible organizational pattern. Thus, the hypnotherapist develops an experiential state of ignorance and becomes the "hypnotic subject" of the client, "allowing" the latter to "draw" their distinctions onto the therapist's "blank slate." In this way, diagnostic information unfolds naturally through intense interpersonal absorption. Invariant patterns of self-devaluation manifest through observed repetitions, constancies, confusions, shifts, client metaphors, emotion, evaluations, and other processes.

In this process, inductive and abductive procedures are favored over the deductive logics characterizing traditional nomothetic frameworks. The diagnostic experience resembles a Sherlock Holmes mystery or a jigsaw or crossword puzzle; the operator *knows* that solutions exist and becomes absorbed in cooperating with the client to discover them. Trance processes play a central role for both therapist and client, especially in maintaining "autonomy in common-unity."

The diagnostic process operates during the entire therapy. Multiple modalities are utilized — e.g., written descriptions (family history, problem history, goals, etc.); casual conversation; hypnotic explorations; direct questioning; experiential "identification" with the client, etc. The goal is to identify "patterns which disconnect" — i.e., dominant "split co-relations." They are often not immediately obvious, being obscured (and protected) by the well-developed "distraction techniques" of the client. I usually find hypnotic orientation allows me to develop a general "feel" for underlying patterns, since such an orientation allows undistracted absorption. To bypass possible defenses and insecurities, I then "home in" on the pattern via gentle and indirect probing.

Many verbal and nonverbal cues may serve as "red flags" indicating possible "correlational splits." The ones listed below are especially simple and useful, and should give a flavor of the idiosyncratic yet structured nature of such cues.

**1. "Control" intentions.**

Power and control are painful illusions. We are controlled by what we try to control. We are dominated by what we try to dominate. We become what we attempt to violently oppose. Thus, attempts to unilaterally "control" any "co-relation" (i.e., any inter- or intrapersonal relationship) generally lead to vicious and "sense-less" loops of escalating violence. Simple examples of "control" statements:

- I try to control my eating, because I hate my fat body ... I binge mostly when I feel depressed.
- I try to give myself suggestions to feel good, but I can't stop my internal dialogue from filling me with doubts.
- Over the past few months, I keep "catching" myself trying to withdraw and not go out and meet (a prospective wife). ... I have to fight off the depression and make sure to keep going out, because I'll never meet anybody if I don't try. ...
- I force myself to exercise two hours a day ... but often get injured.
- Control is paramount in my life. ... I was and still am controlled by my mother. I like to control my environment, who's in it, and what they do.

In each example, one "part" tries to "control" or "overcome" or "get rid of" its "subversionary" complement. (This implies that the "controller" is "out of control.") The result: Heads you lose, tails you don't win.

**2. Evaluative terms.**

Values are unitary, unconditional, and refer to *being* states; e-valuations are dualistic ("good" vs. "bad"), conditional (e.g., only "good" is acceptable), and refer to *becoming* (i.e., performance) processes. Identification with a "positive" co-relation (state, experience, person, way of being, concept, etc.) necessarily also entails an identity bind to its "negative" co-relation complement: they are two sides of the same coin. Because one cannot exist without the other, one ("good") supports the other ("bad"). The unitary distinction is complementary in form! Thus, I keep lists of a client's "positive" and "negative" evaluations, finding them excellent pointers to key structures underlying a problem process.

The therapist must set aside his own evaluations in order to recognize those of the client. Typically, the "clearing out" process described above will need to be periodically regenerated.

**3. Implied causatives.**

Underlying many problem loops is the belief that a given behavior *causes* a particular (undesired) state of being, and that the opposite behavior (therefore) will cause the desired state. A few examples:

- If I don't force myself to exercise, I'll die of a heart attack (like my father).
- If I don't hold on tightly to someone, they'll go away.
- If I can get rid of my mother's voice (inside of me), I'll be able to listen to what's happening inside.

Figure 3.5 illustrates how such statements generate double-bind loops. (Extended examples of such binds can be found in Ronald Laing's *Knots* [1971].) As with any double bind, dealing with *either* one *or* the other complement is futile. Neither is "true" or "false"; they are "partner" co-relations engaged in a dissociational cycle. The hypnotherapist must accept both complements in working to return them to their circle of autonomy.

**4. Flip-flops.**

Double-bind loops can also be detected by recurrent flip-flops between self-contradicting states. For example:

- My father is a lovely generous man who is a bossy and controlling alcoholic . . . my way was never right in his eyes.
- I must exercise and diet to avoid premature death . . . but when I'm not dieting I'll exercise and when I'm not exercising I'll diet although sometimes I'll not do either although never both.

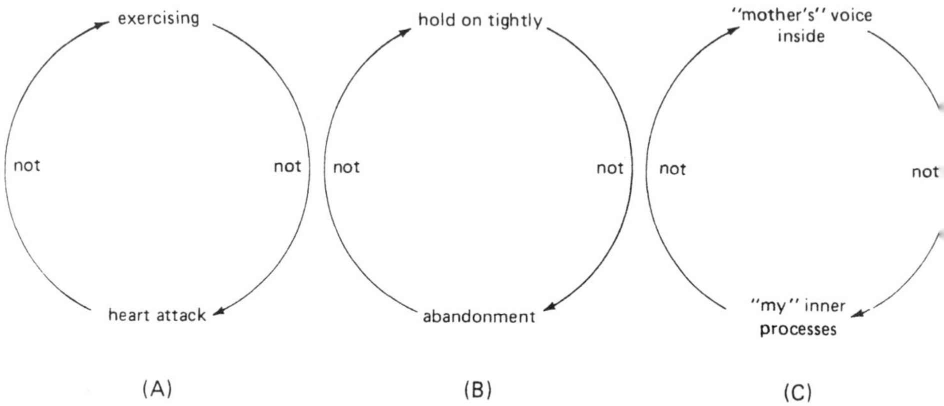


Figure 3.5.
Double binds as complementary "(k)nots."

Flip-flop loops occur in many other ways, of course. A client may promise to carry out a homework assignment and then "forget" or otherwise fail to do so, or a couple may loop between two opposing states. Oscillations (i.e., temporal rhythms) are the basis of all living processes. Problems develop when the content processed in an oscillatory loop becomes fixed in self-contradicting, arhythmic, and disruptive loops.

**5. Hedges and qualifiers.**

Such statements often suggest "split co-operators" arranged in a "front/back" position in which the "out front" actor is "puppeted" by a disbelieving and distrusting monitor. The "front" usually placates while the "back" monitors from its withdrawn "control tower" position. (This pattern is often labeled "passive/aggressive." Whatever the label, remember that the "parts" are one and the same structure.) Examples:

- The family story is that I . . .
- I was mother's favorite, though I didn't consciously understand that while growing up.

- I'll try as much as possible to follow your suggestions.

Clients distinguishing themselves with such statements are often highly skilled in inducing the therapist to accuse them of "resistance" or a related unilateral co-relation. The therapist can bypass any such senseless co-operational struggles by fully appreciating and encouraging the client's ability to maintain control and to not fully believe or respond to therapeutic communications. In other words, loop with the pattern.

**6. Constants.**

Assuming that the unity of any distinction is expressed (e.g., actualized) in complementarity of form, the *fixed and invariant* presence of a belief, behavior, attitude, experience, etc., suggests that its complement, if not also clearly presented, is unconsciously dominant. Thus, the intimidating person typically feels insecure; the forever cheerful person with a constant (usually frozen) smile is sunk in underlying sadness; the person who accepts everything accepts nothing. These fixed positions are usually maintained by induction (or reduction or seduction) of others — spouse, friend, enemy, therapist, client, etc. — into the complementary role. Therapists' observations of their own fixed patterns with a client may be useful diagnostic cues in this regard. For example, in a recent session with a seemingly fragile middle-aged woman, I discovered my facial muscles sore from smiling so reassuredly (as was she). This "quick detection" of a "minimal cue" revealed a mutual induction effective in distracting our attention from a painful experience.

Constancies are sometimes difficult to recognize, since that *which is constant becomes unconscious*! As Bateson (1979) and others have emphasized, we perceive differences. Thus, that which never changes in a person's expressions often goes consciously unnoticed. I find hypnotic perception extremely useful in this regard, as it "draws" me to invariances in a person's expressions. These invariances may seem irrelevant or trivial, yet they often prove important.

**7. Absolute quantifiers.**

This class of expressions is well-known to most therapists. Examples:

- I never would think of leaving a relationship.
- I should stop telling myself what I should be doing.
- I'm always the one that everybody can count on.
- I must succeed or I'll always be unhappy.

Such quantifiers indicate "time-frozen" correlations that forbid risking participation in the probabilistic world of temporal interactions. Thus, the events marked by "time-frozen" quantifiers will be experienced in a self-devaluing, dissociated fashion.

**8. Emotions.**

To reiterate, emotions ("away from motion") may be considered as image/cognition/feeling condensations which symbolize an event's relevance to self-identified goals, beliefs, values, etc. (Gilligan & Bower, 1984). (For example, anger might translate generally as a perceived violation of one's integrity.) Emotion is evidenced by multiple cues which can be seen, felt, and heard: a rhythmic shift, pupillary dilation, temporary motoric inhibition, increase in arousal, etc.

Tuning to emotional processes is essential to recognizing the personal values of the client in response to ongoing hypnotherapeutic communications. As Erickson emphasized:

> Keeping well and clearly in mind his actual wishes the author casually and permissively (or apparently permissively) presents a wealth of seemingly related ideas in a manner carefully calculated to hold or to fixate the subject's attention rather than the subject's eyes or to induce a special muscle state. Instead, every effort is made to direct the subject's attention to processes within himself, to his own body sensations, his memories, emotions, thoughts, feelings, ideas, past learnings, past experiences, and past conditions, as well as to elicit current conditionings, understandings, and ideas. . . . in the therapeutic use of hypnosis, one primarily meets the patient's needs on the terms he himself proposes; and then fixates the patient's attention, through adequate respect for and utilization of his method of presenting his problem, to his own inner processes of mental functioning. (Haley, 1967, pp. 498–499)

The client's emotional cues instruct the hypnotherapist how to maneuver in this way — when to stop or start or continue, when to lighten or intensify, focus or disperse, etc. A seemingly innocuous word or topic in an extended hypnotic discourse may stimulate happiness, sadness, anger, etc. The hypnotherapist makes note of the correlation and may immediately or later circle back to investigate it more fully. As a general rule, the hypnotherapist seeks to have clients absorbed in emotional processes without indulging or consciously focusing on them. (This may be described as the essence of a therapeutic trance.)

Breathing pattern is an important variable in emotional expression. If the client's breathing is rhythmic, I generally have complete confidence in his or her ability to autonomously explore and value the experience. On the other hand, inhibited or irregular breathing invariably has self-devaluing (dissociational) consequences. In such cases, the hypnotherapist's responsibility is to absorb the client into an interpersonal loop where self-valuing processes can be achieved.

**9. Confusions or discontinuities.**

Experiential shifts of any kind in either therapist or client may be diagnostically meaningful. For example, the therapist might discover in acknowledging his or her own confusion the deft inductions a client successively uses to disorient self and other; the same skill can then be used as the basis for transformational processes.

Relatedly, idiosyncratic cues may signal the onset of a client's dissociational pattern. One client would twirl his thumbs when he started to withdraw into an intrapersonal loop. Dissociational markers for other clients have included neck muscles becoming extremely tight, scratching the arm of the chair, slight tilting of the head, increasing tempo of speech. (All constrict their breathing.) These are naturalistic ideomotor responses and hence minimal and repetitive rather than gross and voluntary in nature. They indicate how and when a client unconsciously withdraws into self-devaluing loops, and are thus of primary importance to the Ericksonian hypnotherapist.

Other common shifts of potential diagnostic value include sudden changes in topic; spontaneous and rapid development of, or emergence from, trance; a series of questions by the client; shifts in rhythm, tempo, attention, or posture.

**10. Hypnotic observations.**

In hypnotically tuning to the client, the hypnotherapist may be surprised to find idiosyncratic and seemingly irrelevant cues "pop into" awareness. Experiential observation often reveals some significant pattern to which one's unconscious has drawn attention. This was discussed earlier, so it will not be elaborated further here.

In summary, these are a few of the patterns that can be used in unfolding awareness of a client's unique organizational tapestry. Many other patterns can be observed (idiosyncratic habits, emphasized words, stories the client tells, any repetition, etc.). Again, the key idea is that diagnostic information is best obtained from orienting fully and nonevaluatively to the client rather than to some predetermined constructs. Clinical training and professional skill is essential; so is allowing the client to determine how one's therapy skills will be applied.

It may be wondered whether these patterns are too general or vague or elemental. I find this to be their strength, i.e., they indicate where and when a client's constraints are but don't specify their content. The Ericksonian approach assumes that the client can do this much better than any model. Although many would disagree, diagnostic ("knowing through") models seem to be used more as shields protecting (and thereby deepening) a therapist's insecurity than as processes for serving the unique needs of the client. (As Brown [1979] observed, expansion of reference generally correlates with contraction of awareness.) I believe that it is absolutely essential for the therapist to feel secure and autonomous in the therapeutic correlation. As in any interpersonal relationship, this need cannot be satisfied by denying (i.e., dissociating from) personal "response-ability."

The patterns described above enable the therapist to satisfy the dual "response-abilities" of (1) experientially absorbing *as a person* in a context of *being*, and (2) actively operating *as* a *therapist* utilizing sophisticated skills and techniques. Thus, the described diagnostic patterns assume a hypnotherapeutic context distinguished by Ericksonian principles and processes. It is difficult to imagine their value being realized in non-experiential contexts.

### *A General Procedure for Hypnotherapy*

The Ericksoman hypnotherapist generates the structure of a therapy from the structure of a client's processes. The client's "theory" of how the world works becomes the therapist's "theory" of how to work both "inside" ("a part of") and "outside" ("apart from") the client's world. Many strategies can be used to guide this paradoxical process. Outlined below is one such procedure I developed for therapy and teaching purposes. Space considerations necessitate a selective presentation that is suggestive rather than complete. The model is illustrated with one of my therapy cases, a psychiatrist who could not urinate in public restrooms. I trust the reader to elaborate with his or her own content.

**1. Develop process description of time-frozen relationship problem.** To reiterate, this can be done in many ways. Preliminary information I find especially important to secure includes family history; present living situation; description of problem (when it started, where and how and with whom it occurs, where and how and with whom it does not occur, why it is a problem, etc.); previous solution attempts; assets, strengths, positive associations; boundary definitions; etc.

In the case of the psychiatrist[6] (whom we'll call Phil) with the "bashful bladder," inquiry disclosed:

- He was 37, married for 8 years with no children; very successful professionally; excellent writing skills; good extemporaneous speaker.
- Phil and his wife lived 200 miles apart, ostensibly because of professional commitments; immediately after marriage, Phil lost sexual attraction to his wife, though they seemed genuinely good friends (like brother and sister); Phil could urinate around Eileen "even more comfortably" than when by himself; he had periodic affairs with women (none of them clients) who admired his professional talents.
- The urination problem apparently had persisted over 30 years; mother would bring young Phil to Hollywood studios for screen tests, and when he was amidst other auditioning children she would loudly ask if he had to urinate; many different psychotherapies (including hypnotherapy) had failed; Phil claimed to be very responsive to hypnosis, and proved to be overly so (i.e., he would rush into trance and withdraw from any interpersonal connection).
- His parents were both Jewish immigrants from Russia; father described as a writer, trusting, lazy, uncommitted, out frequently with cronies; mother described as misunderstood, untrusting, unliked (except by Phil); family had unspoken rule that bathroom was never a private space; father would spend hours at a stretch on the toilet reading the newspaper.
- Unacceptable experiences (self-disidentifications) included: expressing anger at anybody (except himself and his father); being lazy; failing;

[6] I have altered some incidental details in my description to protect the privacy of the client.

being unreliable (e.g., not honoring commitments); abandoning his mother (or wife).

- Problem process included constant worrying (about someone hearing him urinate); clamping down on abdominal muscles when trying to urinate (facial expressions as in constipation); eyes darting around; self-berating internal dialogue; occasional success via distracting attention by reading.

**2. Ensure that description contains no pejorative expressions or clinical diagnostic terms.**

All processes are equally valid and thus "value-able" in their essence; they assume different functional values when contextualized in some action frame. Thus, "deframing" descriptions is essential to the Ericksonian cornerstone principle of utilization, which assumes that *everything* the person is doing is exactly what they should be doing. A "deframed" description is one holding no evaluative connotations (either "positive" or "negative") for either therapist or client. The potential of a process to be evaluatively positive is equivalent to its potential to be evaluatively negative. Thus, you will know you have a non-evaluative description if "positive" (i.e., acceptable) instances of its expression can be generated as easily as so-called "negative" (unacceptable) instances.

**3. Identify "split" complements in description.**

That is, list all oppositional relationships indicated by the client. Some that were salient for Phil:

a. mother vs. father
b. mother vs. wife
c. failure vs. success
d. public performance vs. private performance
e. not getting angry at others (except father) vs. berating self
f. commitment to being with wife vs. not being with wife
g. sexuality with wife vs. sexuality with admiring women
h. urinating around wife vs. not urinating around anyhody else
i. declared identification with mother vs. declared disidentification with father

**4. Generate deep structure pattern that seems central.**

Once multiple "splits" have been listed, I usually spend time contemplating what co-relational patterns seem centrally thematic. (Stated in another way, these themes are the structurally invariant patterns whose expression is essential for maintaining the organizational identity of a system.) Not surprisingly, I typically find correlations clustered in complementary or triangulated patterns. In Phil's case, the interrelated ideas of private/public expression, child/adult "con-fusions," and failure/success outcomes seemed pervasive.

Once identified, central patterns can be degenerated into their components and transformed into a general deep structure representation. For example:

> PERSON(s) (child, mother, father, illicit lover) PERFORMING (successfully, unsuccessfully) {BIOLOGICAL} FUNCTION (sexual, urination, parenting) in SITUATION (private, public) with ATTENTIONAL STRATEGY (images, sensations, motor patterns, internal dialogue. perception. memories, cognitions).

Figure 3.6 illustrates how the general frames can be represented by closed loops, with a frame's members also clustered in "k(nots)." This sort of representation can illustrate undifferentiated correlations bound such that all members of a frame are accessed when one of them is addressed. Thus, the "person" performing the (urinating) function may be conceptualized as a "boy/mother/father" family constellation. All of these "family members" should be addressed if hypnotherapeutic communications are to be effective. This can be accomplished in physical or imaginal (hypnotic) actuality; the "pattern which disconnects" is equally present in the intrapersonal and interpersonal systems.

Note that each member of a deep structure category can be expressed in many ways. Different linguistic tokens emphasize different perspectives of a multidimensional idea, pattern, or being. (The "maps" are not the territory.) Thus, "child" could be replaced in the person frame with "boy," "baby," "son," "brother," "son of a child's grandparent," etc. *Each token shades the meaning of its context in a slightly different manner.* By gradually substituting different tokens for an expression in the interweave of hypnotic communication, the pattern (and hence the meaning) of the overall tapestry of the representational structure can be unconsciously altered.

The deep structure loops also can suggest attentional patterns that are problem-relevant. For example, the experience of physical sensation and whether it was generated by external or internal references seemed relevant to Phil's situation and thus a potentially good entry point for indirect hypnotic interventions, as is noted below.

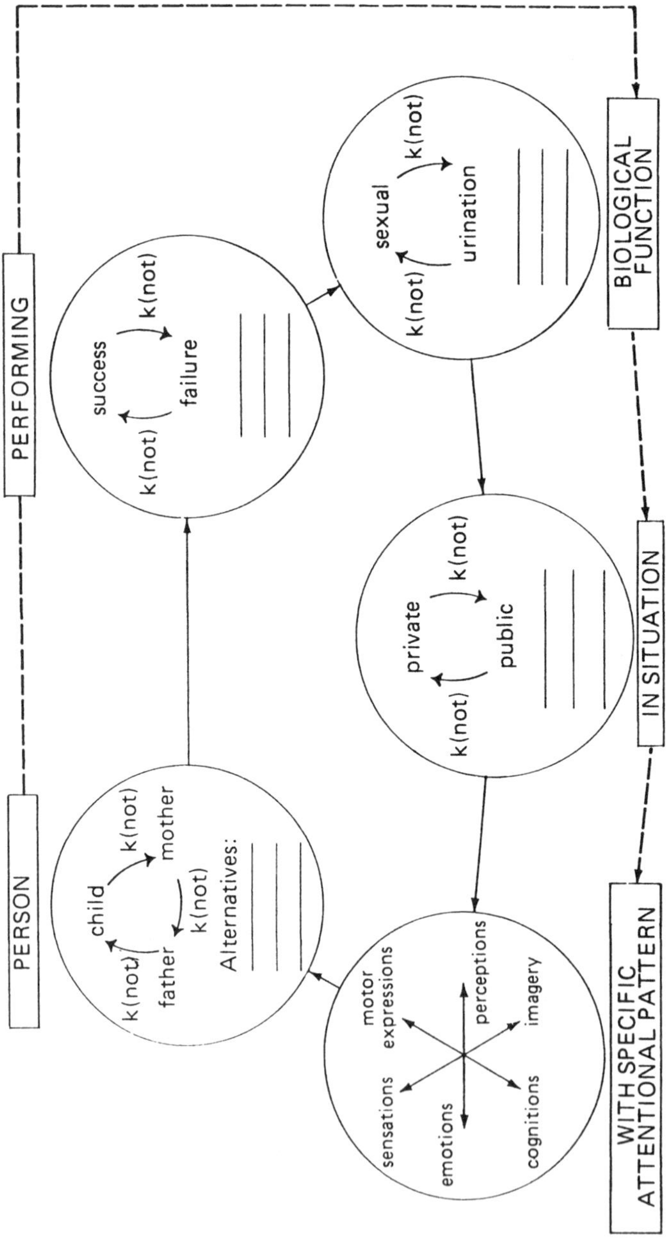


Figure 3.6
Deep structure loop representation.

**5. Generate for various correlational loops examples of a correlational process with equivalent potential to be useful or not useful.**

Again, the point here is to "deframe" descriptions so they are nonevaluative context-independent expressions. This can he accomplished by first translating a "negatively" framed problem process (e.g., "failing at urinating in public") into a "deframed" expression which is nonevaluative and context general (e.g., "the value of not succeeding in expressing a biological function in public"). The therapist can then generate examples of when expressing this general process may be self-valuing and when it may be self-devaluing. The "symptom" is thus revealed as an essential skill that should be appreciated and actually amplified (e.g., differentiated) rather than rejected. Its actual value derives from its actualized context; thus, shifting its context transforms its value.

The nonevaluative description also constitutes a "re-source" description from which multiple hypnotherapy strategies can be generated. I think it is this fundamental level of pattern which Erickson had in mind when emphasizing hypnotherapeutic communication as a process of communicating simple ideas in a variety of different fashions.

**6. Identify idiosyncratic client patterns (conscious processes, concerns, styles) that need to be included in any hypnotherapeutic strategy.**

For example, what might interfere with trance development? With carrying out homework assignments? With cooperating straightforwardly? Each person will have different patterns that will thwart straightforward strategies (e.g., a standardized hypnotic induction). The Ericksonian hypnotherapist gladly accepts such patterns as the changing topological ground on which all therapeutic communications are molded. A few of the issues I had to keep in mind in Phil's case were:

a. He needed privacy. He needed to experientially participate in public (i.e., with me) while maintaining autonomy. Initially, the slightest attempts to focus on his personal experience triggered a "self-dissociating trance withdrawal." This suggested that a central hypnotherapy strategy should be dissociational processes. (To distinguish therapeutic dissociational processes from those already experienced by a client, full absorption in the "interpersonal trance" — e.g., client entranced with eyes open — should be ensured before intrapersonal trance is encouraged.)
b. He needed intellectual absorption. Phil was a highly intelligent man

who enjoyed unusual ideas. Hypnotherapeutic ideas were most effective when "seeded" among hypnotic communications that were highly complex, shifting frequently among many esoteric "far-out" topics, referring to childhood experiences periodically, and paradoxical in nature.

c. He needed interpersonal contact. It seemed essential that some or all members of the "family system" (mother, father, wife) be included to connect Phil's private and public worlds. His parents lived 3,000 miles away, with his father in a rest home. His wife lived 200 miles away and was more available, so I included her in some of the sessions.

These few examples emphasize the complete *acceptance* of idiosyncratic patterns. Once a pattern is absorbed into the *interpersonal* loop, hypnotherapeutic strategy shifts to expanding and unbinding the constraint. Thus, hypnotic communications with Phil initially were interspersed among "far-out" intellectual concepts; later, "close-in" experiential processes became the focus. Thus, the absorption of a process is used to gradually develop its complement.

**7. Generate stories which emphasize multiple possibilities for balancing correlations in self-valuing fashions.**

The general idea description (step 4) can be used along with other processes in this regard. Strategies for constructing and delivering stories vary widely. For example, Lankton and Lankton (1983) and Gordon (1978) present highly structured formats for Ericksonian story-telling. My preference is to operate in a much less predetermined fashion. I think of stories as vehicles for interpersonally conveying general ideas and developing general processes through unconscious experiential channels. I generally do this best by holding in mind some simple generative ideas that can be hypnotically interwoven in elaborate and repetitious ways with the ever-changing ongoing processes of the client. I use free-form structures such as the 6-statement balance loops (outlined earlier) to chunk and return to basic themes.

I usually jot down before a session some stories from my personal experience that are likely to (a) absorb the client's general interests, (b) map without conscious mediation onto some aspect of the problem, and (c) function as a trance induction (or deepener) as well. The following are a few story themes I noted before a session with Phil. They suggest how any learning or idea can be organized and reorganized in an infinite number of fashions:

- Learning the elemental units of the alphabet and learning to combine and recombine these elemental units to spell out new and different meanings (e.g., one's name, a nickname, a city, a favorite sandwich, "relief").

- Learning elementary muscular relationships in learning to write without undue tension: learning to combine words into sentences into paragraphs into stories into books, and learning to "rewrite the right rite right without any lefts right except for the middle third"; my experience as a martial arts instructor and learning differentiation of sensations and muscular orientations; spending time at my word processor to form new meanings in private; a writer's block and the circle around it.
- The embarrassment and self-consciousness I felt at my first prom; wondering what others would think; where did the (pin) hole "open up"; remembering my parents' stern warning; having to learn "undercover" about "under the covers"; learning to withdraw into an altered state; listening to angry voices (on rock music); always maintaining a hold on what was important; etc.

**8. List hypnotic phenomena, processes, and strategies that can absorb the problem process and then expand and balance its structure.**

To do this, you might imagine the client as already in a "deep trance" induced and maintained by their intrapersonal and interpersonal patterns. That is, the symptom may be regarded as self-devaluing, spontaneously generated trance phenomena. Using this frame, one can ask: Which hypnotic phenomena are salient? Which are not? (Amnesia, ideomotoric responses, age regression, age progression, automatic talking, etc.) How does the person withdraw when threatened or under stress? How does he or she enjoy himself or herself? What sorts of processes does he or she absorb in? (Reading, sports, business, music, etc.) Identifying how a person naturalistically generates his or her "reality" (i.e., dominant constraints) will indicate what hypnotic processes will be effective. The following are a few of the hypnotic processes developed with Phil:

a. *Ideo-dynamic processes.* I especially focused in great detail on ideosensory processes (sensation dispersion, constriction, displacement, etc.); ideo-imaginal processes (e.g., letting images come and go autonomously while maintaining security); and ideocognitive processes (e.g., internal dialogue). In training clients in such processes, it is usually best to orient away from the problem content until experiential learnings have been realized.

b. *A "Trance-parent" (transparent) Self providing "SuperVision" and guidance.* This was a modified version of Erickson's "February-man" technique used to fill developmental gaps in a client's experience (Erickson & Rossi, 1979).
c. *The pleasurable "void state" of the Middle of Nowhere.* This technique was suggested by his common reference to urination as "voiding." The state was initially described as a relatively neutral yet intensely absorbing universe of "empty space." Details added gradually included "that absolutely amazing and puzzling discovery" of little holes and passages which could "open and close before a blinking eye could wink twice" and oscillate so successfully that one could not fail to be proud to be engaged in that "trance-mission" from those "United States of Consciousness" in which each state had its own governor. Thus, the hypnotic "void" state served multiple purposes, including (1) the establishment of a general context for autonomous and secure self-exploration and (2) a specific form in which indirect suggestions regarding the urination process were embedded.
d. *Hypnotic dreams.*
e. *Trance with eyes open and focused.* Phil learned to develop hypnotic tunnel vision in various ways, including complete fixation on his hands. Posthypnotic suggestions emphasised that he could "focus fully on the task at hand," i.e., attentionally absorb when in a public "stall." In a related process, Phil learned to "image" his (actual) hands with a "steadfast gaze" so that he would "only vaguely" feel the "private secretions of sensation" in "peripheral regions." This process was instrumental in solving the urination problem; the tunnel vision disenabled the access of panic-triggering images and related disruptive processes.

**9. Generate homework assignments which satisfy requirements of step 8.**

I find it especially important to identify and "prescribe" processes the client habitually engages in that might "undo" therapeutic progress. Phil was given many homework assignments, a majority of them in the form of posthypnotic suggestions (since he was most responsive to dissociational trance processes). A few of them were:

a. *Privacy.* Among many related prescriptions, Phil was instructed both in trance and waking states that he should withhold at least one secret each week.

b. *"Be-rating processes."* Phil reported constantly "berating" himself for failing to urinate. I chided him at length for failing to "be rating" himself in more diverse fashions. His natural confusion at this paradoxical expression was utilized to secure his cooperation in developing a "multiple-modality system" so that he could "be rating" how well he "succeeded in failing to adequately be-rate himself as well as how well he failed at succeeding in finding ever new ways to critically orient to himself and then some."

c. *Self-hypnosis.* Practicing self-hypnotic processes was deemed an important aspect of therapy, as Phil desperately needed an experiential context for enjoying secure privacy. I made some trance tapes for him, taught him several self-hypnotic processes, and assigned a variety of specific tasks (e.g., practicing tunnel vision).

### 10. Review all generated material to ensure intention is to experientially cooperate with a human being rather than to operate on a category or concept.

It is easy to deeply absorb in generating and using patterns, sometimes forgetting that the living being is the only real source of change. For ethical and practical purposes, it is therefore useful to periodically check that orientation to the *person* of the client is paramount.

### 11. Reiterate loop if needed.

The general procedure outlined here is really a rough framework for multiple session therapy. Thus, it can be reiteratively used as long as the problem(s) remains.

## CONCLUSION

I have chosen in this chapter to paint in broad strokes some primitive distinctions for a generative autonomy approach in Ericksonian hypnotherapy. This work was motivated significantly by an increasing conviction that traditional models are hopelessly inadequate for representing Erickson's contributions. This chapter is an initial attempt to elucidate the bare bones of an alternative paradigm emphasizing generative principles of common-unity, complementarily, and multiplicity. The ideas are fleshed out and extended in other works (in progress). I invite the reader to respond with such an understanding, and look forward to common-unity participation in refining and modifying the views advanced above. In doing so, I would like to bring closure to this writing with the following beautiful passage from T. S. Eliot's *Four Quartets*:

> We shall not cease fron exploration
> And the end of all our exploring
> Will be to arrive where we started
> And know the place for the first time.

# Chapter 4

# Coevolution of Primary Process in Brief Therapy[1]

> An aged man is but a paltry thing
> A tattered coat upon a stick, unless
> Soul clap its hands and sing.
>
> — W. B. Yeats

When I met Milton Erickson in the mid-1970s, he was an aged man leaning upon a stick, beset by physical illnesses sufficient to make any man paltry. But far from tattered, Erickson exuded a strength and wisdom that touched and inspired many around him. Part of his influence owed to remarkable technical skills: Better than just about anybody, he studied and learned how to communicate therapeutically. But something else about Erickson, call it "soul" if you will, was even more powerful than his technique. You could not help being impressed by the ways he thought, the ways he looked at you, the ways he spoke. Simply stated, his approach to psychotherapy was highly unorthodox and highly effective.

While some of Erickson's style was idiosyncratic to him and therefore of little direct value to us, much of it reflected highly original ideas about psychotherapy. Taken together, these ideas constitute a context for psychotherapy that is quite different from traditional approaches. This difference in context can significantly affect how technique is used and received: Techniques of

[1] This essay appeared previously in J. Zeig & S. Gilligan (Eds.). 1990. *Brief therapy: Myths, methods, metaphors.* New York: Brunner/Mazel.

Ericksonian psychotherapy may have a positive effect within one context, but may be misused and have negative effects when applied within a more traditional context. This idea was suggested by Gregory Bateson during a 1976 interview with Brad Keeney:

KEENEY: You're saying that people who go see Erickson come away with a craving for power?

BATESON: Yes! They all want power.

KEENEY: Is there something about seeing (Erickson) that induces this power hungriness?

BATESON: Well, it's the skill which he has of manipulating the other person which really in the long run does not separate him as an ego dominant to the other person. *He works in the weave of the complex and they come away with a trick, which is separate from the total complex, therefore goeth counter to it and becomes a sort of power.* I think it's something like that. (Italics added)

I agree with Bateson's comments, and find them especially relevant to the current state of Ericksonian psychotherapy. At this point we have many sophisticated techniques: We know how to induce hypnotic trance in many ways, how to give indirect suggestions, and how to weave marvelous metaphors. We know 101 ways to assign homework, how to paradox and counter-paradox, and so forth. At the same time, I believe we have considerably less sophistication regarding the personal context of the therapist applying such techniques. More attention has been paid to what "suggestions" therapists give clients than to what suggestions therapists might give themselves to best work with clients. There has been greater emphasis on joining and utilizing the client's unconscious processes than on tapping into the therapist's unconscious creativity. And there has been more focus on how therapists may influence clients than on the reciprocal effect of clients on therapists.

Such an imbalance is unnecessary and perhaps dangerous, for it fosters the illusion that experience resides exclusively within the client, thereby denying or ignoring the therapist's participation at every level in the relationship. Such a dissociation gives rise to further illusions of power and attempts to control others.

This "goeth counter" to the spirit and example of Erickson's work, and may result in ineffective therapy. To avoid such peril, I believe it is important to emphasize how the therapist may participate, in Bateson's words, within the "weave of the total complex" of the therapy relationship.

That's what I'd like to do in this paper. I'd like to first describe some suggestions that therapists may give themselves to help them participate fully and effectively with clients. Then I'd like to describe a case history that will hopefully provide some sense of what kind of a therapy arises from giving one's self such suggestions.

## ACCESSING THE THERAPEUTIC SELF OF THE THERAPIST

To begin, let us imagine a therapist sitting in his office, waiting for a client to arrive. This therapist, like most, is conscientious, hard-working, and concerned. He wants to do a good job. He has read 143 of Erickson's success stories, has attended 31 workshops within the past five years, and has listened to 92 different hypnotic inductions (including a few Ronald Reagan speeches) in the past year. Yet sitting in his chair, waiting and wondering, a sudden realization overwhelms him: All this is not enough! The knowledge, all the information in the world, is not enough to make him effective. He must have a way to use this knowledge, to access this information while immersed in the therapeutic relationship. He must be able to tap into not only his own resources, but those of the client, for both will be needed for successful therapy. The question is, how can he do this?

When I need to shift into such a state, which is every time I begin a session, I find it helpful to first give myself a series of hypnotic-like suggestions. These suggestions are meant to be self-dissipating; that is, they should fairly rapidly disappear from conscious thinking and move into unconscious thinking, to reappear only when I'm stuck. The purpose of using such suggestions is to develop a way of being that will allow techniques and solutions to arise from the integrity of the relationship, rather than from me as an individual.

### *Cooperation*

The first suggestion is, *cooperate*. By this I mean something different from what my father (and perhaps yours) meant when he said, "You'd better cooperate!" The underlying idea here is that therapists and clients co-create realities together; each deeply and unavoidably influences the other. By appreciating this mutual influence, therapists can take advantage of it. They can set aside the limiting and erroneous assumption that the therapist is responsible for developing all techniques, resources, and solutions, and instead find ways to join with the client so that both contribute equally.

A helpful image here might be the potato sack race that most of us have participated in at a picnic or county fair. In such a race, you and your partner each have one leg inside the sack and one leg outside. When synchronized with your partner in this three-legged race, progress is made; when you're out of rhythm, both of you fall down. The situation is similar in therapy, where both therapist and client have one foot inside the system and one foot outside. In this view, progress is made by co-operating *with* rather than operating *on* another person. The client has ways of being, as does the therapist; the task is to find ways to blend those patterns so that two "I's," rather than one, focus together to provide a depth vision of possible futures. Neither "I," neither point of view, is superior to the other; but working together, "apart from and yet a part of" each other, they constitute an effective team.

### *Experiential Participation*

A second suggestion therapists can give to themselves is, *experientially participate*. That is, do not confine yourself to an analytical mode; find ways to get out of your head and into the interpersonal connectedness of the relationship. Rather than being merely an outside observer or an inside participant, become an observer/participant immersed in what Mary Catherine Bateson (1988) calls "disciplined subjectivity". This of course is one of the major suggestions Ericksonian therapists give clients. It is based on the idea that the analytical mind is basically conservative; it votes for Ronald Reagan every time! It tends to see things from one perspective and acts to preserve that perspective. This is fine in many instances, but not when recurrent problems are indicating a need for a change. In such instances, a deframing into direct experience is called for. While we generally agree that it is important for clients to do this, we sometimes forget that it is equally important for therapists also. As Erickson commented:

> Too many psychotherapists try to plan what thinking they will do instead of waiting to see what the stimulus they receive is, and then letting their unconscious mind respond to that stimulus. (In Gordon & Meyers-Anderson, 1981, p. 17)

By shifting into a receptive, experiential mode, therapists are modeling the creative state that they are asking clients to experiment with. The general attitude is, The water's fine; come on in and try it at your rate and in your own style. An experiential mode also lets therapists sense the client's reality from multiple perspectives, something crucial to being helpful.

In the tradition of Ericksonian psychotherapy, hypnotic processes are a major means for shifting from analytical rigidity to experiential fluidity. Both clients and therapists can use and benefit from them, albeit in different ways. As Erickson noted:

> If I have any doubts about my capacity to see the important things I go into a trance. When there is a crucial issue with a patient and I don't want to miss any of the clues I go into a trance . . . I start keeping close track of every movement, sign, or behavioral manifestation that could be important. (Erickson & Rossi, 1977, p. 42)

I devoted an entire chapter in my book (Gilligan, 1987) to talking about how therapists can use hypnotic processes in a responsible fashion. All I'd like to emphasize here is that using them can really improve both the sensitivity and influence, the receiving and the giving, of your communication.

### *Future Orientation*

In experientially cooperating with clients, therapists need to have some clear sense of intention. In this regard, a third helpful "mantra" is, *orient to the future.* This is a basic value that distinguishes Ericksonian psychotherapy from the primary orientation to the past emphasized by traditional approaches. It is also differs from the primary focus of most clients, who enter therapy fixed on a troubling past. Thus, I emphasize this basic value of future orientation in initial interview with clients, and then spend a lot of time and effort making it experientially alive during the therapy. One way I've been doing this lately involves literally hypnotically hallucinating the client's future self in the room. It's a sort of three-ring circus: one ring is the therapist, a second is the client system, and the third ring is the future self. I use conversation between the first two to generate the third, guided by the general underlying question, "What does your desired future self look, sound, and feel like?". Once the future self is hallucinated, I treat it as an actual human presence and look to develop a balance experiential connection between it, the client, and me. Experiencing this 3-in-1, 1-in-3 paradox not only regresses me to childhood learnings in Catholic schools, it allows me to feel confident about trusting my unconscious to contribute to the therapy.

This is partly because orienting to the future self serves as a positive constraint; it provides an image of achievement around which the unconscious can weave patterns. It moves experiential communication from a wide-open free association to controlled spontaneity. By expanding the therapist's attention, it also reduces the likelihood of getting dragged into the undertow of some relationships. For example, most of you have probably experienced getting lost in a relationship with a borderline or depressive personality. Part of this owes, I think, to the instability of a dyadic relationship. By sensing a "future self" as fully as you sense the client's presenting self, you can be "a part of yet apart from" the client's present reality. This will allow you to support and utilize where clients are while at the same time orienting to where they can also be.

### *Solutions*

A fourth suggestion therapists might give themselves is, *think in terms of solutions rather than problems.* Clients present problems, emphasizing what they can't do; Ericksonian therapists organize in terms of solutions, in terms of what the client can do. The basic difference here has been nicely described by Joseph Chilton Pearce. Pearce (1981) pointed out that each of us is born with a set of "neural injunctions", or what we call in hypnosis, "irresistible suggestions". Regardless of name, nationality, religion, politics, race, or whatever, you *will* respond to these suggestions. They include "walk", "talk", construct a world image, and generate a self-image of yourself within that self-constructed world. Each task involves primary and secondary processes. For example, the primary path in walking is, simply, to walk; secondary paths include balancing, shifting weight, and falling. As long as your attention remains tuned to the primary process of walking, falling is a solution, not a problem; it is essential to learning to walk. But if primary attention becomes somehow misdirected from walking to falling, problems become dominant. Pearce (1981) describes this as the movement from the "little f" fall to the "big F" Fall from biblical grace. To move back into one's "good graces," then, involves reorienting to solutions, i.e., to the developmental skills and challenges a person is facing.

### *Resources*

A related suggestion is, *think in terms of resources rather than deficits.* The general question is, How can I use my processes and patterns and their processes and patterns, whatever they may be, as the basis for therapeutic interaction? A good rule of thumb is to claim as a resource any experience or skill involving emotion, either positive or negative, since emotion indicates the self is involved in the process (Gilligan, 1982). In the client's experience this might involve clearly positive resources, such as the memory of a success, an empowering symbol, or a positive figure in the person's life. Symptoms, however, qualify as equally powerful resources. For example, a depressed client complained of an nagging inner voice that recurrently incanted, "You can't do it. ... you can't do it. ... you can't do it." Approaching this "tape loop" as a potential resource, trance was initiated in the following way:

> John, there are many things that should and could be done, but we both know that *you can't do it!* What do I mean by that? Well, I'd like you to sit there in that chair and look at me without blinking your eyes. But I bet *you can't do it!* I'd like you to *not listen* to my voice, but you probably *can't do it!* I'd like you to try *not* to think of *not* listening at an unconscious level, but *you can't do it!* I'd like you to not *signal* by lifting a finger when *you're ready* to go deeper into trance, but you can't *do it*, can you not now?

These suggestions, offered in an intense fashion, absorbed John's attention and were further used as an element of the solution.

Just as the client's ongoing processes can be regarded as resources, so can the therapist's. For example, I was working with an elderly Irish gentleman whose legs were, in his words, "howling at him." It was a strange and intense pain that baffled the neurologists, occurring precisely from the knees down and being unresponsive to medicine and psychological interventions by other specialists. While I felt confident that hypnotic pain control could be achieved, every method I introduced — age regression, age progression, dissociation, shifting the locus of sensation — failed miserably. During these efforts, a 15-year-old memory of the last time I saw my Irish grandfather, right before his death, would periodically filter through my awareness. I wondered what Grandpa Jack was doing "visiting" me, then quickly concluded that I was distracted and thus dismissed him to try to concentrate more on the issue of pain.

However, further efforts failed and Grandpa Jack continued to return. Finally, I responded to the "minimal cues" indicating that somehow I was "off," finally gave up my fixed frame of assuming that pain was the issue, and surrendered contemplatively to the recurrent image of Grandpa Jack. Suddenly, it dawned on me: dying was the issue here, not pain. So I began to softly share stories about my grandfather, including his last trip back to Ireland and his death. As I did, the man's body softened for the first time and tears welled up in his eyes. Thus, Grandpa Jack was the key opening the passage to therapeutic progress.

What I'd like to suggest is that everybody has their Grandpa Jack. By thinking in terms of resources, therapists can discover how their ongoing process provide many resources helpful in working with clients. This, of course, makes for better therapy.

### *Context*

A sixth suggestion is, *appreciate context as the key to therapeutic change.* This idea here is that all meaning is derived from context, so that when you change the context you change the value of an expression. For example, say someone complains of withdrawing. The question can be asked, "Is withdrawal good or bad?" If you think this is a trick question, you're right: Sometimes withdrawal is useful, sometimes not. It depends on the context. Thus, the challenge is to take that process of withdrawing that's self-defeating in one context and co-create a variety of other contexts, some of which feature withdrawal in more satisfying ways. Maybe she will withdraw into self-appreciation, perhaps she will withdraw for only 10 minutes a day, perhaps she will withdraw into a relationship with a pet or another person. You don't know and they don't know at the outset how they will use withdrawal comfortably and self-supportively; what you *can* realize is that by supporting clients in doing their symptom "more and better," they can find contexts in which it will be a solution, not a symptom.

Another application of contextual thinking comes from the observation that people lose a connection to larger contexts when they experience a symptom, and that this may be what's blocking the natural development of solutions. For example, say someone complains of a migraine headache. In such cases, a question I often ask is, When you have a migraine headache, how do your hands feel? They look at me like I'm nuts and ask, What the hell do my hands have to do with the pain in my head? My response is, Exactly my question! The idea here is that when people develop chronic pain in one part of their body, they dissociate the rest of their body. Or when they develop anxiety, they lose their social connection to others. Or when they access a trauma, they can't access any other memories. In each case, experience is functionally separated from its deeper organismic, social, and psychological contexts. The figure gets dissociated from the ground, the piece from the whole, the conscious from the unconscious, the problem from the solution. A cornerstone idea in Ericksonian psychotherapy is that reconnecting individuals to larger contexts allows change to naturally occur.

### *Multiple Truth Values*

Experimenting with context emphasizes that the primary interest of therapy is constructed meanings, rather than objective reality per se. In this regard, another suggestion is, *appreciate and accept multiple truth values.* Appreciate that your reality, your way of being, your perspective, is not superior to the client's. Both therapist and client are operating in "as if" worlds, acting "as if" the world were this way or that way. Assuming that your "as if" world is better or more accurate moves therapy into a competitive power play; on the other hand, letting two different "as if" realities interact allows new "baby" realities to be born, some of which may be more useful to the person's present needs and challenges.

Another application of truth values has to do with the logic you use to organize your experience as therapist. While most of us have been trained to reflexively use traditional either/or logic, this may not be the best way to promote change. The words of Niels Bohr, the physicist who founded quantum mechanics, are useful in this regard. There are two kinds of truth, Dr. Bohr noted. In the shallow kind, the opposite of a true statement is false; in the deep kind, the opposite is equally true. This logic where something and its opposite are equally true has been pointed out by Freud, Jung, and others to be the logic of the unconscious. It is a logic underlying paradoxical assignments, the logic that allows us to see a symptom as a solution. It is a logic that allows us to encourage clients to both hold on and let go, to change and not change, to appreciate both sides of a conflict. In short, it is a logic of cooperation, a logic of healing, a logic of love.

OK. So now using the logic of realizing that if I want to finish on time, I'd better be moving on, I'd like to just summarize these seven suggestions therapists can give themselves: (1) cooperate, (2) experientially participate, (3) orient to the future, (4) orient to solutions, (5) orient to resources, (6) appreciate context as the key to change, and (7) appreciate multiple truth values. As these ideas integrate deeply into both of each of your minds, I'd like to illustrate one way they might be applied by describing to you the case of someone I worked with periodically over the course of a year.

## CASE EXAMPLE

Maureen entered therapy seeking, in her words, more confidence at work. She was 36, the oldest of five children in a strict Irish-Catholic family, married with no children, and a highly successful businesswoman. She complained of experiencing debilitating fear and stress when making presentations at work, and hoped that hypnosis could help her feel more comfortable in such situations.

Three 90-minute sessions were needed to handle this challenge. In the first session, hypnosis was described as a mastery process wherein experiential resources could be accessed and used for therapeutic purposes, and several light trances were successfully developed. A self-hypnosis process was then demonstrated and assigned as a daily homework task.

In the second session, a deeper trance was induced and suggestions to develop a comfortable state were elaborated. As Maureen accomplished this, I suggested that her unconscious mind access an experiential symbol that would help her revivify and maintain this state when making presentations. It was noted that symbols come in many forms — for example, memories, objects, or persons — and that what she came up with might not make sense to her conscious mind. She was surprised and intrigued upon developing a vivid image of a big friendly bear. I congratulated her and suggested that she hypnotically explore where in the context of making presentations the bear would be most helpful as an ally. After a minute or so of silent exploration, she smiled while describing a big happy bear sitting in the back of the meeting room while she was making a presentation. I encouraged her to continue this hypnotic rehearsal for another 10 minutes or so, and then reoriented her from trance.

This process of envisioning a bear in the meeting room was then repeated. This time, however, Maureen entered trance with her self-hypnosis technique and kept her eyes open throughout the explorations. Both modifications were designed to help her use the process in the target situation. Upon reorienting from trance, she expressed delight and satisfaction in her newly found hypnotic skills. She was congratulated and encouraged to practice each night in preparation for her presentation later that week.

Maureen returned two weeks later in a happy mood. She had made two presentations since the last meeting, and did surprisingly well in each. Initial doubts and fears seemed to disappear after she hypnotically "discovered" a big happy bear sitting attentively and supportively in the back of the room. Whenever she would need to bolster her comfort and confidence during the presentations, a brief and unnoticeable orientation to the bear would suffice. She expressed confidence in continued success, and we therefore agreed that the therapy contract had been satisfied. After reviewing the therapy and talking about how to maintain the changes made, farewells were exchanged and the session ended.

About six weeks later, Maureen called to urgently request another appointment. Something terrible was happening, and she didn't know what it was. It had started several days earlier, with the sudden and inexplicable onset of severe stomach pains. So intense were they that she felt compelled to seek help at the emergency room of the local hospital, where a series of tests and examinations all proved negative. When the attending physician discussed with her the possibility of psychological factors being involved, her concern increased and she decided to call me.

I arranged to see her the next day. Since she expressed great interest in knowing what was happening, I began by asking many questions. I obtained a detailed description of the pain, learned that it was sometimes accompanied by self-mutilating images and severely critical internal dialogue, and that it had occurred (to a lesser extent) on at least several other occasions in the past years. Maureen couldn't connect the symptoms to any present difficulties as she thought her work and family life were going pretty well. She also couldn't attribute them to anything in her family of origin, though she did describe both parents as being alcoholic and physically violent.

Given that the symptoms had a dissociative quality to them, I decided to use the dissociative method of ideomotor finger questioning. After inducing a light trance and using suggestions to establish a "yes" finger, a "no" finger, and a "I don't know" finger I asked if her unconscious mind knew what the pain was about. Her "yes" finger lifted. I asked if it was all right to let her conscious mind know. The "no" finger lifted. I asked if her unconscious was willing to work with me on the matter and let her conscious mind know at the proper time. The "yes" finger lifted. I therefore elaborated suggestions for her to go very deeply into a trance, deep enough to appreciate that her unconscious mind was very intelligent, intelligent enough to be able to summon the resources and develop the means to deal suitably with the challenge at "hand." I further noted how she had a "body" of experiential knowledge, and how her unconscious could express itself through this body in a variety of ways. I pointed out that while her unconscious could express experience through bodily pains, it could just as thoroughly express ideas through bodily *movements* as her *ideomotor* finger signaling showed. I therefore suggested that each night during the week, and also whenever she felt any pains developing, she find a safe and private place to sit down, go into trance, orient to the question, "What healthy needs can my unconscious body of experience express?," and then let herself draw or paint for a half hour or so. When I asked her unconscious if this seemed like a good plan, it signalled yes; when I inquired whether anything else needed to be added, she signalled no. So after a few more minutes, she was reoriented from trance, given the same instructions in a waking state, and bidden good-bye.

She arrived for the next session with about a half dozen paintings, each one intense and extraordinary. We sat shoulder to shoulder, examining the paintings with a shared hypnotic absorption. I found myself orienting to the stomach regions of different painted characters, for they were filled with black or red circles. When I gently drew attention to them, she seemed to plummet into a silent, emotion-filled space, her eyes fighting back tears. I asked her what she was aware of, and she said she didn't know. Tuning to my own inner processes, I became vividly aware of a memory of puppies dying. That's when I consciously realized that the holes suggested a dead baby.

Making sure to remain experientially connected, I paused silently for awhile before softly beginning to describe the memory of the puppies. Her tears began to flow and her body was racked by sobs. For the next 15 minutes or so, she cried and I gently consoled her. Slowly her story came out. Fleeing an abusive home situation at 17, she moved into a commune and promptly got pregnant. Despite her guilt and confusion, she and the baby's father immediately went for a medical abortion, after which he insisted angrily that the situation be completely forgotten, for the baby "no longer existed." She never spoke a word about it though apparently she didn't forget. As we discovered later, on each anniversary of the abortion she had been overwhelmed with severe depression and physical pains.

Sitting with Maureen, I couldn't help but sense the baby's presence in the room, so I softly suggested, "She's still alive!" These words seemed to touch something inside of her, so I continued by gently pointing that while the baby was indeed no longer physically living, her spirit seemed to continue to exist. She nodded silently and tears reappeared, this time more gently. We talked about burial rituals across different cultures, and I suggested that her baby's spirit was still awaiting one. This idea resonated deeply within her, so I suggested that she engage in four preparation tasks. The first was to use meditation and self-hypnosis to find a name for the baby. The second was to spend 45 minutes a day writing letters to the baby, communicating whatever she needed to about her feelings then and now. The third was to make some physical burial symbols to accompany the baby's spirit on its passage to safety. The fourth was to select some living symbols of her commitment to new life.

She returned five days later with the tasks completed. She reported that deciding upon a name and writing the letters were both important and very emotional processes for her. She also showed the baby's outfit she knitted and the paintings she painted for burial gifts, and noted she had purchased two plants as symbols of new life. We discussed details of the ceremony, and she decided upon a nearby wilderness preserve as a burial site. She emphasized that somehow it was very important for her to do this alone, but with my presence as a support and witness.

We met several days later at the wilderness preserve. After a brief meditational ceremony, we walked in silence so she could find a proper burial site. She selected a private clearing near a stream after about a half hour, and I knelt down and waited as she dug a hole, laid out an altar cloth, and arranged the ritual items. Beginning the ceremony with about 10 minutes of intense, focused silence, she suddenly let out a piercing cry, followed by words addressed to the baby about what happened, why, how she felt now, what she wanted for the baby's spirit, and so forth. During this process, the baby was named, the burial gifts and new life symbols were placed in the grave, and a good-bye message was offered. The ceremony ended with about five minutes of meditational silence.

As we walked back to the cars, I let her know how deeply touched and moved I was by the whole event. I also suggested that she continue the letter writing during the next week to express any lingering feelings to the baby or other individuals (e g., family members), and that she plant a new seed in her garden each day to honor new life emerging. She returned the following week with reports of experiencing a deep calm and peace since the ceremony, occasionally joined by waves of sadness. The tasks had been helpful, and she had suffered no physical pains or self-denigrating internal processes. After several follow-up sessions over the next month showed no return of the symptoms, therapy was terminated.

I wish by this time, some six months later, that I could end this story like some of Erickson's case histories, namely that the client was seen at a casual social gathering with six children, expressing a little bit of the symptom for old time's sake. But I can't. I've seen Maureen again in therapy, this time with her husband regarding some interests and issues around getting pregnant. They're not pregnant yet, but they're practicing, and that's what important.[2] More important, I think, is that Maureen feels hope for the future and a deepened confidence in her ability to handle life's challenges.

This, I think, is what therapy is all about. My intention in describing this case has been to illuminate how an Ericksonian approach may be especially effective in this regard. The case illustrates some key ideas in this approach: (1) therapy as cooperation between therapist and client; (2) therapy as involving the unconscious processes of both therapist and client; (3) unconscious processes being expressed in both inner trances and outer experiences such as rituals; (4) techniques and solutions being co-created; (5) future orientation and resources as the primary tools; and (6) how context determines meaning and how context can be shifted, such that a scream can be a symptom or a solution.

---

[2] Author's note: Several years after the original publication of this chapter, Maureen gave birth to a beautiful little girl.

# Chapter 5

# The Fight Against Fundamentalism: Searching for Soul in Erickson's Legacy[1]

> I'm certainly glad I'm not a Jungian.
>
> — Carl Jung

> I would never belong to a club that would have me as a member.
>
> — Groucho Marx

One of the most interesting things that could be said about Milton Erickson is that he did not practice Ericksonian psychotherapy. He rejected theory, frameworks, and set techniques. His writings usually emphasized a few generative principles, then concentrated on describing specific cases where these principles were creatively applied. The effectiveness of his work inspired many, though few of us seemed to take his atheoretical claims at face value. Instead, we proceeded on the assumption that of course there was a theory or a framework, it was just hidden or unstated. This assumption conveniently allowed many of his students, myself included, to "helpfully" explain what Erickson was "really" doing. A whole new field of Ericksonian psychotherapy was born, as the intricacies of Erickson's patterns were written about and

[1] This essay appeared previously in Jeffrey K. Zeig. 1994. *Ericksonian methods: The essence of the story*. New York: Brunner/Mazel.

promulgated at a dizzying rate. Twelve years after Erickson's death, this "field" is gathered here in Phoenix, ostensibly around the theme of addressing "the essence of the story."

I would like to suggest that the essence of Erickson had to do with things like soul and aesthetics, and that this essence is becoming increasingly obscured by the ever increasing "stories" or models purporting to reveal what Erickson was "really" about. I don't think this has anything to do with the myth-makers, of whom I have been one. I agree with Jeff Zeig's insightful observation that one of Erickson's great gifts was attracting and mentoring bright and dedicated students. Rather, my suggestion is that the way Erickson operated was so non-traditional that attempts to describe him in traditional terms, such as a particular framework or set of techniques, are woefully inadequate and misleading.

If you read the various "stories" or books about Erickson, it seems that they are not talking about the same person, but about many different persons. Therein I believe is an extraordinary essence of Erickson: He operated within the ancient and venerable tradition of the Magician Healer, a master shape-shifter who adapted at deep levels to whomever he was addressing — patients and students alike. He was like an aikido master in his centered presence, accepting and using whatever patterns were presented in order to reconnect persons with their own centers. He drew upon his extraordinary skills and experience uniquely in each case, changing not only the patterns of the patient or student but also his own form simultaneously. In other words, he operated flexibly on two levels simultaneously — the level of communication patterns and the deeper level of the personality applying the communication pattern.

This extraordinary skill is, I must admit, somewhat difficult to address in written form. However, I would like to try to do so, in hopes that it may open new ways to sense the essence and the story (or stories) of Erickson's legacy. I'll begin by suggesting the figure/field (or figure/ground) distinction as a generative principle for psychotherapy. This distinction will be used to draw a difference between therapy approaches based on fundamentalist philosophies and those organized around aesthetic principles. A case from Erickson will be used to illustrate an aesthetic approach. Finally, four generative principles for practicing such an approach will be elaborated.

## THE FIGURE/FIELD DISTINCTION

When you took your first psychology course in college, you probably learned about the figure/ground concept, represented in Figure 5.1. The idea is that

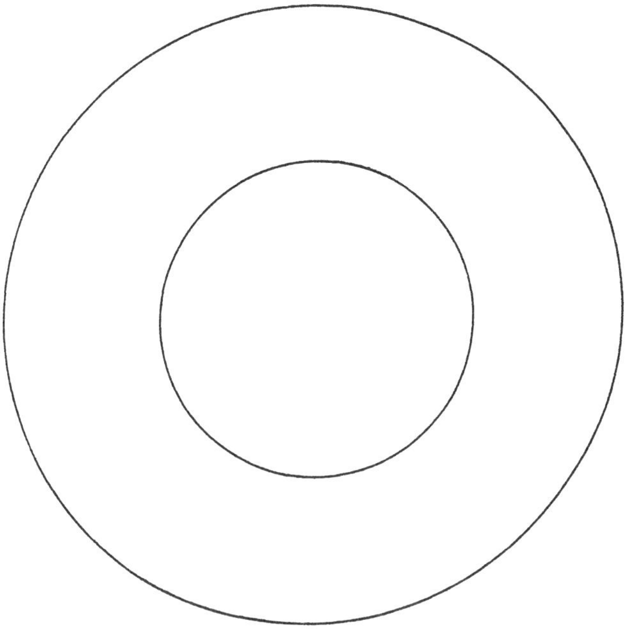

Figure 5.1.
The figure/field distinction.

you perceive something only against a background different from that something. Thus, if you see something moving, it's because the movement is in relationship to a field (including yourself as an observer) that is not moving in that way. Similarly, you hear a sound only because it's different from that which preceded and that which follows it. (Interestingly, if the same sound is presented continuously, your brain habituates to it and you don't hear it any more.) As Bateson (1979) put it, we sense "differences" only insofar as that something is different from something else.

This basic idea is a generative principle for therapy. We might call it the "little circle/big circle" approach to life. The "little circle" is what we focus on (what's in our "conscious mind"), while the "big circle" is the larger context in which it is held (what's in our "unconscious mind"). There are a number of different examples of this figure/field relationship. If the little circle is the "text" — the story or description of things — the big circle is the "context" (all the values, experiences, intentions of the writer/reader). If the little circle is the conscious mind, the big circle is the unconscious mind. The little circle might be an individual, while the big circle is the social system within which that person is in relationship. If the little circle is a single experience — say, a trauma — the big circle is the entire life experiences of the person. If the little circle is a diagnostic category, ego-state, or frame of reference — such as depression or anxiety — the big circle is the larger context of all the person's ego states and frames of reference.

A central idea in this approach is that an awareness of both circles in the figure/field distinction is crucial. (In fact, I will be suggesting that the Self is the integration of these two domains.) As individuals, we feel empowered and competent when we have a sense of both our individuality and our connectedness or a sense of belonging to something bigger. Similarly, we feel more able to deal with a difficult experience when we maintain a sense of connectedness to what Erickson called the vast array of (other) experiential learnings.

At the same time, if our experience of the "little circle" becomes disconnected from the "big circle," bad things happen. As the Spanish poet Antonio Machado (1983, p. 147) remarked:

> In my solitude
> I have seen things very clearly
> That were not true.

One striking example of the effects of figure/field disconnection is the experience of trauma. Here an event occurs that knocks a person from connectedness to his or her body, community, and other experiences. The victim often feels isolated, disempowered, and out of relationship to both inner and outer worlds. When one is in such a state, it seems that no other possibilities exist: The traumatic event is the person's identity.

I call this a fundamentalist approach to life: The text is "read" as the one true description of reality. That is, there is objective truth and it is singular. No other possibilities are contemplated. The world breaks into some version of the inside "us" against the outside "them." A primary premise is that there is "original sin," that is, there is something wrong with one's core essence. Control and violence become dominant means of dealing with the world. As Erickson repeatedly stressed, we therapists traditionally operate as fundamentalists. We start with the premise that something "out there" in the client is wrong; we use our model or theory as the fundamentalist text to "diagnose" or tell us what exactly the person is doing wrong (and what he/she should be doing as signs of "true" mental health); and we try to control the relationship with the intention of "converting" the client (or "sinner") to the light of mental health. The point, to echo Erickson, is that we try to reduce the person into the Procrustean confines of our "little circle" and lose connectedness to the "bigger circle" of the Self and its unique values, experiences, and interests. When this happens, attempts to solve the problem actually have the unintended effect of creating new and bigger problems (cf. Watzlawick, Weakland & Fisch, 1974).[2] The suggestion here is that recurrent problems indicate a disconnection between whatever is being referenced in the little circle — whether it be a person, a body pain, an undesirable behavior, etc. — and the rest of the experience in the big circle.

An alternative to fundamentalism is what Bateson (1972, 1979; Keeney, 1983) called aesthetics. Aesthetics focuses on neither the figure nor the field, but rather regards them as the warp and woof of a single relationship pattern. Bateson (1979) called this "the pattern that connects." He asserted that neither the conscious nor the unconscious was capable of producing wise or artistic expression: The "pattern that connects" the "little circle" (ego) and the "big circle" is the key.

As an aside, I would like to suggest that while this view is consistent with how Erickson acted, it is different from how he talked. Erickson emphasized that the goal of hypnotherapy was to move consciousness from the limitations of the conscious mind ("the little circle") to the creativity of the unconscious ("the big circle"). However, I think Erickson's description did not always fit his actions. He certainly saw how by talking to what he called a person's "unconscious mind" some extraordinary changes would result. However, I think that Erickson, operating as a quintessential participant, committed the predictable error of not including himself in the description. In other words, the generative pattern was neither the patient's nor Erickson's unconscious mind in isolation; it was the aesthetic fit between Erickson and his patients that made the difference.

Gregory Bateson, who sent a number of people (including myself) Erickson's way, suggested something of what I'm trying to get at when talking about Erickson and his students during an interview with Brad Keeney (1977):

---

[2] The idea that conscious purpose distorts consciousness and thus leads to faulty adaption was central to Gregory Bateson's (1972) thinking.

KEENEY: You're saying that people who go see Erickson come away with a craving for power?

BATESON: Yes! They all want power.

KEENEY: Is there something about seeing [Erickson] that induces this power hungriness?

BATESON: Well, it's the skill which he has of manipulating the other person which really in the long run does not separate him as an ego dominant to the other person. He works in the weave of the total complex and they come away with a trick which is separate from the total complex, therefore, goeth counter to it and becomes a sort of power. I think it's something like that. (p. 49)

This "weave of the total complex" is the aesthetic field of which I speak. In contrast to a fundamentalist focus, aesthetics is not tied to a model, theory, or set of techniques. The relationship itself is the text, and its organicity means that it is forever changing. Working effectively within this field requires rigorous training in a tradition (such as hypnotic therapy), but the specific techniques arise from this ever-shifting ground; thus, their form and meaning are also constantly changing. Obvious examples of working in this way are playing jazz or writing novels. When such an approach is used in therapy, curiosity and fit predominate as organizing principles, rather than control and manipulation.

Technique is thus seen quite differently in an aesthetic context. In a fundamentalist approach, for instance, metaphor comes to be regarded as a clever technique for manipulating a person's "unconscious mind" to change its ways in a manner presumed by the therapist to be superior. It is an error-correction device performed by a privileged expert from the outside in. It usually deteriorates rapidly into an approach where you are thinking, "What stories do I tell for depression or for anxiety?" rather than, "How do I cooperate with and empower *this* unique person at *this* unique moment?"

In contrast, an aesthetic approach works from the outside in and the inside out simultaneously. In joining a person rather than filling a conceptual framework, the therapist shifts from manipulating someone "out there" to cooperating with someone with whom a connection is felt. Patterns and values are felt not only in terms of their symbolic values but also in kinesthetic terms such as contour, texture, and numinosity. (As someone once remarked, aesthetics is born as a discourse of the body.) Stories arise from an interest in validating and expanding these patterns, so their expression can be more variable and more connected to a sense of well-being. A metaphor is thus not a causal vehicle for change but rather a possibility for expanding the ways a person can, as Bill O'Hanlon says, "do and view" what they're already "up to."

Other differences between aesthetic and fundamentalist approaches are equally startling. Take, for example, Erickson's suggestion to "trust the unconscious." A fundamentalist would hear that as saying the "unconscious" is a sort of Savior or Messiah, the All-Knowing and All-loving Father or Mother or Inner Child who, if we give ourselves over to it completely, will lead us to the Promised Land where we will live happily ever after. One's self would presumably be seen as passive and on the sidelines, taking in the drooling mouth or full-body levitations of one's amazingly hypnotized body. Of course, some people, therapists and clients alike, are drawn to this fantasy, and see hypnosis or stories or indirect suggestion as the magical wand that heals. Others adopt a cynical, senescent attitude, criticizing "trust in one's unconscious" as a dangerously irresponsible challenge to the monolith of control-driven thinking. Each response would be sharing the same literal, reductionistic understanding of "trust the unconscious."

Trusting the unconscious means something quite different within an aesthetic approach. It suggests an artistic process of becoming a part of something bigger than your ego while maintaining your individual center in the process. In the case of therapy, it means letting go of fixed scripts to join a field where you have connectedness to your self *and* to your client(s) *and* to some shared purpose or intent. You are constrained, in the best sense of the word, to feel and follow the ever-shifting fit between people having a conversation about creating, a future that works for the client(s). While this requires tremendous letting go and being guided by something "bigger" than one's conscious mind, it also requires considerably more concentration, rigor, and compassion than fundamentalist approaches. Thus, the aesthetic understanding of "trusting the unconscious" is more like a saxophonist playing jazz, a dancer feeling the music, or Magic Johnson leading a fast break.

## THE AFRICAN VIOLET QUEEN: WORKING WITH A PERSON, NOT A PERSONA

Having brushed in broad strokes the outlines of an aesthetic approach to therapy, I'd like to turn now to some of the ways it might play out in psychotherapy. Let me begin by offering a beautiful case example which is especially helpful in illustrating the figure/field distinction. This is Erickson's case (reported in Zeig, 1980) of the African Violet Queen of Milwaukee. The woman's nephew, a Detroit physician, had been seeing Erickson as a psychiatry patient. He mentioned to Erickson his concerns about his aunt, a 52-year-old wealthy woman who lived alone in her large house in Milwaukee. The woman had never been married and was not very socially active. She ventured out of her house only to attend church services, and her family grew increasingly concerned that she was depressed and suicidal. She apparently had refused to seek help and the nephew, upon hearing that Erickson would be in Milwaukee on a speaking engagement, asked Erickson if he might pay the woman a visit. Erickson agreed to do so.

As traditional therapists, we would probably form an immediate answer to the underlying question of, "Who is this woman?" From a fundamentalist view, this response probably would be organized in terms of a "depression" that needed "treatment," whether in the form of medication or metaphors. Depression would be the name of the little circle, and the big circle of the rest of the person's life space would probably be ignored or dealt with as secondary at best.

Forever a nonfundamentalist, Erickson approached the situation in a different way. He arranged to meet the woman in her home and got her to give him a tour. He observed that (1) she was socially isolated and emotionally flat, with a passive and obedient response style, (2) she expressed a deep sense of commitment to her church community (she attended services regularly, though she never talked or made contact with others), and (3) she grew some beautiful African violet plants in the sunroom of her house. Appreciating these and other descriptions as equally valid, he became curious about how this "big circle" of distinctions might increase the woman's participation in the community.

He got the woman to raise many more African violets. He then directed her to give one of these plants to individuals or families in her church community each time one of them experienced an important transition event, such as a marriage, death, birth, leaving home, illness, or job change. You can imagine what happened both to her inner and outer worlds. As Erickson noted, she became "too busy to be depressed." At the same time, others began to respond to her in warm and affectionate ways. She became quite active in the community and earned the appreciation and attention of many people. When she died some 20 years later, many mourned the loss of the woman who had come to be known as the "African Violet Queen of Milwaukee."

What's remarkable to me about this case is how Erickson worked with a person rather than treating a problem. Instead of reducing her to some "little circle" of mental diagnosis or metaphorical description, he approached her as a unique person with a variety of identities, values, and interests. He demonstrated that while persons stuck in "problems" typically restrict their attention to a single "little circle" or frame, therapists looking to empower widen their lens to include the big circle of multiple distinctions. Therapy thus becomes a conversation that uses distinctions of both the little and big circles, especially the shifting relationship between them, to empower solutions that are already developing.

## SOME GUIDELINES FOR AESTHETIC PRACTICE

An obvious question at this point is how one learns this type of therapy. Unfortunately, this is a little like asking how one learns to live life: There is no set way. Each person must find his or her own way, informed in part by different traditions that suggest different possibilities. To see what possibilities arise from an aesthetic tradition, let us return to our figure/field distinction. Four aspects of this relationship are relevant. The first is the little circle, which in hypnotic terms is known as the conscious mind. It contains the dominant focus of attention. We will refer to this as the dominant story or persona with which the client identifies and/or by which the therapist describes the client. For example, the dominant story might be that the client is depressed or a trauma survivor or a borderline personality.

A second aspect of the figure/field relationship is the big circle, which in hypnosis is the unconscious mind. It represents all that is a part of the person but not presently consciously attended to. In the case of the African Violet Queen, this included the African violets and her commitments as a church member.

The third aspect is the combination of the little circle and big circle, which might be called the Self. This aspect often goes unnoticed, since it is not connected to doing or having, but rather with being. Erickson (1980b) referred to it as the "vital beingness of the self that is often overlooked" (p. 345).

The fourth aspect is the life energies pulsating through the person. These are the experiential learnings that are challenging the person at a given time. To paraphrase Bly (1981), someone inside tries to teach us only one or two things each day. As we will see, these teachings include loving, fighting, healing, blessing, dying, and all the other great archetypal forces in the world.

These four aspects of the figure/field relationship translate into four intervention principles:

1. Sense the Self.
2. Make room for the dominant story/persona.
3. Include nondominant stories/personae.
4. Get that the person is "up to something big."

Let's look at each of these principles in turn.

### *1. Sense the self.*

The Spanish writer Ortega y Gasset once was talking with a friend about why he loved a particular woman. He remarked that from a psychological point of view, one might suggest that he loved the woman because she reminded him of his mother (or perhaps *didn't* remind him of his mother); or because she fulfilled some need in him; or because they were polar opposites, and so on. Ortega y Gasset rejected such conjecture as wholly irrelevant, saying instead that he loved this woman precisely because she was *this* woman and no other. She was who she was and no one else. It was *her* that he loved, not her story or her psychology or her differences or similarities.

Connecting with a person at this level is possible in many contexts, and I think it is a central organizing principle for working, in Bateson's words, in the weave of the total complex. It is about seeing a person not in terms of a historical past or a problem or even a solution. It is about sensing and aligning with the soul of a person who doesn't think in terms of "change" and doesn't need mental constructs or your latest epistemologies, but rather is felt as a sense of being in community. When such a being "shows up," good things happen.

In an aesthetic tradition, feeling and relationship connectedness, not mental precision, are the primary guides in such an endeavor. These are not emotional feelings, but rather something less personal and ego-driven. It is the feeling an athlete or musician or any other artist must sense in order to let things happen with controlled spontaneity. It is not a feeling of an inner state or an outer state, but of a relationship field that includes both self and other and perhaps something else.

Usually, we are so busy trying to manipulate each other and avoid our anxiety that such a connection is not sensed as a possibility. However, it shows up clearly at special times in each of our lives. You may have experienced it when holding a new baby in your arms, or when sitting with a dying person. In such moments, the masks and the stories fall away and you are left experiencing the incredible uniqueness and humanness of the persons involved. This may also happen when you experience great art, at special moments in a friendship, in a hypnotic trance, when gardening, or perhaps when walking in the woods. These activities constitute what I call "traditions of the aesthetic," for they move one from a state of doing to an aesthetic state of being. Of course, one may still be active during such events; it's just that it feels like it's all happening without conscious dominance. You may gently steer at times, but you cannot aggressively control. It is at this "intersection of the timeless with time," as Eliot (1963, p. 198) called it, where you "fall in love" with life and with the beingness of the person or the vision of the artist.

I am suggesting that this "falling in love" process is central to an aesthetic approach. It provides a centering context where the therapist can "not know" and "not do," to use Erickson and Rossi's (1979) idea. This releases the therapist from the compulsiveness of "trying to help" or "trying to change" the person and allows him or her to experientially "get" that the client doesn't need to do anything in order to be OK. This aesthetic connection allows one to sense the client's wholeness, center, and experiential vitality. This connectedness is the ever shifting "creative unconscious" that one feels and follows in aesthetic psychotherapy. At this level, people are not seen as having problems or doing inappropriate things; rather, they are experienced as being unique and extraordinary, "up to something big." They may wish to express themselves differently in the world, and you may support and challenge them to get the details of their life in order, but they don't need to do anything to be OK. They already are and always will be.

*2. Make room for the dominant story.*

Once this contextual connection is developed, the therapist is able to make room for the dominant story. This is what's inside the little circle, what the client is often exclusively focused on. It may also be referred to as the dominant persona, the presenting problem, the presenting self, or the ego-state from which a person is operating. In psychotherapy interviews, it typically is organized around a single identity theme, such as:

1. I am depression.

2. I am a helpless victim.
3. I am trauma.

Like any story, this identity will have a beginning (that is, what happened to cause the present state); other characters involved (especially antagonists, such as parents, perpetrators, or a symptom such as anxiety); dominant actions (symptomatic behaviors); an emotional tone (e.g., tragedy); and an implied future ("Things will always be like this").

This dominant story is the fixed frame that gets imposed upon an experience, so that whatever comes up continues to be viewed and interacted with in predictable, fixed ways. Thus, while a dominant story contains essential experiences vital to a person, it also prevents the person from freely discovering effective ways to interact with these experiences. Therefore, an essential goal of aesthetic psychotherapy is to deconstruct a story, so a person can experience what's inside of it without being bound by fixed ways of understanding or responding to it. This "deconstruction" or "deframing" is the same process that a hypnotic induction seeks to accomplish in psychotherapy: freeing a person from frames and reconnecting him or her to life without story. Thus, this aesthetic approach is somewhat "anti-narrative"; it sees narrative descriptions as ultimately secondary to the primacy of the person who cannot be reduced to any story.

It is easy for therapists and clients alike to get caught in the story. In a psychotherapy conversation, the therapist is often implicitly invited into the story as a heroic rescuer who will help the traumatized client in some noble way to overcome some bad processes. Once inside the story, however, the therapist will lose any sense that the person is much more than the story, and conversation will be limited to trying to fix a persona rather than talking with a person who is capable in many, many ways.

There are a variety of ways to know one is lost in the story. Perhaps the easiest is when you feel caught in the undertow. Every therapist has had the experience of looking at the appointment calendar and getting that terrible feeling of "Guess who's coming to therapy?!" Similarly, when you find yourself thinking of a client primarily in terms of a traditional diagnosis — "This patient is a borderline," or "This guy is chronically depressed" — you are in danger of losing a vital connection to the person and his or her multiple identities. The challenge is to make room for these dominant stories, knowing that sometimes they need to be heard, sometimes they can be utilized, but always they represent only one description of a person. Many others exist, and the task of psychotherapy is to make room for some of these others as well. Again, the story of the African Violet Queen is instructive. Erickson made room for the depression story and worked in the bigger field of the person at the same time.

When one is talking with a client, it is helpful to note when the story is beginning. Cues include explanations ("I am this way because of the past"), feelings that have a scripted quality, disconnection from the relationship connectedness, and feelings in the client or therapist of helplessness. At such points, it may be helpful to stop listening to the story and reconnect with the person via nonverbal channels.

When I first started studying with Erickson, he advised me to work with schizophrenics. I secured a couple of volunteer positions, one in a locked ward of a large mental hospital and the other in a halfway house for adolescent schizophrenics. I thought I would practice hypnosis with these patients, but it turned out that their inductions and stories were much more hypnotically potent then mine! In other words, I would end up much more "tranced" in such conversations. When I related this to Erickson, who worked extensively with schizophrenics, he laughed and advised me to develop a meaningful relationship with the patient's left ear. I asked him to elaborate, because after all I needed a big solution for my big problem. When he refused, I felt I had no alternative except to develop the most meaningful relationship with a left ear that had ever been developed.

I went back to the halfway house, where the schizophrenics were lined up, waiting for my return, ready to practice all their latest hypnotic techniques. As I sat down with the first person, he wound up for the delivery and began his schizophrenic "pitch." I found myself deeply absorbed with his left ear, an experiential connection that grew as he continued his story. What was amazing was that I was no longer listening to the content, I was staying with the relationship! A wonderful feeling of calm elation filled me, as I realized that no matter where the story went, I was just sitting in the room with this person. I could make room for the story, without losing my center or connectedness to the relationship!

As I practiced developing this sort of connection with other clients, it was a wonderful thing to discover that such a two-level relationship allowed me to sense that the person was not the persona, but much, much more. This appreciation allows conversations to include important information from the little circle while continuing to blend it with resources and other possibilities from the big circle, all in the service of moving consciousness from an identification with a position or story to a centering within a person. Again, this is what a hypnotic induction looks to accomplish in therapy. It frees the person from the learned limitations of a frame and connects him or her with the generativity needed to show up and deal with the "now" of a given situation.

*3. Include nondominant stories/personae.*

The third principle of an aesthetic approach involves expanding the conversation to make room for the many other possible descriptions and resources of the person. Steve de Shazer (1985, 1988, 1991) has contributed immensely in this area, with his suggestions for psychotherapy conversations based on what a person is doing when the problem isn't happening ("exceptions") or what the person might be doing if the problem were solved ("miracle questions"). Indeed, the whole emerging emphasis on solution-focused and solution-oriented questions looks to shift the conversation from the little circle to the big circle.

In my own practice, I often move to the big circle by holding what I call "contemplative questions" about the client. For example, I might wonder what he looked like when he was born or what he will look like at the moment of his death; or what he looked like before the problem became a dominant story or will look like after the problem is solved. I especially like to wonder what the opposite persona to his dominant story looks like. For example, if the person presents as a selfish and uncaring persona, I look for his extraordinary compassion and vulnerability. Once I experientially sense this "other self" by both seeing it and feeling it, I look to speak to it. For example, I might compliment the person on his extraordinary compassion, adding that probably he receives such compliments regularly. If he says he doesn't, I might gently chide him for being so shy, adding that surely his extraordinary vulnerability and loving nature is obvious to others. Delivered in the proper way (usually involving a blend of what we will describe below as Lover energy with Trickster presence), it usually accesses curiosity as well as vulnerability, and sometimes sadness. Now, both the dominant persona (which might be reframed as "caring about one's self") and the complementary nondominant persona (which might be called "the incredible longing to connect with others") are both in the aesthetic field. Of course, the person is neither of these personae, so the conversation now becomes how the Self can be responsible for both of these needs in the service of something bigger. This leads us to our fourth principle, namely:

*4. Get that the person is "up to something big."*

In aesthetic terms, this is an inevitable, normative learning that would have to be faced regardless of history or circumstances. In other words, over the course of your life, whether or not you like it, you will need to master challenges that come from someplace much deeper than your conscious mind. You cannot control such experiences, but you can cooperate and learn from them. Trauma or other crises may precipitate them and shape and color their meaning, but such learnings will challenge each person in various ways throughout life.

Examples include forming and transforming a self-image, a social identity, a sexual identity, a community, and so forth. Many skills are important in these and other tasks; the point here is that people are constantly engaged in such primary, normative learnings. Both therapist and client often focus on the "mistakes" incurred during such times, thereby committing what Pearce (1981) has called the "error-correction error," which is akin to primarily focusing on the falls incurred during the process of learning to walk. Such focus on secondary processes disconnects consciousness from what Pribram (1971) has called the deeper "image of achievement" that relentlessly calls us to "walk, walk, walk." It's easy to lose awareness of this primary level — in hypnotic terms, we would say that we lose touch with the unconscious and become overly identified with the error-correction control-driven orientation of the conscious mind. Therapeutic conversations in the aesthetic tradition thus look to dissolve the storied frameworks of the conscious mind and return persons to an experientially felt sense of their own inner voices, their own inner images, and their own feelings. With these connections, it is possible to navigate the important learnings of life.

One way I've been working with this process in recent years is through what might be called "archetypal traditions of learning." The basic idea, developed by Jung (1964) and addressed more recently by Pearson (1989) and Moore and Gillette (1990), is that we have stored in our unconscious different patterns of learning, developed over thousands of years of experience. Each of these traditions has a positive side and a negative side, depending on whether they are grounded or ungrounded within the Self. The central idea is that you need to come to terms with these energies, or they will come to terms with you in the forms of their dark sides.

The four archetypes I've been working with are the King/Queen, the Lover, the Warrior, and the Magician (see Figure 5.2). The King/Queen provides blessings and a sense of one's place(s) in the social world; its dark side is tyranny and curses. It is the inner voice that tells you in the best way that you belong in the world, that you are special and have something important to contribute; or that you have no right to exist or no abilities or competencies or future.

The Lover deals with passion and communion; when unintegrated or abused, its dark side is addiction. So its energies draw you to connect and join and surrender to something bigger than yourself. When not grounded within the Self, it is expressed as addictive communion with drugs, food, people, or some other pseudo Lover.

The Warrior energies are concerned with boundaries, commitment, and service. They help you to declare your values, your interests, your sense of Self. They keep you focused and committed in relationships. They detect bullshit, reflect attacks, and help you to fight for integrity and for your voice to be heard and respected. When unintegrated, Warrior energies are expressed as rage and invasion of others.

The Magician energies focus on transformation (the death of one identity and the birth of another), enchantment, and healing; the dark side is deception and trickery, and the dark spells of symptomology. You encounter these energies especially at times of identity shifts, or during traumas, or in trance. Magicians know the paradoxical, image-symbolic, storytelling language of the underworld. Erickson was a beautiful example of the Magician archetype, all the way down to his physical wound due to polio, purple outfits, and hypnotic language. In its dark form, the Magician is into deception of self and other; it is a bullshitter, chameleon, distracter, seducer, and cheap reframer.

The important thing is that *none of these archetypes is you.* As Jung repeatedly emphasized, the most important archetype is the Self, which is the unique *you* that is waiting to be claimed and developed. When the Self is sensed, the different archetypal learnings coalesce as unique expressions of you. You continue to integrate the powers of love into your life. You develop the Warrior skills of setting boundaries, declaring values, making commitments, cutting through deception, and fighting for integrity. You learn the Magician skills of persuasion, enchantment, reframing, storytelling, and navigating developmental transitions. You cultivate the inner King and/or Queen that give blessings to self and other, and you sense how people and patterns fit and belong in a just order.

When these archetypal energies are not connected with the Self, they continue to challenge you nonetheless. However, now you are left mired in their

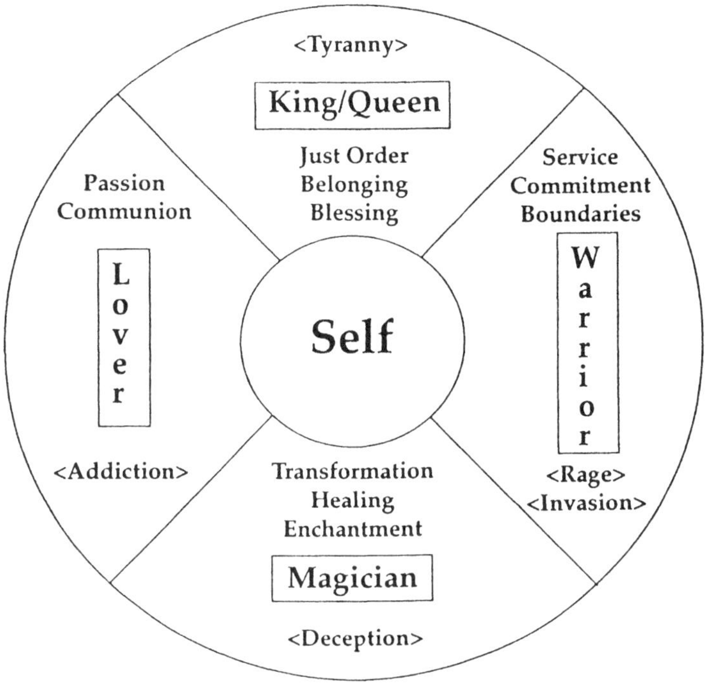


Figure 5.2.
Some great traditions of learning:
King/Queen, Warrior, Lover, and Magician
adapted from Moore and Gillette, 1990.

dark forms — addiction and anxiety, self-denigration, rage and boundary-breaking, and the dark trances of symptomology. Thinking in terms of these archetypes can help therapists sense how even (or especially) when clients are caught in any of these processes, they are deeply engaged in some important archetypal process. By sensing what this process might be, the therapist may support a person in claiming it and expressing it with more variety, responsibility, and integrity.

To accomplish this, I have been using what might be called "listening questions" for each tradition. These are not questions to be answered cognitively; they are internally held in a focused, contemplative way while one is talking with the client, in the same way that a hypnotic subject is encouraged to allow ideas or associations to develop with relaxed concentration, experientially felt connectedness, and curiosity. As the poet Antonio Machado (1983, p. 143) suggested: "To talk with someone, ask a question first, then — listen."

For the tradition of the Lover, the listening questions are:

1. For whom/where is this person's passion or love connected?
2. For whom/where is love being withdrawn?
3. As this person connects with his inner Lover, what might his future look like?

From the Warrior tradition, the questions are:

1. This person is fighting for something important — what is it?
2. Where are more boundaries needed?
3. As this person connects with her inner Warrior(s), what might her future look like?

The questions for the Magician archetype are:

1. What major shift in identity is occurring? From what to what?
2. Where are the unattended wounds that need to be addressed?
3. As this person connects with the Magician energies, what might his future look like?

And the King/Queen questions are:

1. What is this person's place(s) in the world — personally, socially, professionally? (That is, where is she special?)
2. What blessings are needed?
3. As this person connects to the inner King or Queen, how might his or her future be different?

As the therapist reflects on these questions, any responses arising are not taken as truth, but as suggestions about how the symptom may be seen as a solution. The value of a description is entirely in the client's response: If the person stays cognitive and intellectual, it won't make a difference. If the therapist's response accesses some deeper experiential response in the client — a trance, an emotional feeling, a disruption — it's a keeper. Further conversations then look to keep a person engaged at this experiential level-again, merely intellectual discussions will make a mockery of the archetypal traditions — with the intent of encouraging the person to claim the power so that it may be developed in responsible, satisfying ways.

The three questions asked for each tradition enable three intervention ideas central to Erickson's legacy:

1. You're up to something big! (*Compliment*)
2. You can do it even "more and better." (*Expand*)
3. As you continue to do it, many possible learnings will develop. (*Suggest possibilities/open imagination*).

Thus, for example, a male perpetrator of violence might be acknowledged as having big-time involvement in the Warrior archetype, albeit in its dark, immature forms. Invitations to responsibility, as Jenkins (1990) has called them, are then developed that encourage and challenge the person to identify and expand his images of an inner Warrior (many may be initially imaged as rageful fathers or Rambo-like sociopaths). As more responsible, integrated Warrior energies are connected, they can be blended with those of the King (who is in charge of directing the Warrior) and the Lover (who softens and balances the Warrior). Again, the person is none of these archetypes, so you continue to talk directly and encourage him or her to "show up" in a responsible way.

Similarly, a person with suicidal thoughts might be seen as engaged in the death and rebirth cycle of the Magician tradition. In this way, the voice that says "I don't want to live this life anymore" may be regarded as having great integrity. It is, of course, a highly dangerous situation, since the person (and the culture) usually stories such ideas in terms of images of suicide. The challenge is, therefore, to develop a ritual space that constrains the person from physically acting while making room for the deeper psychic process of death and rebirth. In terms of the latter, I might say to the suicidal client something like, "There's something inside of you that says a death is needed. I hear that voice and believe that voice . . . I think it speaks with great integrity . . . something may indeed need to die inside of you." When delivered in an experientially sensitive way, such a message typically absorbs and relaxes a suicidal person, as it is often the first time someone has spoken directly to the relentless death-seeking voice and validated it as vital to Self-development. Further conversations seek to develop ways to allow this inner voice to help in a self-affirming though difficult psychic death process. Since the Magician energies are especially familiar with altered states, ritual and trance are common features of this conversation.

As with any therapeutic process, the therapist works at each step of the process to ensure adequate safety and maintain experiential participation. The client's inner processes guide the action, but the therapist is responsible for creating a therapeutic context where new meanings and possibilities arise. Of course, many other techniques are used along with the archetypal processes. The goal in therapy is not to develop archetypes; it is to help a person live life in a more satisfying fashion.

## SUMMARY

What I have tried to do is suggest how therapy might be conducted within an aesthetic approach. Central to this approach is the figure/field distinction that recognizes not only the little circle of a person's conscious mind and the big circle of the unconscious, but also the Self that permeates both and the archetypal energies that move through the entire system. We have seen that when consciousness is reduced to a position or a story, fundamentalism follows and bad things happen. When consciousness spreads both inside and outside whatever circle of distinction has been drawn, the art of living one's life well is possible.

In closing, I want to return to the main theme of the Congress, namely the essence and story of Erickson's legacy. I am suggesting that the essence is *not* a story; it's something more organic and much less describable. Stories are the "sweet nothings" that we whisper into each other's ears as we go about the bigger business of showing up in life in a direct way. They may help us to make meaning and focus attention, but once we identify with them, we become rigid fundamentalists.

I believe Erickson's legacy was one of freeing therapists and clients alike from fundamentalism. I have suggested various ideas about how fundamentalism might be discarded in favor of an aesthetic approach. Of course, all these suggestions are more "sweet nothings" waiting to create the next generation of fundamentalists. The challenge remains as before: how to enjoy the stories while still sensing that the essence is something else altogether. Thus, I would like to leave you with the exhortation of the poet Antonio Machado (1983, p. 149), who said: "Wake up, you poets: let echoes end, and voices begin."

# Part II:

# Applications and Demonstrations

# Chapter 6

# ACCESSING UNCONSCIOUS PROCESSES[1]

GILLIGAN: You've asked to come up here and volunteer for some explorations on a particular issue that you have in mind. Would you mind briefly describing that to the others?

CONNIE: Yes. I take comprehensive exams in September, and I'm a very good student, but I tend not to have any sense of knowing what I know; and I have to integrate three years' worth of material. And when I take exams, ordinarily I go into trance, so I don't remember later what I've written or have any sense of really knowing that information when I'm not in trance.

GILLIGAN: Now, you do well on your exams in the trance?

CONNIE: Yes.

GILLIGAN: Now, what do you think concerns you then about not doing well, or apprehension that you may not do well, on the coming test if you went into a trance?

CONNIE: Because this requires a great deal of integration. To study for one exam means to memorize maybe 80 pages. That's not a difficult task ...

GILLIGAN: Oh, no. I'm sure everybody in the audience agrees with you. [laughter]

---

[1] Transcript of a demonstration given in Dallas, December 1982, at an Erickson Congress. The subject was a participant in the conference. Dr. Gilligan interviewed her briefly on the preceding day.

This essay appeared previously in Stephen R. Lankton and Jeffrey K. Zeig. 1989. *Extrapolations: Demonstrations of Ericksonian therapy*. Ericksonian Monographs No. 6. New York: Brunner/Mazel.

CONNIE: Over time, over time, but three years' worth of material, I don't trust myself to be able to integrate that much. And the kind of questions they ask are questions that will cover many courses.

GILLIGAN: So you think you would like to forego a trance on exam day?

CONNIE: No, no. I think I would like to go into trance when I start studying in June and just stay in trance until the exam. [laughter]

GILLIGAN: You don't live in California, do you?

CONNIE: No.

GILLIGAN: I think I know where that's legal. [laughter] Okay. Now you've had a lot of previous trance experience.

CONNIE: Uh huh.

GILLIGAN: Any with me?

CONNIE: I did a workshop with you in Chicago, but I didn't work with you individually.

GILLIGAN: Do you remember the group? Did you experience a trance as a member of that group? What position were you in at that time?

CONNIE: I was a student.

GILLIGAN: And your body position?

CONNIE: Oh, that position. [she adjusts her posture]

GILLIGAN: Okay, now what I would like to do, I think, is demonstrate for the others and offer for you some communication regarding how dissociational processes can be used in various ways. Now, if I am correct in hearing you and talking with you earlier, one of the things that you would like to do is to be able to experience dissociation, and yet have some assurance that the integration will be able to manifest itself on test day.

CONNIE: In fact, as I'm studying, I would like to have some secure sense that I was utilizing the time well.

GILLIGAN: And right now you experience dissociation without much conscious awareness about what happens. Is that par for the course in trance experiences for you?

CONNIE: What do you mean?

GILLIGAN: Is that what typically happens in all situations when you develop a trance?

CONNIE: No, it would depend on how deep the trance was.

GILLIGAN: Okay. Now, do you experience hand movement in trance?

CONNIE: Uh huh. [Yes]

GILLIGAN: And you have a "yes" finger? [pause; the index finger lifts up] [After a lull, there's laughter.]

GILLIGAN: Now that goes to show you we're both sitting here in front of a large audience, right now. And you can *look* at me *here* and *hear* me *here*; recognize for *now* that out *there* are *them*; recognize also that you needn't *hear* there; involved perhaps *now*, however, it is the case. [pause; looks at hands again] And a "no" finger? It is as if you have experienced . . . You've got the ability consciously to respond. You've also got the ability to unconsciously respond . . . and you can develop the awareness to recognize the difference between the two. Now a moment ago, I asked about the "yes" finger, and there are two types of lifting: A right finger begins to jerk, just like the hand, *up*. And also then, effortful voluntary movement. And both can really complement the other, as long as they don't compete. Now, how do you feel right now? [Connie develops eye fixation on her hand, with body catalepsy.]

CONNIE: Relaxed.

GILLIGAN: Relaxed. And what are you aware of developing in visual awareness?

CONNIE: I'm aware of your face . . . and the light . . . and my eyes to my right primarily.

GILLIGAN: And has my face begun to change yet?

CONNIE: No.

GILLIGAN: Has the feeling in your hands begun to change yet?

CONNIE: Yes, there is a tingling in my right hand.

GILLIGAN: A tingling in your right hand? And has the feeling in your feet begun to change yet?

CONNIE: They're tingling.

GILLIGAN: Do you enjoy that tingling?

CONNIE: Sure.

GILLIGAN: Has the feeling in your eyelids begun to change yet?

CONNIE: No.

GILLIGAN: Has the feeling in your chest begun to change yet?

CONNIE: Heavy.

GILLIGAN: And your visual awareness? [Connie continues unblinking eye fixation, suggesting tunnel vision.]

GILLIGAN: And your left hand? . . . Now, one of the suggestions that I would like to offer is that you have a variety of different experiences of trance already under your belt. One of the nice things that you can do is be able to reorganize certain hypnotic responses so they occur in a complementary fashion. Whether it's the feet, and the sensation may be *right* and *left* foot *changing*; or whether it's the hands, and feeling *right* and *left* hands *changing*; or whether it's my face, and the lighting on my face *changing*, the fact of the matter still remains: You *really* can continue to *wonder*, to question. You really can continue to recognize that it's important, to hold out just a little bit, and it's important also to wait [weight], wait [weight], wait on the one hand. And on the other hand to recognize that a sense of urgency is sometimes a product of the moment, and all moments are transitory.

I know, for example, that in the past week, past month, past year for that matter, I've been completing my doctoral dissertation. I know that in the last month I sat rather intensely . . . in my office . . . at my word processor . . . and typed over and over and over and over and over again. And my *hands* began to feel that they were *operating independently*. I didn't have to think, "Where's the i on the keyboard?" I didn't have to think, "Where's the return on the keyboard?" I didn't have to think, "Where's the delete?" In an automatic way, I utilize those different elements as keys to translate thoughts. What a nice thing about modem technology, word processors, that you can really reorganize on the spot. I know, for example, that in writing my doctoral dissertation, I wrote. [Connie begins to close eyes]

GILLIGAN: You shouldn't go too quickly now, Connie. [eyes flutter and remain open] That's a tendency that should be avoided. You really don't have to leave. You can let the situation alter of its own accord. Or you can use the word processor. You establish different documents on different records. I know that in my 150 page dissertation there are many different documents. Fifteen pages of references, figures, tables, introduction, experiment 1, experiment 2, 3, 4, 5, 6, and general discussion. Well, it came time to print it out for acceptable copy. I had to use document link on the word processor. Never could do that on the typewriter. [pause] One of the wonderful things that you can learn is to be able to *respond selectively*. Now whether it is that hand that's operating independently, or whether it's your *eyelids* blinking *up* and *down* independently. *Down again* independently down, independently. Or the feet *tingling*. You can recognize what is that metaphor, and recognize a symbolic alteration. Sometimes very fitting. And people have idiomatic phrases. "If the shoe fits, wear it." Well, what happens if the shoe does not fit? And you can be able to outfit yourself . . . with clothing proper not only for mundane expression, not only for transitory expression, but a symbolic expression of reorganization in a manner that is appropriate for you as an individual. And so you can let yourself *become aware of visual realities*, and you recognize also that a kinesthetic development, a somatic development can also be par for the course. You can be able to really enjoy . . . a birdie, an eagle. And recognize that you can *score* . . . *soar* . . . *score* with the best of them. And you can do that in so many different ways, Connie. I know, for example, yesterday Jeff Zeig telling me of his newly acquired hobby of learning how to fly glider planes. And he described to me how exhilarating it was just to be able to go along all by himself. And he started out with a lot of investment, with a lot of guidance, supervision. But soon Jeff's at the control all by himself. And he invited me to learn about gliding. I didn't know if it was going to be appropriate. I certainly could imagine being able to *glide from a perspective up on high* and be able to *look down* and see all those different patterns and all different combinations and connections of urban and rural . . . a patchwork of farming, of smokestacks and playing fields, of little boys and girls playing ball, of men and women going to work, and the ability of really being able to enjoy the perspective gained from hang gliding. As I already told Jeff, "I don't know. I certainly will think about it." And that brought a lot of conscious orientation. . . . But there's some fear involved; some anxiety involved.

Now, I know another experience, in growing up, my brother and I were very close. Everywhere my brother went, I went, dressed in the same clothes, red cardigan sweaters going to Mass every Sunday. My brother is several years older. And all the time, the term "the boys" was used to refer to him and me. And growing resentment, a growing recognition of the need for awareness between the two. My brother and I turned into fierce competitive individuals who wouldn't give each other the time of day. I had to learn to *separate* with an awareness so that I could engage in tasks that were interesting for me, he and his. We both stopped wearing red cardigan sweaters. It wasn't until I learned about unconscious response, that I began to recognize how many different *needs for autonomy* and different expressions of autonomy one can have. Oh, a nice *uplift* that one can be able to develop from psychological experience of recognizing reorganization of *different*, sidetracks of *different*, symbolic instances of *different* manners of being able to express differing, opportunities for *difference*, experiences of *dissociational intelligent autonomy*. And whether it is finger *twitch*, lift *up*, hand *up*, press down [hand begins to levitate], whether it is memory from the past, childhood memory. Whether it is *tingling*, alteration, auditory perception. Whether it is onset shortly of dream as soon as hand *lifts*, only as soon as you recognize *own* way, own time. And you really can recognize what is a metaphor.

And if you live in California, you recognize contrast: mountains and coasts. And going up the coast you can recognize how fog can obscure a view, a very beautiful contrast. Growing up in San Francisco, it's hard sometimes to see only a block away. *You can't see beyond that block.* I took my initial education in San Francisco and then Santa Cruz. Both very foggy and both really obscuring vision beyond one block. And luckily, I moved to Palo Alto . . . *take a trip.* Move a distance away, still close enough to the old learning institutions. But one thing very nice about Palo Alto . . . *never foggy.* You can see for a *long* way, and it's always nice to know that in any environment, there's always more *beyond the block.* And your unconscious really *can* demonstrate, Connie. And recognize that you really *can* let yourself develop that depth of trance, really *can* let yourself recognize that there *can* be concerns, there *can* be doubts, there *can* be worries, should be, will be, always will be, but along with that the unconscious response perhaps imperceptible at first [hand jerks up] . . . *that's right, a little bit more,* Connie, enveloping all in good time. As you can operate in good time. You really can *have a good time.* And recognize those manifestations, different realities, can, should occur, with a mixture of different life experiences.

I know that in training martial arts students I learned the joy of pain and pleasure. I learned the satisfaction derived from frustration and completion. And I learned the necessity of contact and withdrawal. I learned the importance of *holding on, letting go.* And at a martial arts studio, a casual observer often asked after an intense test, "How can you possibly test so hard and not really have unpleasant feelings about it? Are you throwing kicks here, throwing punches there? You're integrating everything seemingly. Different combinations punches and kicks, right hand and left hand, right leg, left leg. And how do you do that?" [pause] I know that in training martial arts students you drill them in ways they can enjoy. For example, you can number a hand left hand 1, right hand 2, left foot 3, right foot 4, and you have them jog in place, dance around in place, and listen to the instructors call out the numbers: *1* and the *left* hand there has movement; 2, *right* hand; *1, 2,* a combination of different movements; *1, 2, 3,* left hand, right hand, left foot; 4, 2, 1, right foot, right hand, left hand; 1, 3, 4, left hand, left foot, right foot; 1, 3, 4: *and the middle third,* the center of the integration also predominant, but always keep them running comfortably. You work up a sweat. You should. And you *discover different combinations*. They can be generated from different formal forrns that you have learned. And so rather than going through Pinon 1, Pinon 2, Pinon 3, Pinon 4, Pinon 5, and going through all the different forms, you put them together in different combinations. And you learn in martial arts the importance of combinations in formal forms and placing 24 movements together. And their predicted sequence and taking them apart again. Every student will come in and look and want to throw a jump . . . spin . . . reverse kick, right off the bat. Especially the youngsters who come in, adolescents, will want to do exactly what the black belt is doing, will want to know: How do I throw a jump, double spin, kick? And they demonstrate the fact that if they throw that too fast, too quickly, they are going to land right on their butt.

And so you stress the importance of being able to take a little time not only before a test, but before each workout. And really let yourself limber up physically, limber up emotionally, limber up physically. Are you ready to let your muscles stretch? Because in letting those muscles stretch, what your body is learning to do is to discriminate different muscle groups. . . .

Individuals first come in and throw a punch with the entire body muscles bunched up and tense. Mental awareness is very focused and violent. They really have little power and are off balance. You learn with stretching. You learn through forms. You learn through combinations, *1, 3, 2,* and continue on, exploring all the different permutations: *1, 1, 2, 1, 3, 4, 1, 1, 1, 1, 1, 1, 1, 1,* one, won.

And it really is nice to know that "won" can be in the past tense, and you really can know it can be a *present* in the *past* tense, and know that which was then a *present*, can become now again in the future an utter actuality. And whether you wear white, yellow, green, blue, purple, brown, black, you really can recognize those different combinations of training as opportunities to discriminate, to *strengthen associations*, and gain flexibility. And sometimes individuals express surprise when they find out I have a black belt. They say you don't look overly muscular. I really have to tell them that *you don't have to overpower it*. You learn to operate in accord with *internal rhythm*. You learn to operate in accord with flexibility. And you let those violent, muscle bound people lunge right by. Let all those anxieties drift right on by. I recognize that *1, one, won, I* . . . is a result of repetitive and yet flexible and intelligent investigation.

And your unconscious really can operate in accord with the present needs, and present understanding. I know, for example, that working at Stanford University, a colleague approached me, asked me if I thought that lucid dreaming was a psychological possibility available to anyone. I said I didn't know. It sounded like an interesting research project, and I consented to help him out devising methodology for a lucid dreaming. And so the contemplation of the question: *How do you develop a lucid dreaming state?* It was something that had to be thought over. Food for thought, not only in dreams; food for thought when I was studying other methodologies as well. And I worked with the experimental subjects and trained them to *develop a very deep trance*, and operate in a very deep trance . . . and *let the unconscious do the learning* [Connie moves head slightly] make the adjustment, head *down, up, over* to areas of learning that were going to be important. And I gave those individuals suggestions so they could practice lucid dreaming. And they had at least six dreams every night. I didn't know which one, which dream in the first week was going to be devoted to lucid dreaming. And how can you have a lucid dream and forget that it was lucid? And over the weeks, a development of higher frequencies of lucidity, of awareness of dissociational processes, of awareness of the function of dreams, of the awareness of the ability of the unconscious to integrate, to develop, to explore, to combine learnings in various experiential ways appropriate to the needs of the entire self. You can *feel* it. *You can feel it. You can feel it.* [long pause] And a tiny seed. And yet the beauty of a rose, of a bud, and the patience . . . of letting that bud . . . open up at the appropriate time. And now, that the enjoyment of any rose is occasionally tempered by a thorn. What else is new?

And so my colleague at Stanford mapped out the frequency of reported lucid dreams in a number of subjects and found that all his subjects could learn lucid awareness of dissociational processes. And dreaming really is only one way the unconscious can operate. And you can be able to occupy your time in gardening; you can occupy your time learning martial arts; you can occupy your time at a word processor; you can occupy your time running around the track; you could operate and occupy your time worrying, but always, always, always you can let remain across all of that transitory reality, the recognition of the autonomy of the unconscious. The security and trust.

I know, for example, that an individual, a friend of mine, was studying for a premedical exam. I was very very concerned that she was going to be overwhelmed by the anxiety, because in one day of MCATs she was going to have to go through biology, chemistry, literature, reading comprehension, physics, and *she didn't know how she was going to be able to do it all.* I told her, "I don't know either exactly how *you'll do it.*" But I do know your unconscious can *get to work.* And your unconscious can . . . *take care of it.* And she worried and worried and studied and worried and studied and worried, and got up her hopes and studied some more, and got discouraged and studied some more. Had a snack and went for a walk, studied some more, worried and took pleasure in a TV show, worried, studied, studied, and enjoyed *relaxation trance*, *deep trance*, worried a little bit less, but still some. And the *right* to worry, to be *left* with a *middle third of security* all the while, no matter which side of the issue you do explore. And recognition in doing so, that always, always, always the unconscious has a lot more capacity than a 56K word processor. And has a lot more functions than simple deletion, or return that you can press on a typewriter: Return, Return, Return. Until you hear that chatter in a typewriter; it can be very annoying and distracting. I know, for example, that I used to write on a typewriter, and didn't think I could think without all the chattering of the keys. I didn't realize how useful a word processor can be, and how much more useful it was to be able to see my results on the screen in front of me. And so I told my friend studying for her MCATs that her unconscious could get to work. And she found herself thinking back to *childhood experiences*, very pleasurable, *very secure experiences.* And she had some very friendly dragons. Other people heard about that and said, "*Dragons friendly?*" And her dragons were very friendly. Her "Prince Charming." And she could use those dragons to slay all her other obstacles, and she was very delighted to recognize that those dragons could sit on her shoulder and she'd still have all of the burden on her shoulders, and with the dragon on her shoulder there would be no room left for other associations. That is, you don't want to get too close to a dragon. [pause]

Now when a kitchen gets too hot, you know what you need to do. And so you can recognize, you can let your unconscious *cool things.* Everybody does have their own style, Connie. And so I don't know exactly how it will happen for you. I know, for example, one day a group of black belts were standing around, and I began to talk about how I control pain by experiencing it as heat and allowing it to emanate out and escape from my fingers and toes; and that is a way to control pain. And Rodney, a third degree black belt, said "No, whenever it gets painful for me, I just think of my girlfriend." He said, "I let myself experience the pleasure of being with my girlfriend, and then that pain is enjoyable tingling of a degree that I can't share with you here." And Chris, a second degree black belt, said that his body got completely numb and he felt very detached. And you really can learn combinations appropriate for the situation. Based with one situation, a *1, 1, 1, 2, 4, meta 4*; 2 ... 4 ... 3, *meta 4*; 4, *meta 4*; 5 ... symbolic alteration; *6* ... flexible combinations; 7 ... a lucky day; *8* ... the experience of a good meal, and the satisfaction of knowing that you can nourish yourself more than once a day; *9* ... *10* ... *10* ... really can attend to unconscious needs; *11* ... a repetition that provides a new meaning ...

And Gregory Bateson used to point out that one plus one is not always two, sometimes three; and he would joke that he would put a wife and a husband together, one plus one sometimes you got three. And you talk about putting two patterns against each other, and you'd get a third pattern. And I pointed out that you can put one beside another one, and get eleven. *And whoever heard of a psychological baker's dozen anyway?* Well, you can skip some that are not important, and continue on in that progression. And you can let the unconscious take care of things. And I like to take every night a substitute for the prayers I used to say when I was a youngster. I thank my unconscious in drifting off, and I acknowledge the unconscious is a smart cookie, and I begin to orient to a different state. But no matter what state that you orient to — Massachusetts, Arizona, Texas, California — you really can recognize the unconscious as a bonafide citizen of the United States of Consciousness. What a nice thing to know ... that you can enjoy that citizenship and let your vote count on election day and feel the satisfaction of bringing home a winner.

And so in a moment, Connie, I'm going to begin to count backwards from ten to one, as I do you can reorient from trance. Bring back only that which is appropriate to bring back. 10 ... 9 ... 8 ... 7 ... 6 ... 5 ... 4 ... 3 ... 2 ... [eyes open] And you fill in the rest!

CONNIE: Uh huh.

GILLIGAN: And you recognize what its present tense is ... And what its future tense will be ... People say that there is no negation ... that can be demonstrated unconsciously. Would you subscribe to such a hypothesis?

GILLIGAN: Uh huh.

GILLIGAN: So would I, but with one exception. You can reject anything. [long pause] Now how does your right hand feel?

CONNIE: Fine.

GILLIGAN: Are you surprised?

CONNIE: No.

GILLIGAN: Take a deep breath. [long pause] And how are you feeling?

CONNIE: Fine.

GILLIGAN: Take your time in reorienting back fully. I know this can be an unusual situation here. You don't have to force yourself to orient back out into the group at large until you feel appropriate about doing so. Okay? [Connie nods head] And I want to thank you very much. [Turns to audience]

GILLIGAN: I'm willing to open the floor in a Moses-like fashion to any comments or questions from the "peanut gallery," if you don't mind. Any questions? I think we have time, for a couple of minutes, if there are any? If you do, you'll have to come up to the microphone.

GILLIGAN (*to Connie*): Feel free not to answer if you don't want to.

MEMBER OF THE AUDIENCE: What was the purpose of the hand motions that you did, and were you aware of hand motions, and what happened when you noticed them?

GILLIGAN (*to Connie*): Do you want to give your impression first? And then I'll make up my answer. [laughter]

CONNIE: I felt a real command to raise one hand or the other, and I was keenly aware the whole time that I wasn't doing it, as far as I know. And I just had to allow that to be, but it was real uncomfortable, because it seemed that became the criterion of the trance; so I was going along with everything else, on the *one hand kind of dissociative* . . . [laughter]

GILLIGAN: I hope the relevance of that to the issue at hand is clear. Quite seriously, one of the things that you want to do — first of all, I introduced a lot of suggestions, not knowing exactly how the person is going to respond to them, and rightfully so, because people, I think, really are unique and will respond according to what's appropriate for them at the moment. This process that I am talking about, reversing certain patterns, is just one of a number of different ways of communicating that idea that I was seeding throughout the entire time, about establishing different patterns, that there's an expectancy of one thing happening, and a real intense hoping that one thing would happen. Yet I was talking about reversal of patterns. Now there were some ideomotoric responses in the hand, not a full hand levitation, and that really doesn't concern me. In fact, it's very nice response that can be utilized, because in the goal state that Connie has, there's going to be plenty of frustrations encountered. So a question becomes: How can I utilize their response as part of the therapeutic goals that are set up? And so, it's a good way to distract and orient and focus their attention, displace the failure onto the hand so that they can work independently at the same time. And also keep them aware, hoping something is going to happen ... and begin to teach them to have dissociated awareness, which was one of my prime goals here.

BOB PEARSON: I think most of you know who I am. I followed Milton Erickson around like a little puppy dog for many years. And let me say to this group, that you have just witnessed the finest example of the embedded metaphor on a spontaneous basis that I have seen in many many years. Thank you, Steve.

GILLIGAN: Thanks, Bob. [applause]

GILLIGAN: Well, I think that's a good place to end. [laughter] Thank you all very much.

## COMMENTARY BY STEVE GILLIGAN

My initial contact with Connie as a volunteer subject came the day before the demonstration. She was among several individuals at the conference who asked if they could serve as the subject. She reported having attended a large 5-day training course of mine in New York City earlier in the year, and expressed an interest in using hypnosis to help her pass some upcoming comprehensive exams in psychology. I selected her because her goal seemed straightforward and addressable within a single session, and because she seemed to be a good hypnotic subject.

### *The Initial Interview*

We met later that day for an initial interview. My thinking was organized around three basic questions: (1) What does she want? (2) What does she perceive as resources and obstacles to what she wants? (3) What are her customary patterns (of thinking, acting, feeling, etc.)?

What she wanted was clear and simple: to pass her comprehensive exams in psychology. She thought this would entail being able to prepare effectively, to relax during the test, to develop an experiential state (e.g., trance) optimal for test performance, to integrate diverse areas of learned information, to relieve any anxiety, and to still "inner chatter."

Among her resources were an excellent hypnotic ability, a solid knowledge base (that is, she knew the material), and a good history of taking tests. Her perceived limitations included a fear of failing, anxiety about integrating multiple areas of learned information, and a self-castigating internal dialogue. Other patterns included an attentional style of intense focused absorption, modest body catalepsy while thinking, and skills of dissociation.

### *Planning the Session*

Once relevant information had been gathered, the next step was to think about how it could be used as the primary basis for the hypnotherapeutic work. Following this basic Ericksonian principle of utilization, I first translated each identified goal, resource, obstacle, and life pattern into a "simple idea" or "resource frame," then contemplatively identified various hypnotic phenomena and stories that would exemplify these ideas in a therapeutic fashion. This included jotting down the following:

1. *You have the ability to prepare at an appropriate rate* (stories: stretching and warming up for martial arts, students wanting to do too much too fast; hypnotic processes: interspersal of counting).
2. *You can relax during the test* (stories: hypnotic absorption during writing of dissertation, "reducing chatter" by shifting from typewriter to computer; hypnotic processes: deep relaxation, hypnotic alteration of sensation).
3. *You can develop lucid dissociational awareness during the test* (stories: Zeig's glider plane rides, lucid dreaming research; hypnotic processes: spatial dissociation, ideomotoric responses, hypnotic and posthypnotically suggested nocturnal dreams).
4. *You can integrate and reorganize many different areas of learning* (stories: computer "document link" processes, friend's medical exams, learning martial arts combinations; hypnotic processes: bodily dissociation of parts, with consequent reintegration into whole body experience).
5. *You can reduce anxiety and inner chatter* (stories: strategies of pain control; hypnotic processes: confusion and deep trance).

This list indicated a basic plan for the session: to hypnotically convey that each aspect of the target situation was an unconscious resource or ability that could be used and expressed in a variety of therapeutic ways. In other words, the hypnosis would revolve around affirming, activating, and making flexible each of the subject's relevant processes so that she could discover her own way of passing the exam. Of course, the plan was considered suggestive rather than mandatory; it was assumed that the actual hypnotic communications would include only some of these ideas, stories, and processes, while also including other references that rose "spontaneously" during the exchange. In this way, the plan was focused, yet not rigid, allowing coherence but also creativity.

### *Getting Started*

By the time we began on the following afternoon, I felt well prepared. Setting my sheet of notes on a chair next to me, my first concern was to experientially connect with myself and with Connie. This is always my initial intention, since the effectiveness of my hypnotic work seems to depend in large part on the presence of an "interpersonal trance" (see Gilligan, 1987).

The presence of a large audience helped to focus my attention inward, and as my body became hypnotically absorbed, I extended my field of nonverbal awareness to include Connie. The sense of nonverbal connectedness with myself and with the client is essential in my work; without it, I would not feel sufficiently able to trust "unconscious" processes to "do their thing." When I am connected in this way, images and words seem to "come to me," rather than being effortfully created by my analytical processes. Whenever I feel stuck or otherwise off center, I shift attention immediately to reconnecting with this nonverbal interpersonal field. I consider it much more important to therapeutic success than what is being said verbally.

It was not difficult to establish a sense of experiential absorption with Connie. As we nonverbally connected, I became intensely curious about how trance would develop, how her conscious processes could be paced and depotentiated, and how the central intention of passing the comprehensive exams could be hypnotically addressed in a variety of helpful ways.

### *Developing Trance*

After asking a few preliminary questions to establish the purpose of our work together, I decided to develop trance via questions regarding previous trance experiences. Connie adjusted her posture and developed mild catalepsy, which I utilized by introducing the general idea of hypnotic dissociation and the specific suggestion of ideomotor finger response. She responded positively to this suggestion, which I ratified and framed as an instance of unconscious autonomy.

This process of unconscious responses was then extended to the areas of tunnel vision and body sensation. These suggestions were made because it seemed that she was already developing such responses; that is, her bodily catalepsy and fixed eye focus were outer indicators of inner bodily changes and visual alterations.

This initial interchange is typical in that the suggestions for hypnotic phenomena are primarily requests for the subject to amplify already occurring experiential responses. Thus, the hypnosis is elicited rather than imposed. This makes it easier for the therapist and more therapeutic for the client.

### *Introducing Ideas*

A major purpose of developing trance in therapy is to enhance receptivity to new ways of thinking and behaving. Thus, Connie's development of trance indicated to me that she was ready to receive key ideas and suggestions. Much of the demonstration can be seen as involving the hypnotic communication of such ideas. Typically, an idea was emphasized (e.g., "You have the ability to integrate different areas of learning") and then an experiential example in the form of a story or a hypnotic phenomena was provided. These two levels of hypnotic suggestion serve to emphasize a general ability while also providing multiple experiential reference structure for expressing that ability.

One of the key ideas in hypnotherapy is that an idea becomes therapeutically potent only when it is experientially sensed as significant — when it is translated into some personally meaningful event. In this view, a major purpose of hypnosis is making ideas "come alive" in the body, so that they become realized in actual expression.

### *Utilizing Ongoing Responses*

To ensure this "felt sense" of the presented ideas, the hypnotherapist needs to observe and utilize the subject's ongoing responses. One way to do this involves periodically "pacing" nonverbal responses ("You're doing this," "You're doing that"), thereby including the subject's body as an integral part of the conversational field.

A related technique is to frame language suggestions in terms of already occurring responses. For example, at the beginning of the session Connie developed ideomotoric finger movements, so I emphasized how she could "wait [weight]" on the one hand and "recognize" things on the other hand. At another point, Connie moved her head, whereupon I noted how she could let her "unconscious do the learning . . . make the adjustment . . . head down, up, over to areas of learning that were going to be important."

A third technique is to observe bodily responses indicating analytical movement (e.g., arrhythmic movements, eyebrow furrowing) and respond with techniques that depotentiate such interference with hypnotic processes. This was a major purpose in periodically using the overloading and confusing statements involving numbers and rapid shifts of topics. Such communications were designed to ensure that Connie didn't try to figure things out consciously, but rather would allow her unconscious mind to do the learning while in trance.

### *Concluding Remarks*

While the above remarks suggest a great deal of thinking and strategizing on my part, it is important to emphasize that my actual experience during this hypnotic session (and most others) is decidedly unanalytical. While I train myself rigorously and try to prepare well for each client, the actual work is characterized by a deep sense of being an observer participant. My interest is in discovering a cooperative partnership both with my unconscious and with the client so that the negotiated goals of the relationship can be realized in some unique and mutually satisfying fashion. Preparation and hard work is essential in this regard, but so is creativity and trusting the unconscious. When a balance between these two is realized, effective therapeutic work is often the result.

I believe that this happened with Connie. The videos clearly indicate the development of a therapeutic trance in both of us, and follow up reports were equally satisfying. Specifically, Connie passed her exams with high marks and is now a practicing therapist.

## COMMENTARY BY JEFF ZEIG, PH.D.

The therapeutic use of indirect (multilevel) communication is probably the outstanding contribution Milton H. Erickson made to the health sciences. Therapeutic anecdotes were often a vehicle in which multilevel messages could be embedded. One striking example is Erickson's case of Joe and the tomato plants, where on the social level he discussed how a tomato plant grew, while on the psychological level he interspersed suggestions of pain control.

Embedded within a story (which could be something as commonplace as the growth of a seed into a tomato plant, or the process of a child learning to write the letters of the alphabet), Erickson used hypnotic language, including presuppositions, embedded commands, misspeaking, confusion technique, nonverbal methods, symbolic communication, directed truisms, and word plays, to build a wealth of positive associations to elicit from within the patient's personal history resources (previously unrecognized learnings) to accomplish therapeutic goals. When sufficient associations were elicited, salutary changes in behavior would be forthcoming because of the ideodynamic effect whereby thoughts become actualized in behavior. For example, when one thinks about a lemon, one can begin to salivate. This ideodynamic effect is especially strong during trance.

If Milton Erickson was the inventor of therapeutic multilevel communication, Stephen G. Gilligan is the poet laureate. In this particular therapy, Gilligan is extraordinarily facile at guiding associations by weaving psychological level messages within anecdotes and through using hypnotic language. Gilligan is confident, witty, and respectful of the patient with whom he works. His concentration is intense and approaches the remarkable concentration of Erickson. Careful study of this transcript will provide even the expert in Ericksonian techniques the opportunity to learn more about the language of hypnosis. More than that, the tape needs to be viewed to experience the wealth of nonverbal techniques that Gilligan uses to provide therapy. It is no wonder that Erickson's longtime student Robert Pearson remarks at the end of the tape that this is the "finest example of embedded metaphor I have seen in many years."

There is an additional aspect of the technique of hypnotically embedding messages that has not received as much attention in the literature as it should. One of the "laws" of communication is that the effectiveness of therapeutic messages should be judged by the response of the subject, not merely by the cleverness inherent in the communication. Erickson used one-step-removed methods in concert with *eliciting responsiveness*. During the initial phase of induction, Erickson would build responsiveness to multilevel communication. For example, to elicit eye closure, Erickson might have suggested, "The next time I say 'now' ... close your eyes ... NOW!" Erickson often hesitated and softened his voice when he said the words, "Close your eyes," to make them a command. He would gradually "train" patients to respond to such subtle messages. Also, he would use cues that were more overt and perhaps confusing, as in the example above where the second "NOW" unexpectedly followed as both a pregnant command and as an intended indirect cue. Usually, Erickson would not proceed with therapeutic multilevel techniques until he demonstrated, during induction, observable responsiveness to general indirect suggestions. It was as if demonstrated responsiveness to general indirect techniques was a cue that the induction period of therapy was over and the therapeutic period of therapy was to begin.

Erickson often discriminated between the induction phase and the utilization phase of treatment, but he never clarified what signaled the end of induction and the beginning of utilization. Here is one way of making a distinction: When demonstrable response is garnered to the multilevel communication during induction, induction is over. It is as if the patient indicates: "Okay, I'm open to working with you. The door is open to my constructive unconscious. I will let you influence me." Therefore, Erickson would work during induction to elicit to the maximum extent possible the patient's responsiveness to minimal cues. Once initial responsiveness to indirect methods was established, the therapy could begin.

In Gilligan's techniques, one can see the technique of building responsiveness to minimal cues. For example, early in the induction, Gilligan closes his eyes in a suggestive way. Subsequently, the patient blinks in response to Gilligan's cue and eventually closes her eyes. The importance of building responsiveness to minimal cues before eliciting therapeutic associations cannot be overemphasized. Casting seed onto the ground is not apt to lead to a good harvest unless the ground has been adequately tilled and fertilized.

Hindsight being 20/20, there are other options for treatment that could be pursued. For example, in this phase of his development, Gilligan emulates his mentor by using Erickson's voice tone and rhythm of speech. When Gilligan met Erickson, Erickson was an infirm man with a speech defect due in part to the residuals of polio. Gilligan modeled Erickson as a way of learning his teacher's methods. In retrospect, it might be more beneficial to use his own voice rather than Erickson's. As Gilligan has evolved over the years, he has developed his own voice.

Also, there is some overload for the patient. There is no possible way she can absorb, even unconsciously, all the multilevel messages Gilligan provides. A more targeted intervention may have been just as effective. Moreover, it would have been good to have some "follow-through." Gilligan's setup and intervention is masterful, but, perhaps due to the limitations of time, we do not get to see the follow-through. For example, there could have been some "process instruction," perhaps through another story, at the end of the induction to provide suggestions for how to use the elicited resources. Alternately, there could have been some "future pacing" in which she practiced using some of the resources via mental rehearsal.

A final critique has to do with Gilligan's alembical method. If the masterful use of complex multilevel technique is necessary for successful treatment, we are in trouble, because only a few can aspire to Gilligan's poetic use of language and techniques of influence.

## Chapter 7

# The Therapist as Variety Generator: Developing Solutions with Depressed Clients[1]

Life is a series of solutions waiting to be discovered. These solutions are successful responses to the developmental challenges of living: walking and talking, working and loving, separating and joining, and so forth. To succeed in these areas, one must individuate, or grow to be more unique as an individual, for ultimately the solutions to these developmental challenges are distinct for each person. The path of discovering solutions is thus a circuitous one, replete with uncertainties, false starts, dead ends, and falls. As long as one's image of achievement (e.g., walking) remains primary, such falls actively contribute toward solutions (cf. Pearce, 1981). But whenever such "errors" garner primary attention, one becomes misdirected into "error correction errors" (Pearce, 1981), thereby setting the stage for a self dominated by problems.

It is at this point that therapists sometimes enter the scene. What they encounter are individuals oriented more to problems than to solutions. Such individuals may be observed "viewing and doing" (O'Hanlon & Wilk, 1987) things in the same way, time after time, while complaining that such invariant patterns are involuntary and undesirable. Caught in this predicament, individu-

[1] This essay appeared previously in Michael D. Yapko. 1989. *Brief therapy approaches to treating anxiety and depression.* New York: Brunner/Mazel.

als may evidence little connection to the resources needed to direct attention to the future and positive achievements.

Faced with these presentations, therapists may be tempted to believe them. They may orient to clients primarily in terms of deficits rather than assets, problems instead of solutions, the past more than the future. Such views advance images of clients as incompetent, sick, or "broken," and suggest therapy as a process in which the primary tools for change are the therapist's presumed wisdom and skill. In this approach, therapy proceeds by the client learning to adopt the therapist's reality, with significant deviations from this "progress" framed as the client's "resistances."

For example, let us say a client arrives in the office with a complaint of depression. His verbal reports emphasize social withdrawal, sleepless nights, listless days, poor appetite, and so forth; while his nonverbal behavior features sighs, slumped body, soft speech, and slow tempo. The therapist searching for problems and deficits will not have far to look: The client can be diagnosed as having "depression" and therapy can be constructed as a process for eradicating this undesirable entity.

Such an impression, though easy to develop, may not be the most efficacious for promoting therapeutic change. It may unwittingly deepen an orientation to the client's shortcomings and reinforce his or her sense of inadequacy. It may foster an unbalanced and inaccurate representation of the problem residing in the client and the solution in the therapist. Furthermore, it may organize the attention of both therapist and client around "errors" rather than "solutions."

This chapter advances an alternative view in which therapist and client cooperate in order to develop solutions. Each is seen as possessing essential resources that, when operating together, provide an extra dimension in much the same way that two eyes focusing together yield perceptual depth (cf. de Shazer, 1982). Primary attention in this approach is to solutions, resources, the future, and unconscious processes (Gilligan, 1987). Problems, shortcomings, the past, and analytical processes are seen as secondary processes that may contribute to solutions. At the same time, it is assumed that difficulties arise whenever these secondary processes are given primary emphasis.

This approach would generate a different "reality" in the case of the client complaining of depression. Operating from the premise that the focus of therapy (e.g., what is going to be talked about) is negotiated (O'Hanlon & Wilk, 1987), the therapist would orient attention toward developing a mutually acceptable image of achievement regarding the client's future (Gilligan,

1988a). Various techniques might be used to engage both the therapist's and the client's unconscious processes in this endeavor. For example, the client might be asked to think on a smaller scale, or hypnosis might be used to develop a state of psychophysical "centering" and to enhance imaging abilities (Gilligan, 1988a).

As a sense of the desired future cooperatively emerged, experiential resources for developing it would be identified and utilized. Such resources are derived from different domains: social (e.g., relationships with other people), psychological (e.g., a powerful symbol), and organismic (e.g., bodily states) (Gilligan, 1988b). They include pleasant processes (e.g., memories of successes or satisfying achievements) as well as unpleasant ones (e.g., symptoms), since both involve the emotional connections needed to absorb and motivate a person. For example, the depressive symptom of social withdrawal might be appreciated as an essential contribution to a desired future of social connectedness. The therapy task would thus be to discover ways that withdrawal, along with other resources, might lead to social competency. This would likely involve having the client "do the symptom more and better," that is, in a greater number of ways and with a greater quality of self-involvement. Thus, this cooperative approach does not view a symptom as "bad" or something to be eliminated. Rather, it is seen as a valuable contribution to the primary goal of developing a satisfying future. Techniques are used to enhance the way the client is expressing the symptom, so that it is reconnected within the overall context of the whole person. Hypnosis is used as an outstanding tool both for amplifying primary processes and for "deframing" and reframing expressions (Gilligan, 1987).

In this cooperative approach, one of the major roles the therapist plays is that of "variety generator." That is, it is assumed that problems develop from rigid fixation to one way of doing and viewing things. In this view, solutions emerge when the client is able to "do and view" in a variety of different ways. The remainder of the chapter explores ways in which the therapist can facilitate this process. Generating variety in psychophysical states is first explored, followed by an investigation of other parameters that may be similarly varied (e.g., images of the future, intensity of feeling, time, place, social others, and cognitive frames).

## PSYCHOPHYSICAL VARIABILITY

When clients complain about depression or anxiety, they are usually stuck in an unchanging bodily state. For example, Brenda entered therapy with complaints of depression featuring a chronic feeling of "black heaviness" in her solar plexus. A major problem with such persistent feelings is that, like any other physiological process, a habituation response develops which blocks orientation to novel experience (Pribram, 1971; Siddle, 1983). That is, the more a person remains in an unchanging state, the less that person is able to perceive stimuli in an active fashion. Thus, the chronic bodily state of a depressed or anxious person blocks change, for it deadens the person to direct connections with inner as well as outer worlds. Consequently, a major initial intervention with Brenda, as with other such clients, was to reactivate and vary bodily sensations, thereby enabling such feelings to reconnect with intrapersonal and interpersonal creative responses. An examination of how this may be done with a hypnotic procedure is presented, followed by an overview of complementary homework tasks.

### *Hypnotically Altering Bodily Sensation*

Hypnosis is a very effective tool for reconnecting a person with direct experience of bodily feeling. It is a naturalistic process that allows individuals to reclaim and further develop skills of self-healing and self-expression. It can be used to absorb and redirect attention, amplify experience (e.g., bodily sensations), connect and change nonverbal states, and enhance a sense of aliveness (see Gilligan, 1987). All of these processes are relevant to the revivification of bodily feeling. This section explores a ten-step hypnotic procedure for accomplishing this.

**1. Develop experiential absorption.**

Hypnosis is not an intellectual or conceptual process; rather, it is an experiential immersion in balanced primary process. To enable this process, attention first needs to be absorbed and experientially oriented. One way to do this is with straightforward suggestions, delivered with appropriate nonverbal absorption:

> And so, Brenda, I understand that one of the things that's going on is that you're feeling a sense of heaviness in your body, especially in your

solar plexus. And I take it that you'd like to be able to feel differently, is that true? [Wait for response.] Good. I support that, because I know it is possible to feel a variety of different sensations in your body. The question, of course, is how to allow that to happen, how to experientially remember different possibilities. To answer that question, I'm going to ask you to participate in an experiment, a very simple and safe experiment. The experiment involves first allowing yourself to take a few deep breaths and relax. You don't have to move ... you don't have to talk ... you don't have to try to do anything at all except remain absorbed here with me and here with you and hear me here suggesting possibilities there for your unconscious to hear there and develop now at your rate, in your own style ... that's it ...

If these sorts of suggestions do not adequately absorb attention, the therapist usually needs to enter the client's reality a bit more. This might involve identifying and experientially elaborating the content of the person's ongoing awareness. In depressed individuals, this might be a repetitive voice chanting, "I can't do it. ... Nothing will work," or an overwhelming bodily feeling of emptiness. The emotional attachment to such contents makes them ideal for developing trance. For example, the following approach was used with another depressed client:

You don't believe it is possible ... you sense that no one thing will work ... and I disagree and I agree ... I believe it is possible ... and I believe that no one thing will work ... and you don't believe it is possible ... and I don't believe it is possible for just one feeling to work ... and we are different and yet we can agree on certain things ... and we are the same in other ways, yet we can disagree on certain things ... you don't believe it is possible, and do you also believe that feelings can develop and remain independently of belief? ... do you believe that the heavy feeling can operate independently from your conscious concerns? ... I believe, and we agree and we may disagree that no one thing will work ... at least two of us, at least two feelings ... a feeling of heaviness that is traditional, and who really knows what we should believe about a companion feeling ... I don't know and you don't believe it is possible ...

These communications, delivered in a soft, sensitive, yet intense manner, served to absorb the person's attention. Like all effective hypnotic communications, they did not deny the person's present reality but suggested how that reality could be expanded in different ways.

**2. Distribute attention to three to four areas.**

Once therapist and client are experientially joined, attention is distributed across three to four areas of the body. The idea here is that the analytical mind organizes experience in a linear, sequential fashion, whereas the experiential mind is capable of simultaneous, parallel processes. Shifting attention to multiple foci thus diminishes the former and augments the latter, thereby naturally developing a receptive trance. A straightforward version of the technique is evident in the following transcript:

THERAPIST: ... and so as you continue to hear my voice here, what a nice thing to know that your unconscious mind has an unconscious body ... and that unconscious body can communicate in its own way in so many different ways ... and what do I mean by that? Simply this ... Your hands [look meaningfully at hands] ... your hands can communicate *yes* or *no*, your hands can communicate with feeling, your hands can communicate *yes* or *no*, your hands can communicate with sensation ... and I don't know *which* sensation might begin *now* to develop in those hands ... the *right* hand ... or the *left* hand ... *sensation* ... *heaviness* ... or perhaps *lightness* ... I don't know ... all I know is that your unconscious mind can *let your unconscious* body *communicate* in a way that's right for you ... And how do your hands feel now?

CLIENT: A little heavy.

THERAPIST: That's right ... your unconscious can initiate and develop and work with a *feeling of heaviness* in your body ... And you don't know and I don't know how that feeling might *spread* or *intensify* ... all I know is that you really needn't let your hands hog all of the action ... because you've got a variety of *different body sensations* available ... and as you *hear* me *here* unconsciously with me, your ears may also begin to *develop sensation* ... everybody's entitled to the pleasant surprise of *comfortable ears* ... your hands can be *there*, feeling that heaviness, and your *ears* can be *there*, discovering their ability to develop sensation ... and how do your hands feel now?

CLIENT: The heaviness is moving up the arms.

THERAPIST: That's right ... your unconscious really can have *moving* and *secure sensations*. And how do your ears feel?
CLIENT: I don't feel my ears.
THERAPIST: You don't consciously sense your ears yet. You really can let some feelings recede and others come forward unconsciously, a little more. And as your unconscious body experiments with shifting sensations, shifting feelings, shifting priorities, I'm wondering about your unconscious ability to develop sensation in your eyelids ... That's it ... even as they *blink* ... *blink* ... *blink* ... that's it ... we can both wonder what feelings develop in those eyes unconsciously moving *up* and *down*, *up* and *down*, up and *down* ... your unconscious can learn to respond to certain behavioral cues with automatic satisfying feelings ...

As Gilligan (1987) described, the nonverbal communications accompanying such suggestions should be congruent with the suggested feeling. For example, a feeling of lightness is suggested with upward inflections and soft tone, heaviness is mentioned with downward inflections and a sinking voice, and so forth.

In this way, attention is shifted to at least three areas of the body. This. reorganizes awareness in the body, from a diffuse yet chronic feeling in a symptom area (e.g., chest or stomach), to a shifting and alive pattern of sensations in different parts of the body. In a very real sense, this brings the experiential body back into relationship in the world, a crucial development for a person wanting to change.

**3. Emphasize the hypnotic response as a mastery ability.**

As with any hypnotic development, the therapist ratifies any sensation alterations and frames them as general mastery abilities that may be used in different ways (e.g., for symptom relief).

That's right ... you really can let your unconscious mind and your *unconscious body* respond ... you don't have to try to understand it ... you don't have to try to control it ... because you can *comfortably enjoy* the knowledge that *sensation can develop* in your body in a variety of different ways ... *your unconscious mind has the ability to express a variety of different sensations* ...

**4. Elaborate the mastery theme in multiple dimensions.**

Having introduced the key mastery theme ("your unconscious has the ability to experience a variety of sensations"), the therapist now elaborates the variety of ways in which mastery may experientially develop. Different parameters include:

- *what* (numbness, tingling, warmth, coolness, etc.)
- *when* (now, five minutes, when your unconscious is ready, etc.)
- *how* (slowly, quickly, surprisingly, comfortably, etc.)
- *where* (arm, head, wrist, stomach, etc.)
- *with whom* (all alone, with therapist, with spouse, etc.)

For example:

> And so as you continue to experientially sense that ability to express sensation in a variety of different places . . . what a nice thing to know that you can do so in *many ways* . . . for example, your unconscious body can develop sensations of *heaviness* or *numbness* . . . very real numbness . . . or lightness . . . real *lightness lifting* now . . . so many different possibilities, some of which you will say "no" to, some of which you will say "yes" to, each of which you *can respond to* in a way that fits the needs of the self . . . the needs of the self . . . the *sensations of the self* . . . expressed over time . . . your *unconscious really can* work over time . . . developing *sensations now*, a little more . . . a little bit later . . . a little trance later in those areas where you want, you need to *develop new sensations* . . . at those times, in those places with those individuals, in those areas that best fit your overall development as a human being . . .

**5. Receive and ratify feedback in hypnotic frames.**

During the course of hypnotic explorations, the therapist continually observes and occasionally inquires about the client's ongoing responses. Each response is defined as a legitimate unconscious response and encouraged to further develop.

If the client can talk while remaining comfortably in trance, this can be done straightforwardly. For example:

THERAPIST: And what sensations are you aware of now?
CLIENT: [pause] The hands are very heavy.

THERAPIST: Your unconscious is continuing to develop that feeling of heaviness in the *hands*, Brenda, the hands, *all in the hands*. [This is a suggestion for a lifting of the heavy feelings in the chest.] That's right, your unconscious really does have the ability to develop that *heavy sensation* in your hands ... and who really knows *how* and *when* and *where* that comfortable heaviness, that secure heaviness, will continue to develop ... perhaps the heaviness will *move up* the arm ... perhaps it will spread to the head slowly ... I don't know ... all I know is that your unconscious can *let that feeling develop* in a way and at a rate that is meaningful for you as an individual ...

If talking tends to disrupt trance, a "refractionation" technique (Gilligan, 1987) involving a series of brief trances might be used. That is, a five to ten-minute trance might be followed by a five to ten-minute discussion of the client's responses, followed by a deeper trance utilizing the information, followed by further waking state feedback, and so forth.

Another possibility is to request that ideomotor finger signals indicate when sensation begins to hypnotically develop. When a finger lifts, the hypnotist then proceeds with general ratification:

> That's it ... your unconscious really can express itself in so many *comfortable ways* ... your unconscious can recognize and communicate the onset of useful sensations in a variety of fashions ... and that sensation that is beginning to develop can really develop comfortably ... perhaps it will *spread* ... perhaps it will *intensify* ... perhaps it will remain the same ... I don't know ... all I know is that you can enjoy discovering how your unconscious mind can activate and utilize sensation for your own developmental learnings ... and you can learn so much from that feeling ...

Note that these general communications apply to virtually any sensation development.

**6. Elaborate hypnotic responses: stories.**

During the course of a therapeutic trance, it is common for a client's attention to gradually narrow from multiple possibilities to one or two actualities. Thus, the client usually responds to the many suggestions given by the hypnotist by developing a few responses that are especially meaningful. These responses can be elaborated as resources relevant to the therapy goals. For example, the depressed client described above presented complaints of heaviness in the chest and, in a parallel fashion, responded hypnotically with heavy hands. The therapist can use the hypnotic response (heavy hands) to experientially change the symptomatic response (heavy chest). An excellent technique in this regard involves the use of metaphorical stories that symbolically suggest pathways for change. For example:

> And as those hands continue to develop that special feeling of heaviness, what a nice thing to know that your unconscious mind knows so much about developing new relationships and new learnings . . . and such learnings can happen in so many ways . . . For example, Mary and Joe were going to have a baby . . . They came to see me, and you could note all the changes that had already occurred in her body . . . her body image was no doubt changing as well . . . and Mary and Joe wanted to use hypnosis to have that baby . . . they wanted to use hypnosis to feel comfortable, to stay comfortable, to allow the life deep within Mary to continue to grow and emerge at the right time . . . so I said to them, "That's right, you really can learn how your unconscious mind can work for you in many different ways" . . . And Mary was especially concerned about handling any pain during the delivery . . . and so I asked her where she sensed she needed help with developing comfort and security in her body . . . She indicated her belly, so I let her know in no uncertain terms that she really shouldn't discriminate against herself, that she really had a whole body of possible learnings to draw on and that there was no need to emphasize only that area . . . that any place of discomfort could be joined by other areas of comfort, to *weave a new pattern* of perhaps puzzling but nonetheless compelling *comfort and absorption* . . . Mary developed a nice *deep trance* and I continued to emphasize that the feelings in her belly should be joined and modulated by the feelings in other parts of her . . . and she discovered in trance that her hands could begin to be numb and tingling at the same time . . . she learned in trance how to let the feelings in her hands connect with the feeling in her stomach, to let the inner feelings move outside when needed . . .

This story further elaborated how peripheral resources (hands) could be joined with troublesome areas (belly) to generate new responses. In doing so, it provided the client with experiential opportunities to reconnect and reframe the feeling in her solar plexus to the healing properties of the whole body.

**7. Future pacing.**

Once a hypnotic resource has been linked to a symptomatic response in trance, posthypnotic suggestions are given to ensure that linkage will generalize to other situations. The general idea, related directly or indirectly (e.g., stories), is that when the symptomatic response occurs in the future, the new hypnotic resource can be simultaneously activated to provide a more satisfying experience. For example:

> And so it is satisfying to know that the unconscious can apply learnings in so many ways, in so many areas, at so many times . . . And I really don't know when, and you consciously don't know when, your unconscious will decide to apply these new learnings in those situations where you need them . . . perhaps your unconscious will select out a time tonight, when you feel safe and secure, to begin to activate the comfortable sensations of heaviness in your hands, not to mention your chest, not to mention your sense of lightness, not to mention your chest, not to mention your solar plexus . . . begin to activate those new feelings of heaviness to connect you with a center of comfort, with a center of hypnotic learning, with a center of breathing deeply and comfortably, with a center for dreaming . . . I don't know if it will be tonight . . . whether you will be alone or with others . . . all I know is that your unconscious mind can take the time to learn from those feelings of heaviness in a way that surprises your conscious mind . . .

Thus, the suggestions predict the return of the symptomatic response (heaviness), but within a therapeutic framework of the new learnings. This is the common Ericksonian technique of claiming the symptomatic response as grounds for therapeutic learnings.

**8. Self-appreciation.**

Before concluding trance, several minutes of self-appreciation can be suggested. Besides being a therapeutic process in and of itself, it provides a transition between trance and the waking state.

> And so as you continue to consolidate these new learnings, as you continue to allow your unconscious mind, with each breath you take, to know a little deeper that you really can trust and develop your future in accord with inner needs ... what a nice thing to know that you can take a few moments of clock time, all the time in the world, to simply enjoy yourself ... to thank yourself ... to feel that sense of security ... that sense of knowing that you can always return to this place of comfort ... this place of learning ... this place of appreciating the needs of the self and trusting the resources of the unconscious mind.

**9. Reorient.**

Reorientation is now accomplished in a straightforward fashion:

> And you can keep those resources as you begin to allow yourself to slowly reorient out of trance, back here into the room ... taking all the time in the world in the next several minutes ... perhaps wanting to count from 5 to 1, to allow yourself to gradually reorient ... gradually reorient ... gradually orient ...

**10. Post-trance suggestions.**

Most subjects remain in an extremely receptive state for five to ten minutes after trance is formally ended. This period is an excellent time for gently emphasizing key ideas. As Gilligan (1987) discussed, techniques for accomplishing this include stories, jokes, and embedded suggestions. As in any intimate relationship, the underlying connection between therapist and client is maintained, even as attention gradually expands to include other stimuli and topics.

§

In using this ten-step method, the therapist should remain sensitive to the cooperative nature of the hypnotic relationship. Though both therapist and client share an interest in increasing the client's ability directly to experience bodily sensation, neither knows exactly how this will happen. As Erickson (personal communication, 1977) noted:

> All I know (during hypnotic work) is that I've got an unconscious mind ... and they've got an unconscious mind ... and we're sitting in the same room together ... therefore, trance is inevitable ... I don't

know how . . . I don't know when . . . I don't know why . . . but trance is inevitable . . .

Similarly, the therapist uses this method with a deep confidence in the client's natural ability to experience bodily sensations. The 10-step method is one guide for realizing this ability; another is the client's values and ongoing responses. Blending the two by modifying the method to include the client's contributions will produce the best results.

### *Complementing Hypnotic Work with Tasks*

As a rule, work done in trance should be balanced by work done outside of trance (Gilligan, 1987; Lankton & Lankton, 1983; Yapko, 1988). In this regard, the above hypnotic method may be complemented by tasks designed further to reconnect the depressed or anxious person experientially. For example, the author typically directs such individuals to join some sort of *movement classes*, such as dance therapy, Feldenkrais lessons, yoga, or martial arts. Since it is virtually impossible to be depressed or anxious when immersed in gentle, rhythmic movement processes, such classes are very helpful in reuniting mind and body. Another type of task concerns *social activities*. Following Erickson's (in Rossi, 1980) premise that the social environment provides innumerable opportunities for therapeutic growth, clients are asked to wonder (in and out of trance) about which social resources (persons, places, things, events) might be helpful in developing desired solutions. For Brenda, the depressed client described earlier, tasks included (1) going to the park every other day and (2) becoming involved in an extensive job search (writing letters, getting interviews, and so forth). For another client with similar goals, regular communication with his wife and children became important. Such straightforward tasks are often essential to consolidating and extending the resources revivified in trance.

Another type of task is self-hypnosis. The author teaches most clients self-hypnosis, and then directs them to use this skill to further learnings developed in the sessions. For example, Brenda practiced the hypnotic sensation alteration process nightly for 15 to 20 minutes, developing a ritual that replaced her depressive routine. Self-hypnosis may also be used to rehearse performances in upcoming events (job interviews, family meetings, social gatherings), and to imagine different futures.

Other types of tasks worth mentioning are those that are silly, paradoxical, ambiguous, or otherwise unusual (Lankton & Lankton, 1983). Such tasks may be especially useful in disrupting the rigid mental sets characterizing depressed or anxious individuals. For example, Brenda was given the assignment of carrying around two books, one a heavy and exceedingly dry treatise on depression, the other an edited volume of futurist predictions. Each time she felt depressed, she was to hold the books and sense which one felt more "familiar," then decide from which she would like to read a page. The task puzzled her, and also began to orient her more to thinking about the future.

These and other tasks build on the bodily feelings revived by the hypnotic method. They provide avenues for depressed and anxious persons to channel their attention and opportunities to increase their social participation. In doing so, they constitute important therapeutic techniques for steering individuals back onto their primary path of developmental growth.

## GENERATING VARIETY IN OTHER PARAMETERS

Thus far, how therapists may operate as variety generators in the area of bodily sensation has been examined. Of course, this principle of "do it more, do it better" can be applied in other areas as well. This section overviews how variety may be generated in some of these other areas.

### *Images of the Future*

Earlier it was noted how the vision of the future held by a person influences his or her experience and expression in the present. Unfortunately, depressed and anxious individuals are typically attached to a singular, unsatisfying image of the future. This image is often based on past failures so that, to paraphrase a pop philosopher, such individuals are navigating down the freeway of life with eyes rigidly locked on the rear-view mirror. Thus, the task of the therapist is to orient attention back to the road leading to the future. It is often difficult to do this straightforwardly with clients in waking states, since their rigid response sets render them impervious to considering or committing to new possibilities. The best interventions, therefore, bypass the limits of the conscious mind.

An excellent method in this regard is the pseudo-orientation in time technique developed by Erickson (1954), wherein it is suggested that the desired future has already transpired. The client is then asked to "review" the experiences that have enabled this satisfying future to develop. One version of this technique (see Gilligan, 1988a) involves hallucinating a "rainbow arc" of crystal balls. Hypnotized clients first envision a positive future state within a "crystal ball" located in the lower right peripheral field. They then regress to an early memory that their unconscious selects as useful in developing the future crystal ball. The regression memory is placed in a crystal ball in the lower left peripheral field, and a slightly later memory (relevant to achieving the future crystal ball) is then accessed and placed in the next crystal ball in the left-to-right arc. In this way, a series of "memories" from early childhood to present to "future" is developed as a bridge leading to the desired future state. It is an excellent technique, as it allows both a vision of a satisfying future and a means to frame depressing events as leading to that future. Thus, depression is used as a vehicle of growth rather than as an enemy to be purged.

If clients have difficulty generating a sense of the future while in trance, a process one might call parallel hallucinating may be used. This method, a modified version of Erickson's (1964) "my friend John" technique, involves therapists using their hypnotic abilities to "hallucinate" the "future self" of the client in the office, alongside the therapist and client. This future self is introduced into the conversation, with the goal being to elicit contributions from the client on the topic. For example, Patrick was a young man unresponsive to suggestions for imaging a desired future. As he continued to complain about feeling hopeless, the therapist selected a spot in the office and became curious as to how a satisfying future self would appear. An image gradually emerged, and the therapist continued in the following way:

CLIENT: . . . so I just don't feel I have any support.

THERAPIST: [with intense absorption to spot in room] Do you know what color hair she has?

CLIENT: [disrupted and bewildered] What?

THERAPIST: [maintaining absorption] Her hair? It looks beautiful to me. What do you think?

CLIENT: [still bewildered] I don't understand what you're talking about!

THERAPIST: The woman. This woman. [gesturing to hallucination] You do want to have a relationship, do you not?

CLIENT: [looks sad] Yeah, but what are you doing?

THERAPIST: I'm asking the unconscious to look into your future, and I seem to see you with someone you can trust.

CLIENT: [looks very absorbed but still sad, head drops] That's not possible.

THERAPIST: [looking with hypnotic intensity at client] You consciously don't believe now that it's possible. But I'm here to let you know that it is possible . . . I can see it *there*.

CLIENT: [looking increasingly hypnotically absorbed] She wouldn't stay with me long.

THERAPIST: [continuing to hypnotically absorb client] Yes, you need to think in small chunks. You need to appreciate that some skills do need to continue to develop. You do need to stay connected with resources. And I guess that's why you're here. [client entranced] It's good to know that you have much to learn. Just as it's essential to know what you want. [pause] What color hair does she have?

CLIENT: [pause] Brown.

As this brief excerpt illustrates, therapists can use their own hypnotic abilities to shift primary attention to the future. As a future self is imaged and introduced by the therapist, it can stimulate the client to operate in similar fashion. Note that the therapist acknowledges considerations raised by the client, but does not let them interfere with the primary task of imaging a desired future.

A third method for generating images of viable futures involves "*chunking down*" strategies. This is especially useful with depressives, who tend to think in global, generalized images (Yapko, 1988). For example, Linda was depressed over her inability to actualize any of her future-oriented images, which tended to feature dramatic, life-changing events such as major career achievements and marrying a "Tom Selleck" type character. She was asked in trance to "feel free to limit herself" to decidedly bland and minor images of achievement. These images (e.g., planting a garden, taking a class) provided reference structures for realistic and satisfying changes.

A related strategy is to ask clients hypnotically to generate different "puzzle pieces" of a satisfying future across multiple trances. For example, John, a middle-aged lawyer afraid to make commitments, was asked in trance to let his unconscious reveal just one "puzzle piece" as a clue to a satisfying future. His conscious mind was baffled and disconcerted about the image of a key that developed. This technique was repeated a half dozen times during the following three weeks, with a different image emerging each time. An integrating trance was then developed wherein it was suggested that all the "clues" would fit into a viable image of the future, one that his unconscious could share with him at a rate and in a style appropriate for his overall development. This technique is especially useful with clients like John, whose conscious minds (and their learned limitations) interfere with the envisioning of viable futures.

These and other methods are useful in generating variety when clients are stuck in a single (unsatisfying) image of the future. They do not attempt to take away the limited orientation of the client, but rather expand the range of possibilities to include additional choices.

### *Images of the Past*

Just as depressed and anxious clients become rigidly entrenched in invariant images of the future, so do they attach to singular representations of the past. Thus, the therapist's skill as variety generator also applies to stimulating multiple images of the past. One technique involves hypnotically regressing clients to events before the depressing or anxious process set in. For example, Margaret and Michael entered therapy after 20 years of marriage. Their mutual experience was overshadowed by the memory of Michael's affair and Margaret's attempted suicide three years before. They could revivify few events before this time and felt hopeless about the future. Part of the therapy included regressions to their first meetings together, involving passion, pleasure, and hope. These memories were emphasized as vital resources, and further hypnotic communications involved wondering aloud about how such feelings could "trickle" into the future. Thus, hypnosis was therapeutically used to dislodge the clients' fixation to the tragedies and to reorient them to the resources of having experienced positive times together.

The psychological relationship to one's past can also be hypnotically altered through the age progression techniques noted above. For example, Stella felt depressed after being fired from her job as a newspaper photographer. She was hypnotically progressed a year into the future, and asked to review how her values associated with certain events (such as the job firing) had changed over the past year, as new experiences transpired. As she envisioned herself working as a freelance photographer, she felt thankful about leaving her newspaper position for this new, more satisfying career.

A final technique concerns the type of memories revivified by clients. Depressed individuals all too often orient to sad or somber memories (Gilligan & Bower, 1984). One straightforward intervention is to ask clients, in both trance and waking states, about preferences and pleasures quite unrelated to the symptomatic process. Therapists may interrupt clients' depressive talk with inquiries about favorite flowers, sports, colors, movie stars, and so forth (see Gilligan, 1987). Similarly, clients may be given tasks, such as listing favorite values, and then asked to attend to them actively. In doing so, clients' images of the past become more balanced and their possible futures are expanded.

These techniques assume that the values assigned to the past reflect the values of the self's present state. Thus, shifting the perspective of the viewing state may shift the values assigned to past events. This new representation of the past enables greater freedom in the present and future.

### *Intensity of Feeling*

The intensity a feeling holds may also be varied for therapeutic gain. By learning to increase and decrease intensity, a person gains a sense of mastery and participation in the process (Erickson, 1967). To develop this learning, therapists may use the sorts of rating scales commonly employed in hypnotic pain control processes (Erickson, 1967; Sacerdote, 1982). The author usually introduces several such scales to depressed and anxious clients: the first has to do with degree (1–10) of depression or anxiety felt, the second with the degree (1–10) of security felt. A symptomatic event is accessed and the person is asked: On a scale of 1 to 10, how depressed do you feel? How secure do you feel? Hypnotic interventions such as resource accessing, story telling, sensation alterations, and so forth, are then introduced and the person's ratings again obtained. Just as in the sensation alteration procedure outlined above, the therapist ratifies each ratings shift with general comments about the unconscious ability to change that feeling, and to change that feeling about the feeling in meaningful and appropriate ways.

As a person develops changes in intensity ratings, specific possibilities may be explored. For example, clients may learn to increase and then decrease a feeling of anxiety, while keeping feelings of security constant. The tables are then turned, with security varied while intensity of feeling is maintained. Such operations enable a person to master the process of increasing and decreasing intensity, while also demonstrating how, for example, security may be maintained even when depression temporarily increases. This distinction allows individuals to stay connected with themselves (i.e., not to give up) when a symptomatic event is reaccessed.

For example, Mark developed intense feelings of anxiety before public speaking engagements. He felt such feelings to be involuntary and interpreted them as evidence of impending failure. In therapy he learned to shift the intensity of the anxiety up and down, while increasing his sense of security. This process enabled him to join and remain comfortable with the feelings of anxiety that began to develop at his next presentation.

### *Physical Context*

A person may be stuck in a certain experience by virtue of performing it in the same *physical context* time and time again. This can be determined by straightforwardly inquiring as to where a symptom is expressed. If it occurs in the same place repeatedly, varying that physical context may enable new possibilities to emerge. For example, Rebecca was a middle-aged secretary who complained of feeling "empty and blue." Living alone, her symptoms were most acute each evening when she would plop herself into a chair and stare at the television. A set of interventions concentrated on having her practice "the ability to feel empty and blue" in various physical locations, including in a meditation room at home, at the library, and in the park. Of course, her feelings varied with the context shifts, as they invariably will, and new ways of being then became available.

Another client, Robert, complained of overeating. This frequently involved consuming large amounts of peanuts while watching television. He was directed to build a "goober shrine" in his spare room at home, and was assigned a certain "goober ritual" to practice in front of the shrine upon returning home from work each night. This ritual, which he found hilarious, disrupted his "goober mania," whereupon trance work was used to develop alternate ways of "feeling and filling" his inner needs.

### *Social Others*

A final variable worth noting is *social others*. Therapists may identify who is present when a person feels depressed or otherwise symptomatic. If clients are typically alone, they may be directed to express their symptom with others. For example, Mary was a hardworking professional wife and mother who complained of binge eating. She felt guilty and sad about not spending enough time with her husband, just as she felt depressed about her uncontrollable snacking. She was directed to schedule a 30-minute "binge" walk early each morning with her husband. She was to carry sundry snacks with her during this time, offering them to her husband along with the cryptic inquiry, "Do you want more?" She was then to ask herself the same question while keeping her husband "in the back of her mind." Carried out over a two-week interval, this strategy of "doing her symptom" in a different social context (with her husband, on a walk) elicited a variety of emotional responses from her. She stopped binging and began to pay more attention to her marriage. Both she and her husband cut back on professional commitments and sought couples therapy.

Variability may also be introduced when the symptom is performed by two or more people. Don and Paul were a gay couple expressing dissatisfaction in their sexual relationship. Don would want to "get right to it" and finish sex within minutes, whereas Paul felt he often needed over an hour to open up emotionally. Their different timings would frequently result in disruptive arguments during sex. They were given the simple task of setting aside an hour each evening for an experiment. The experiment would begin with them taking "up to 60 seconds, no more" for a gentle kiss. Don was then to take a deep sigh, walk into his study and lock the door, and spend the next 45 minutes engaged in his pleasurable hobby of reading poetry and writing in his journal. Meanwhile, Paul was to remain on the bed fantasizing slowly and sensuously, knowing in the back of his mind that 45 minutes would not be quite enough time. After 45 minutes, Don was to reenter the room and receive a kiss from Paul, whereupon both could wonder how they might "come together emotionally." This task of social separation enabled satisfying sex to develop for both of them. Interestingly, after a week Paul began to "cheat" and surprise Don in his office before the time was up.

These two brief examples indicate how a fixed social relationship may block the natural process of developmental change. As this parameter is varied, new possibilities reveal themselves and more satisfying ways of being may emerge.

## SUMMARY

In exploring the process of human change, it becomes apparent that many parameters are involved in the construction of an experiential reality: bodily sensation, images of the future, images of the past, and so forth. When these parameters are free to vary according to changing needs and situations, developmental growth is possible; but when they become rigid and invariant, sensitivity to the vital "now" of the experiential self is lost and problems typically develop. In this view, the therapist operates as a variety generator in promoting flexibility and change across different aspects of experience. Although we have identified some of these parameters, many others exist: *time* (when, how long), *frequency* (how often), *cognitive frame* (what it means), *attribution* (why it happened), and so forth. The task of the therapist is to identify those values that are rigidly and dysfunctionally fixed for a given client, and to introduce interventions that will support and expand his or her range of expression. As variability increases, so does the connectedness of the symptomatic expression to its larger (social, organismic, or psychological) contexts. This recontextualization enables the symptom to operate as part of a solution to the challenges of developmental growth. And this, first and foremost, is the commitment of therapy.

Chapter 8

# SOLUTIONS AND RESOLUTIONS: ERICKSONIAN HYPNOTHERAPY WITH INCEST SURVIVOR GROUPS[1]

*by Stephen G. Gilligan Ph.D. & Christine M. Kennedy, Ed.D.*

Until recently, we as a society have hidden from the reality of childhood sexual abuse, especially incest. We have preferred to image childhood molesters as only bums and degenerates. We have assumed that if individuals were good citizens, educated and well-functioning family providers, then they could not possibly also be sexually molesting their children.

The societal "secret" is now being revealed: Incest is a national problem of virtual epidemic proportions. A Planned Parenthood (1985) project estimates that at least one in four girls and one in eight boys is sexually molested before adulthood. The perpetrator is usually a family member or a close friend of the family (Butler-Smith, 1985; Forward and Buck, 1979). And incest happens in families of all educational, intellectual, racial, ethnic, religious, and economic groups (Butler-Smith, 1985).

Denying the problem enables its perpetuation. Incest often continues until it is directly challenged and reported. Furthermore, the patterns of incest are passed on intergenerationally: Molesters are more likely to have been sexually abused themselves as children, as are their spouses (Justice & Justice, 1979).

---

[1] This essay appeared previously in the *Journal of Strategic and Systemic Therapies* 8, no. 4 (winter 1989): 9–17.

This tragic pattern of replication is at least partly due to the secrecy and denial shrouding incestuous relationships.

As might be expected, incest survivors are affected in significant ways by this denial. They find it difficult to trust themselves and others, and they abuse alcohol, drugs, food, and their bodies at an alarming rate (Briere, 1984). They have difficulty in areas such as sexual identity, body image, intimacy, and relationship boundaries (Justice & Justice, 1979). And they are often plagued and depressed by "inner tapes" of self-blame, revulsion, fear and shame. These problems can be so severe that continuing to deny an incestuous event is in some ways more painful and disabling than the event itself.

In acknowledging the pervasive problem of incest and its denial, we are interested in developing solutions to its consequences. One of our approaches has been a group hypnotherapy program in which incest survivors learn a variety of hypnotically-based skills for developing new ways of responding, both intrapersonally and interpersonally. The remainder of the paper is devoted to describing this program. Its general characteristics are first noted, its structure next detailed, and common outcomes then discussed.

## *Characteristics of the Group*

Our treatment approach can be distinguished by the following six features:

**1. Groups.**

Incestuous families often are very closed (i.e., have rigid boundaries) in relation to the "outside" world, and are typically characterized by the keeping of secrets (Alexander, 1985). To the extent this is so, incest survivors feel very cut off from the world around them and have little awareness regarding how tragically common incest is. Accordingly, they believe the usual consequences of incest (guilt, boundary difficulties, self-abusive behaviours, etc.) are idiosyncratic to them as individuals.This misconception perpetuates the problem, leaving individuals with the sense that something is deeply "wrong" with them while discouraging reconnection with a larger (healing) community.

Groups can be part of the solution in this regard. Rather than further isolating the inner processes of the incest survivor (as sometimes occurs in individual therapy), groups allow exploration of intense experiences in a larger community. When individuals hear that their difficulties are shared by others, experiences become depathologized and normalized. And when the difficulties of recovery are experienced as occurring both "outside" (i.e., in other people) and "inside" the person, the massive walls of dissociation separating the "traumatized self" from the larger (healing) community begin to dissipate.

Perhaps most importantly, groups can be utilized to promote cooperative change processes. We view a group as a collective solution team and ask members to participate accordingly. The group therapists operate as facilitators committed to creating resource contexts and suggesting possible solution strategies. Group members are seen as "peer therapists" working with each other to generate greater variety in dealing with life challenges. This involves a balance between reclaiming inner environments (e.g., the ability to feel full bodily comfort and security) and improving social skills (e.g., how to negotiate intimacy with another person).

**2. Mixed genders.**

When we first began co-leading incest survivor groups together, all members were female. This experience stimulated many questions and responses in one of us (SG), some professional and some personal. At times a sense of guilt and shame would pervade regarding the sexual violence that the male community has committed; at other times, a curiosity would arise concerning how other gender relationships could be explored. This was more than a personal issue, in that we believe developmental growth is possible when persons (including one's self) are primarily sensed as individuals capable of many responses rather than as members of a stereotyped social class. This, in addition to the large number of male incest survivors, led us to open the group to men. Having men and women incest survivors in the same group does create certain challenges. For example, many women are initially more hesitant to fully participate (e.g., talking about their experience) with men around. In general, however, such difficulties offset by the distinct advantages of including men and women. Men and women working together as peer therapists generate models of trust and cooperation. Shared experiences of male and female incest survivors deepens appreciation of how incest is a tragic human experience affecting both genders. In addition, discussion of differences in male and female psychosexual identities (and how they are differentially affected by incest) allows clarification of one's sexual identity. (While we have not yet had any gay or lesbian group members, we expect that their presence will enrich these discussions.)

**3. Hypnosis.**

We use hypnosis as a primary technique for solution development in our groups. We emphasize hypnosis as a naturalistic process that enables individuals to reclaim and develop, at their own rates and in their own styles, skills for self-healing and self-expression (see Gilligan, 1987). We do not use an authoritarian model which focuses on one person "putting something inside" another person, for the obvious reason that it doesn't work effectively with survivors of a traumatic invasion (e.g., incest). Instead, we employ a cooperative model in which individuals learn, with themselves and others, to develop an alliance with their unconscious resources. This is done in a variety of formats, including self-hypnosis, group hypnosis, peer hypnosis (in which members/partners are simultaneously hypnotist and subject), and "double inductions" (in which the co-therapists work jointly with a volunteer).

Hypnosis is valuable in many ways. In a general sense, incest itself is a deeply hypnotic, albeit nontherapeutic, experience: It is a profoundly nonverbal, nonrational exchange that produces an altered state characterized by traditional hypnotic phenomena such as "nonvolitional" expressions, somatic changes, sensory alterations, and boundary shifts (Gilligan, 1988b). It is difficult to reach a person in this state through rational, verbal interventions, as its emotional language and logic is so very different from that of "normal" consciousness (cf. Rossi, 1986). Hypnosis utilizes the logic of such primary processes, and thus can be used therapeutically to allow reconnection with them in a safe way.

Hypnosis is especially useful for developing states of inner security. Trance is learned as an opportunity to set aside nagging "internal chatter" and achieve a state of "psychophysical centering" involving a somatic and psychological sense of well being (Gilligan, 1988a). We emphasize repeatedly that individuals can return to this state of inner security to access a sense of safety and self-protection.

Hypnosis can also be used to access resources. For example, time can be spent revivifying pleasant memories or developing "power symbols" (Gilligan, 1988a). Accessing resources is extraordinarily useful to incest survivors, who often regress to trance-like states where few resources are available.

Another application of hypnosis is in changing one's relationship to trance-like phenomena connected to the traumatic event. For example, an incest survivor who experiences frightening "out of body" experiences can learn to perform this hypnotic skill in ways that are comfortable and useful (e.g., for a detached review of key memories). In general, hypnosis enables perceived deficits to be translated into assets (Erickson and Rossi, 1981).

Hypnosis also enables boundary flexibility. We have found this extremely relevant to incest survivors, who often have great difficulty in comfortably setting self-other boundaries. Individuals in trance can learn to "harden" or "soften," expand or contract, and change or stabilize their sensed boundaries. Learning such skills enables participation in relationships in ways that reflect changing needs and values.

Because these various hypnotic skills involve powerful reconnections with an "inner self," they are effective only when a person's rate and style of hypnotic processing is respected. Individuals who are frightened or absorbed in distracting inner processes will be unwilling or unable to participate in hypnotic experiences. Thus, therapists must actively encourage and coach incest survivors to remain sensitive to their unique styles of developing and experiencing trances, so that individual needs are respected. This will often mean slowing down, working with smaller "chunks" of time or material, expanding the trance to include more resources, and so forth.

We consider these sorts of skills — use of primary processes, developing inner security, accessing resources, reframing symptom phenomena, and shifting boundaries — to be central to the developmental growth of incest survivors. While emphasizing the value of hypnosis in this regard, we are aware that non-hypnotic methods may also be used to develop such skills. Thus, therapists not versed in hypnosis may achieve similar outcomes using non-hypnotic methods.

**4. Mastery Orientation.**

Our approach to healing and hypnosis revolves around the theme of mastery of life experiences. Consistent with Erickson's (1948; Erickson & Rossi, 1981) approach, we orient more to solutions than to problems. We view incest survivors firstly as human beings struggling with the same developmental challenges that others face, and secondly as individuals deeply affected by incest and its subsequent denial. Our primary intention is thus to facilitate competency in such skills as the development of self/other differentiation (i.e., boundaries), positive body images, intimacy with a mate, and social participation and competency. To do this, we sort for assets rather than deficits. We emphasize each skill as a right to be claimed and an ability to be developed. The group thus becomes a training ground to actualize these skills.

This is not say that the incestuous experiences of the past are ignored. While we do not primarily focus on or deliberately access such experiences, they often emerge when a developmental skill of, say, intimacy, is being explored. When this happens, such experiences are used to further develop the skill in question. For example, a person may be having sexual problems featuring a reaccess of the incestuous experience. In this case, we would emphasize the important abilities being expressed: withdrawal, body dissociation, intense memories. We would then explore how these abilities could be further developed to include comfortable withdrawal, useful dissociation (e.g., a protective observer), protective numbness, other memories, and so forth. Finally, we would encourage the development of complementary abilities — contact, sensation, present orientation. As Gilligan (1988b) has elaborated, this enables symptoms to be used as important contributions to developmental solutions.

**5. Future Orientation.**

Hand in hand with our mastery approach is a primary orientation to the future. We see the past as a reservoir of valuable learnings and potential resources, and the future as the basis of growth and development. We believe the former is best used primarily in the service of the latter. We thus encourage individuals to orient, at both conscious and unconscious levels, to those desired ways of being. Past experiences, whether pleasant or unpleasant, are viewed as markers on the developmental "path" leading to these satisfying futures. We emphasize that because this path is an individual one, walking it requires sensitivity and flexibility to the changing needs and patterns distinguishing each person's journey.

**6. Context-Connectedness.**

We believe that certain life experiences persist and are felt to be problematic when they have become functionally dissociated from the larger contexts of a person's life, i.e., when individuals involved in unpleasant experiences do not have access to other experiences from their lives. For example, a person may be so overwhelmed by the emotional memory of an incestuous event that a functional amnesia develops regarding other memories and relationships. This cuts the person off from the essential resources needed for change. In this sense, problems reflect a figure/field dissociation, while solutions arise from figure/field connectedness.

Based on these premises, we work to develop solutions by reconnecting individuals to resource contexts. We emphasize three types of contexts in this regard. The first is *social context*, having to do with one's social self as well as social others (family members, close friends, support groups, therapists, etc.). Whereas individuals traumatized by incestuous experiences have usually dissociated from such social resources, we work to reconnect this context so that they may stay with themselves and others.

A second resource field is the *organismic context,* involving one's body and its deep connection to the larger environment. The tremendous invasiveness of incest usually triggers massive dissociation from body and environment. If maintained, this protective mechanism creates many problems, for it denies access to the security and wisdom found in organismic connectedness. Thus, we work to reconnect individuals with their bodies and the environment around them via a variety of training exercises including breathing, movement, physical connection with others, eye focusing, sensation focusing, and body dissociation and reassociation exercises.

A third solution field is the *experiential-symbolic context* involving the psychic-symbol world of memory and imagination. While each person has access to an incredible variety of symbols, each one constituting a potential resource, certain dissociative experiences (e.g., incest) tend to break a person's connection with such resources. For example, a person revivifying an incestuous experience may be unable to also recall other experiences involving needed resources (safety, assertiveness, bodily comfort). Thus, we work to reconnect individuals with their entire field of symbols so that they may reclaim their inner world as a resource field. For example, an incest survivor who would panic any time someone touched her learned to access a memory involving the feeling of confidence and bodily connectedness while jogging. She used this memory as a resource symbol to reconnect with her body in the situations where she had previously dissociated.

### *The Structure of the Group*

We have thus far seen how our mixed-gender groups involve a hypnotically based, future-oriented approach to mastery of developmental skills. We turn now to a more specific description of how the groups are actually run.

### *Group Formation*

The group meets for 10 to 12 weekly sessions, each session several hours long. Membership includes eight to ten incest survivors plus two therapists. Thus far, group members have been white, middle-class heterosexuals ranging in age from 15 to about 60. They are recruited from referral sources, our own therapy practices, and ads in local papers.

Respondents are interviewed and provided with further information, including that the group will include men and women, use hypnosis (especially self-hypnosis) at times as a resource tool, and be organized around certain mastery themes.

*Mastery Themes*

Each weekly meeting focuses on a single mastery theme. The following is a representative sequence for a 12-week group:

1. Accessing security and an "inner center"
2. Envisioning a positive future
3. Reclaiming the past: Power symbols and other resources
4. Sensing and claiming interpersonal boundaries
5. Body image
6. Bodily expression
7. Anger
8. Secrets and disclosures
9. Self-parenting
10. Sexuality
11. Generating altered states without substance abuse
12. Future orientation

*Structure of Sessions*

To explore these mastery themes, we usually proceed in a given session in the following manner.

**1. Introductory centering (5 minutes).**

We start each meeting with a brief experiential centering process. We alternate, with one therapist leading one week, the other the following week, and both the third week. We use permissive communications that emphasize resource development and the need to participate in ways that respect individual rates and styles (see Gilligan, 1987). For example:

> Good evening and welcome. We've got a lot to do tonight, so we'd like to take a few minutes to center our attention for the evening. This will be a "non-denominational" process, meaning that people from all

walks of life can participate. We'd basically like to invite you to take a few minutes to get centered and comfortable with yourself and tune into whatever your needs and interests are here tonight. We suggest that you begin by arranging yourself in a comfortable position. You can keep your eyes open or closed. You can listen to me or not. You can participate in the process fully or partially or not at all. As in any process, you may experience things for awhile, come out for awhile, go back into it, and so forth. And as in all process that we will be exploring, we want to emphasize that you have your own limits, your own needs, and your own pace. More than anything else, we will be emphasizing that in the weeks ahead. So we encourage you to respect your style and proceed accordingly.

With that in mind, go ahead and take a few deep breaths, and get as comfortable as seems appropriate for you at this point. You don't have to talk, although you could and can if you so desire. We encourage you to hold on to the need to attend to your individual needs, and let go of only that tension which you sense as unnecessary ... That's it ... And as you continue to breathe ... as you continue to hold onto important values ... as you continue to let go of unnecessary tension ... you can remain centered and aware in the room here ... [This is repeated several times] ...

And that sense of centering, that sense of awareness, that attention that is yours ... can be used in many positive and safe ways. For example, what a nice thing to know that you have the ability to image resources ... or image pleasant scenes ... or image comforting places. We don't know which place or which symbol is most comforting for you ... it may be the beach ... it may be a friend ... it may something as simple as a color. But whatever it is, we'd like to suggest that you can imagine, you can think about, you can become absorbed in that symbol in a way that allows you to feel comfortable ... in a way that allows you to feel secure ... [This is elaborated for another minute or so] ... in a way that allows you to know that you can stay with yourself during the group tonight and in the days ahead as you discover new ways to enjoy yourself, to develop yourself, to protect yourself ... So why not take a few moments now to sense that image ... to know that you can return to it whenever you need to recenter tonight ... and then when you're ready, take a nice deep breath and come on back out here ...

While these suggestions focus on resource development, those in later sessions also include future orientation, e.g., Erickson's (1954; de Shazer, 1982; Gilligan, 1988a) "crystal ball" projection techniques.

The response to this process is variable. Some people develop and maintain deep absorption; others remain completely analytical; most experience partial involvement. Since incest survivors often compare their performance (unfavorably) to an idealized image of how they should be participating, we emphasize the importance of respecting individual rates and styles of participation.

**2. Group sharing (10 minutes).**

In the first session this involves introductions. We emphasize the value of the group in terms of recovering and reclaiming skills and abilities, while also encouraging each person to find and respect their own style and degree of participation. We introduce ourselves, describing briefly our training backgrounds, our experience in working with incest and related issues, and our interests in the group. We then move around the group, asking each participant to introduce themselves.

In subsequent sessions the group sharing process centers around events that have transpired since the last meeting. This includes successes (e.g., "What we did in group last week really made a difference this week in relating to my spouse"), difficulties (e.g., "I really had a difficult time responding to my boss's criticisms this week"), and surprises (e.g., "My parents visited us last week"). Given time constraints, individuals are encouraged to use the weekly theme issue to deal with emerging issues. (Earlier experience demonstrated that an entire evening could be spent on unstructured "talking about" challenges; we find it much more useful to devote most of the group process to more structured explorations).

**3. Introduction of mastery theme (10 minutes).**

We then make a general didactic presentation of the weekly theme. The theme (e.g., envisioning a satisfying future) is first presented as a general ability needed by every person in order to develop and grow. We note how the connection to this ability is often lost via incestuous invasion, and cite some consequences of such a disconnection (e.g., depression, absorption in the past, fear). When we ask if such symptoms are experienced by any members of the group, they are usually relieved and often surprised when most people raise their hands. Advantages of regaining the ability are then emphasized, and participants are asked if they are interested in developing such advantages. Their agreement is used to devote the evening to reclaiming and developing mastery with the ability.

**4 & 5. Demonstration of exercise (30 minutes) and exercise (40 minutes).**

In the initial sessions this involves a simple demonstration by the therapists with a volunteer, followed by the group breaking into pairs to practice. These exercises have included developing a safe dissociational space (the "Middle of Nowhere"), accessing a security symbol, and developing altered states with another person ("mutual hypnosis").

Later sessions involve more complex exercises carried out in multiple steps, with each step demonstrated by the therapists and then practiced by group members in small "pods." These "pods" usually consist of three people, with one person operating as a "genius," one as a "wizard," and one as a "coach." The wizard guides the genius through the structured experiential process, while the coach closely monitors both people to ensure that security and centering is maintained. If cues (interrupted breathing, postural collapse, muscular tension) indicate that genius or wizard needs to "recenter", the coach gently moves in to help reaccess the security resources that have been hypnotically developed in previous sessions. Also, the two therapists are around to offer supervision and, in the event of emotional accessing, to provide additional therapeutic allies for the tri-pod.

The exercises are, of course, based on the mastery theme of that evening. For example, the theme of generating satisfying futures is explored via the following four-step exercise.

(i) *Envision a satisfying future.*

Trance is first developed. In the demonstration, a general hypnotic induction is used; in the practice pods, wizards guide geniuses in using a self-hypnosis process practiced in the first sessions. Once a person signals (e.g., via a head nod) that a satisfactory trance has been achieved, the therapist (or wizard) suggests the development of a desired future. For example:

> And as you continue to enjoy that feeling of security, what a nice thing to know that you can feel very secure in knowing that your inner mind is an ally that can support you in many ways . . . And so as you continue to hear the sound of our voices, and continue to orient to that feeling of security, what a nice thing to know that your unconscious can

> begin to move into your awareness some image ... a very special image ... of a future event or relationship that you would like to have in your life ... maybe it involves a certain way of talking or feeling or acting at work or at home or by yourself ... I don't know ... maybe it will be a seemingly small change ... I don't know ... all I know is that as you continue to breathe and feel very secure at the very deepest level, you can allow that image of a satisfying future to develop in your mind ... some way of being that you would really like to develop ... and when you find that image in your awareness, please signal by nodding your head ...

Difficulties in accessing typically reflect difficulties in trance development, in which case adjustments are made to enhance hypnotic absorption. For example, some individuals like to hold the therapist's hand in order to ensure a social connection; others like to keep their eyes open. Directly asking the person about what they need in order to feel comfortable is generally the best way to obtain such information.

When geniuses signal the envisioning of a satisfying future, they are asked to take a few moments to memorize the image, and then return back to the room.

(ii) *Access and anchor resource.*

A resource symbol helpful to the achievement of the future is now developed and "anchored". The subject is asked to hold the therapist's (or wizard's) hand, reenter trance, and gently squeeze the hand when a symbol is accessed. For example:

> ... And as you continue to enjoy returning to that inner state of security, you can also return to that image of the future ... and I don't know exactly how your unconscious will guide you to achieving that future ... all I know is that you can enjoy developing that future in a way meaningful for you ... and in that process, really in any process, it's nice to have allies to support you ... allies to guide you ... allies to be with you ... and so what I'd like to ask your unconscious mind to do now is to identify and move into your awareness some experiential symbol, some resource, that will be useful to you in moving toward that future ... it may be a feeling, it may be a visual image, it may be a word or a person or an animal ... For example, one person found

> great comfort and support in remembering her big Dalmatian named "Freckles" ... another person found an image of a pumpkin pie somehow deeply meaningful and useful ... so I don't know what symbol will develop for you ... all I know is that you can sense it developing and when it has fully developed, please squeeze my hand gently to indicate thusly ...

When the person squeezes the hand, the therapist very gently squeezes back to "anchor" the experience. The idea here is to associationally connect the hand squeeze with the resource symbol, so that introduction of one can trigger access of the other. After the anchor has been established, the person is reoriented.

(iii) *Test anchors.*

To check the anchor, the person is asked to go back into trance and pay close attention to what happens when his or her hand is gently squeezed. The same process is repeated again, this time with the subject squeezing the hand of the therapist (or wizard). This step is complete when the person reports the reaccessing of the resource symbol upon each hand squeeze.

(iv) *Claiming a satisfying future.*

With resources in hand (so to speak), the person is now ready to hypnotically rehearse the desired state. Instructions are given to squeeze the hand whenever difficulties arise or resources are otherwise needed. Also, the therapist (or wizard) closely monitors the process, and introduces hand squeezing whenever it seems the person may need the resource available. Hand squeezes are accompanied by suggestions to slow down a bit, to take deep breaths, to sense resources, and to move at one's own rate. In this way a person is paced through several rounds of hypnotic enactment of the future.

We have found that most group members are remarkably competent in moving through these structured processes, especially when the steps are "chunked down" sufficiently and security resources are readily available. Working with peers bypasses barriers a number of incest survivors feel when working with a "parent-like" therapist in a one-with-one therapy situation. It shifts the experience of, and recovery from, incest into a community context where one supports and is supported by others. This social recontextualization contributes powerfully to the healing process.

**6. Group discussion (15 minutes).**

Most group members get very involved in the exercise. While the experiences are still fresh, we orient attention to the value of the learnings in the larger context of people's lives. We ask people to comment on how the target ability relates to present challenges and to identify areas where they would most like to apply it. The discussion often is poignant as members describe how they forgot or lost the target ability in the incestuous relationship. Their emotional vulnerability is supported, while the possibility to reclaim the ability in the present and future is gently reiterated.

For example, we devoted one evening to the issue of boundaries. The exercise involved partners standing and facing each other at a distance. As one partner walked toward the other, the other was to sense when his or her boundaries were physically entered and then respond by raising an arm and saying, "Stop! I need my boundaries." One man described how good it felt to sense and claim his boundaries, noting tearfully how new and different it felt to him. We gently emphasized that this skill was his to claim and use, and then asked him if there were any places in his life that he would like to have available such a skill. When he identified a dating situation, further gentle communications were used to help him hypnotically rehearse how he could sense and establish boundaries in this area.

We have found it very useful to hold open-ended group discussions of the incest experiences after rather than before experiential skills and resources have been explored. The context of self-support and confidence generated from such experiential achievements solves the dilemma of how to have clients discuss painful dissociative experiences without "collapsing" back into them.

**7. Future pacing (5 minutes).**

Beginning to wind down the evening, we emphasize the theme again and note how each person can enjoy exploring it during the week. We suggest there will be successes and perhaps a few failures, and note several ways that difficulties might be handled. We then assign homework to further develop the evening theme. This might involve self-hypnosis, working together with another group member, doing some art work, identifying experimental areas to apply the new skills, and so forth.

**8. Closing induction (5 minutes).**

We close with a group trance as general and simple as the opening process. We usually include suggestions for a return to a "center," a review of the evening's learnings, a symbol to remind one of the learnings, a glimpse of the satisfying future, and a few moments to thank one's self for participating in a way that reflected individual needs. Participants are then reoriented and bidden good-bye.

## OUTCOMES

Based on our observations, client reports, and informal follow-ups (conducted unsystematically with various members from one to eighteen months following the completion of a group) we have been impressed and excited with the changes that group members have made in their lives. One common outcome is what might be called a *normalization of the incest experience.* Group members broke vows of secrecy, shifted responsibility (and guilt) away from themselves, recognized incest as occurring in many families (not just their own), realized that the consequences of incest are experienced by most survivors (not just themselves), and developed inner worlds not dominated by the incest experience. The group seemed to be very therapeutic in this regard. As one woman noted, "I never talked about [these experiences] before. I can't believe other people have also experienced this and can understand."

Related to these shifts is *enhanced sexual identity.* Gender identity, especially as it relates to sexuality, often spontaneously emerges as a topic in group discussions. Such discussions and related exercises seem to help individuals clarify and express aspects of sexuality including body image, physical touching, and gender role. As one man noted, "I have a clearer sense of my identity as a man. I've always known I was male and prefer women, but I've had a sense of shame and self-doubt about being molested. The exercises . . . especially the one on boundaries . . . were especially good [in changing that]."

Another area of change has been the *development of inner resources.* In reclaiming their inner worlds, group members have learned to create safety contexts to which they can withdraw when appropriate. They also have learned to use "power symbols" as resources. For example, one woman reported a long-standing pattern of "emotionally merging" with a television program (e.g., "Dynasty") whenever it featured illicit sex. In the group she hypnotically developed the power symbol of a "future woman" that she could "vibrantly feel" in her solar plexus when needed (see Gilligan, 1988a). When the traditional emotional reaction was triggered several nights later, the power symbol spontaneously "turned on" in her (solar plexus) power center. An intense "tug of war" developed, with the power symbol pulling her into her own body and the television images pulling her into the illicit sex scenes. Suddenly she felt a "pop" as her body fell back into the chair. Euphoria washed over her body as she felt a detachment from the television show and an intense feeling of her own body as separate and whole. This sort of dramatic experience, reflecting the idiosyncratic process of unconscious creativity, is not uncommon during the course of any hypnotherapy.

A fourth common result is *increased intimacy* with one's self, other group members, friends, and spouses. By developing stronger and more flexible boundaries while learning to open to others in safe ways, individuals learn the pleasure and satisfaction of negotiating intimacy with integrity. Often this change comes from differentiating intimate others from the perpetrator. As one woman noted:

> I coped with the molestation by my uncle all these years without ever telling anyone. But when my husband reached about the age my uncle was when he molested me, I couldn't look at my husband's eyes without seeing my uncle. Those eyes. I'm glad I have conquered that and can change it into a workable situation. I don't see those eyes anymore. I actually think it's over.

Other people had similar experiences of "deframing" spouses. Improvements have also been observed in *social competency*. Since the group frequently focuses on actual achievements in ongoing experience, people often report enhanced performance at work and other social interactions. Increased assertiveness and confidence is common, as when a man happily described how he effectively challenged a work supervisor who was abusively "dumping" unwarranted responsibilities on him.

Another type of change has to do with *self acceptance*. Perhaps more than most individuals, incest survivors often have great difficulty appreciating and positively framing their inner experiences. For example, a woman participating in a group hypnosis process of accessing a power symbol was convinced she had failed because her image was fading in and out. We repeatedly emphasize that such individual differences are the rule in private experience, not the exception. We thus strongly encourage individuals to move in "baby steps" and to appreciate the rhythmic balance of unconscious processing (e.g., between contact and withdrawal, focusing and defocusing, inner and outer, and so forth). Accordingly, it is not surprising that individuals report increased abilities to accept and positively frame their experiences.

Other changes have occurred in the area of *substance abuse*. We emphasize that incest survivors have high rates of abusing drugs, alcohol, and food (e.g., bulimia), and strongly encourage any such abuses to be handled, for the simple reason that their continuation significantly hampers change. We point out that the group is probably not a sufficient context for breaking addictions, and thus provide information on various treatment programs. A number of our group members have entered and completed such programs.

Changes in the family of origin have also occurred, though in different ways. Some group members have chosen to remain distant from their families; others have grown closer. Some have deemphasized their family, shifting their attention to other relationships; others have entered into family therapy. That there is no overall pattern perhaps reflects our own position of having no set rule about how to relate to the family. This is something we are reconsidering these days, and we are interested in learning from others in this area. Our present orientation assumes that some individuals may fare best by reconciling with their families, while others may do better separately. Given that we have no set rule for all clients, we try to inform clients of the "pros" and "cons" of each possibility, and then support and encourage them to make their own choices.

A final outcome worth noting is a *premature leaving of the group*. In group of 10 or so people, we usually have one or two dropouts along the way. One woman wanted to read a very lengthy letter from her father in the second session. She was disallowed from doing so and didn't return the next session. Another woman left the group after being challenged by a group member to talk to her mother about transpired incestuous events. While on the one hand we assume that every group will have its dropouts, we are concerned and often saddened when this happens. We are very interested in discovering further ways to minimize such occurrences.

## CONCLUSION

The outcomes indicate that the program has helped individuals to reclaim and master basic abilities essential for growth and development. The diversity of such changes indicates how incestuous traumas deeply affect many areas of functioning. Ironically, this depth of involvement may also provide the impetus and opportunity for equally profound growth in emotional integrity and psychological identity. This is what our group participants have suggested to us, and this is what we are interested in continuing to explore.

# Chapter 9

# AGE REGRESSION[1]

*by Stephen Gilligan and Paul Carter*

## INTRODUCTION

GILLIGAN: You sat in a classroom long ago, and sitting in a classroom long ago you listened sometimes in certain ways. You communicated in special ways to those people around you. Do you know this game: Postman? [whispering something in neighbor's ear and saying "Pass it on"]

CARTER: The subject for this afternoon will be all of us, and we are going to do some work Stephen has been getting to with regression. In traditional hypnosis you give direct suggestions to help someone regress in trance. It may be suggested that he should go deeper, deeper and deeper, and then as I count from 1 to 10 you will get younger and younger. But a regressed state is actually very easy to set up naturalistically, without any formal induction, without even a formal trance really. You can begin to introduce or develop a regressed-like state just by using some of the very powerful associations to childhood by games, songs, different kinds of ways of using your body and any other number of things I have written up there. Either you bring them in and actually do them. You sing a song from childhood or you bring in one of the teachers that you had when you were five years old — or you bring your mother and father in. And did you notice that,

[1] This chapter presents a group trance induction offered by Drs. Gilligan and Carter in a Hamburg, Germany, hypnosis training. It originally appeared as a chapter in H. Klippstein (Ed.). 1991. *Ericksonian hypnotherapeutic group inductions*. New York: Brunner/Mazel.

by the way, even still you might be 40 years old, 50 years old, still when you get together with your mother and father, it's almost like you were six again. They are some of the same parents. In a hypnotic induction it can suffice many times to simply describe or talk about some little songs or some other childhood experiences to set up a regressed state. [laughing] Mogens? Where did we go? [with the game: Postman] Right over there? That's it. What did he say to you?

M.: He's bringing me into a trance.

GILLIGAN: Now, what did he say exactly? Can you remember the words?

M.: He said: you can go deeper — deeper — deeper into a trance.

CARTER: Was there more?

M.: No.

CARTER: Not yet?

GILLIGAN: So much for these brilliant intellectual developments that occur in hypnosis workshops. [laughter]

CARTER: So in any case you can use almost anything as a powerful association for childhood to begin to set up a sense of an earlier time, the environment of an earlier time. The value of doing that is to begin to bring out again childlike qualities, not necessarily specific memories, where that's one focus in therapy: to develop very specific memories. What I'm going to suggest that we focus on this afternoon — certainly specific memories will come out — the focus here is more on developing a quality of being a child again, which can be developed through some specific memories and through some activities of childhood bring out that quality of childhood, meaning the softness, the flexibility, the ability to learn, that tremendous ability that we have as a child and start to limit more and more as we grow up, of being able to learn fantastically complex tasks like speaking a language at a rapid rate compared to later on in life, where that rate seemed to slow down a little bit. That can be available to you again through regressing and developing the childhood kinds of qualities.

GILLIGAN: So we would like to ask you at the outset to think and identify what associations, what ways of being, what games, what songs, what sorts of values do you remember as being associated to your childhood, uniquely associated. What did you learn, think, do, experience as a child that you tend not to experience so much as an adult?

CARTER: So for example sitting in a classroom and the teacher asks a question, and nobody wants to answer, right? [laughter] So you sit there and cannot look straight ahead, hoping that she or he wouldn't notice you.

GILLIGAN: Maybe you have had experiences sometimes of being called upon in the classroom, and you hadn't done your homework properly. And you know that the teacher is going to ask about that homework. And you are able to wonder: Is he going to call on me? And what ways did you use as a child to try to distract the teacher from calling on you, that always seemed to work the opposite way? Somehow the teacher just knew when to call on you.

CARTER: [pointing] The young man over here? Ja? [laughter]

GILLIGAN: [to man] Can you elaborate a little bit?

M.: One way I used was to pretend not being there, which only worked when he didn't look in his book. When he looked in his book and then said: Go on, it's your turn, you are lost. Because he did that anyway.

CARTER: So you made yourself invisible? Hm? But then he called your name from the book.

M.: Yes. So this only worked when he looked into the class.

CARTER: How many of you had that ability as a child to make yourself invisible? Become one of the invisible people? Have you seen that movie? Do you have that movie in Europe yet: "The Enchanted Forest?" Or is it: "The Animal Forest?" It was made in South America. About a family who goes down to South America. And the child is taken by the Indians there, by the invisible people? I guess, you didn't see it. I'm starting to feel I'm the only one who has seen that movie.

GILLIGAN: Change the subject! [laughter]

CARTER: You see, we tried those things, and sometimes people just don't relate to what you are talking about. And whenever you begin a hypnotic induction you often-times start by throwing out an idea like Stephen talked about not doing the homework. Some of you didn't respond, or others of you started responding stronger, which gives you an idea of how to proceed.

If you are working in a group, for example, you put out an idea and you see who responds strongly to that idea. And if you want to focus on that person's development, then you may focus on that idea a little bit more. And then you might want to shift to another topic for a while to see who else may respond to a different idea. It's the same thing if you are working with a family, presenting some different ideas. In any case we will do some things in here, where we present a whole variety of ideas, some of which will probably be meaningless to you individually, some of which you will probably find rather meaningful. You can certainly notice what you respond with and feel free to focus on these things that are useful to you.

What we would like to do is a group induction to give you an opportunity to just experience some changes inside yourself. Before the beginning of this we are going to ask you to take out something to write on, a piece of paper or something. Get one from someone near you along with a pen or a pencil.

GILLIGAN: Your learning task, one that you mastered long ago, is to let yourself master it again in the present.

CARTER: Now most of us as adults believe we are supposed to know everything already. Or at least know most everything, for example, how to write. And because of that it becomes much more difficult to learn. For example, to learn a new language, it's much more difficult, if you think you've mostly taken care of your language learning. And so it's often much more difficult to go through some of the frustrations and changes that go on, when you are learning something new. Many people don't, whether it's learning a new therapy skill, learning a new sport skill, learning a new language skill. Often times we stop. But as a child generally you don't think you are supposed to know everything. That's a good thing to remember. I would like to ask you to be willing to take some time to not know again. To be a little bit like a child again and to just feel what it is like to explore. And part of what helps the child do that is not being concerned about where you are going. See, now as an adult you know, you are supposed to be very successful. So that if you are not that way when you begin, you think, "There is something wrong with me." But as a child you don't know so much what it means necessarily to be that successful, you just enjoy playing with new skills where you are.[2]

| CARTER: | GILLIGAN: |
|---|---|
| | So even as Paul is talking about that topic<br>that really is<br>oriented to the adult life |
| so you can begin to allow yourself to<br>*make that change* | |

[2] Gilligan and Carter now begin to shift into a double induction, wherein both voices are speaking simultaneously.

in a very
simple way
able

So for that purpose what we'll ask
you to do is:
put your pen or your pencil
in the *other* hand, not
the hand you normally
write with, but in the *other* hand.

And what we are going to ask you
to do
not right now, but in a moment,
is to write your name.
And when I'm going to ask you to
take a minute
of clock time to do this
normally you can write your name
in a couple of seconds, so you all
know you can do that.
This is a different task.
What I'm going to ask you to do
is *really slow down.*
Take a few seconds,
actually 5 or 10 seconds for every
letter in your name.
Make it *very very slow.*
Let yourself *watch* each line
develop
*very very slow.*

So go ahead, start and take
a good full minute at least

clock time, about ten seconds

and *wonder* what it would be like to be

to hear the voices
*Listen* to the voices now much more as a
*child.*

I remember, for example,

ten years ago, there was a young boy,
that lived with us. Little Eric was *six*
*years old,*

in the first grade.
Little Eric was learning in the *first grade*
a variety of different things

He was *learning to write* "Eric."
His name was "Eric" with a "c."
He was learning to pronounce

words and letters.
He was *learning* to tell a big A
from a little a,
big B
from a little b.

Big C
from little c,
a p from a q

a t from a u,
from a to c.
And he learned all the tasks and different
things.
And Eric's school had an open

for each letter. Write your name,
your first name.
Mogens,

Barbara, Wolfgang, Maureen.
One letter at a time.

And if you already have finished
more than two letters,
then *slow down.*
Cut your speed in half,

*real slow.*

And when you have finished

your name
if you need more time
take it!
If you don't need more time,

then just below your name begin
to write your address, the number,
street, where you lived as a child,
when you were going to school.
If you can't remember it, then
just write any one you can remember.
And what you wore and where you sit.
Even *where you live now.*

house for all the different parents to visit.

We would *go to the school* and see how
the young children do it.
Open house for first-grade children.

And Eric had Frank, his father.
Paul and I were
like uncles to him as we
were living in the same house.
So the three of us went to that
classroom
together and visited the *first-grade
classroom* in order to
examine, to *explore,* to *discover.*
Little Eric was *learning.*
Now, what do you learn in grade one?
And the seats we walked in were very
small. And the teacher said:
*Please sit in the first-grade seat.* And we
sat down, Frank in one chair, Paul in
another chair, Stephen in the third chair.
And we felt ourselves really *develop
a sense of remembering* what it was like
to learn as a small
child.
And Mrs. Bigger
was a teacher.
And grade one teachers often-times
have
strange-sounding names, the teachers.
*What's the teacher wearing?*

What did the teacher call you?

Write very slow!
Even a little bit slower than you wrote
your name

to make the letters of that and to form
those numbers.
And as you do that
you might begin to *remember* some of
the *feelings* you had

*learning* to write those numbers

and *learning* to write those *letters.*

Then go ahead and finish this address
slowly!
And when you have done
you can put down your pen
and pencils,
let your hands rest on your lap
and close your eyes and
*let your mind go!*

And when you learn those letters
you have to learn the big A
and also the little a, and you
have to learn the printed A
and the cursive A.
And you try to learn the difference
between *A* and *day* and *pay*, and is the
circle on a p the same as the circle
on a d?
The hump on the m the same as the
hump of the n? And learning to write
them not only down, but learning
to write them *in between the lines.*

And how long can you *sit comfortably?*
And who sat in front of you?

And what kind of desk was it now?
And what kind of pencil is it?

And what kind

of feeling to learn to write and *write*
*right* numbers.
Learning the 1, the 2, the 3, and
learning *more and more unconsciously.*
Write right, write!
And Mrs. Bigger showed the different
pictures, *cat,*
*dog,*

the different animals.

And every child had a different animal.
Every child developed a special
relationship.
If there is a rabbit
or if there is another kind of animal.

You are going to develop as a child
a variety of emotional relationships.
You are going to develop as a child
a variety of associations.
You are going to develop as a child
a variety of different understandings.
How to *spell your name,*
different understandings.

How to address that teacher?

And first it's so hard to get
them to stay in between the lines.
And when you finished writing
put your pens and pencils down
and sit back comfortably in your chair

and let yourself go!

We didn't only learn writing as a child.
We didn't only learn counting in
a trance. As a child you learn

You learn to *sing songs*.

You learn a game.

Maybe you learn the alphabet song:
A, B, C, D, E, F, G,
H, I, J, K, L, M, N, O, P,
Q, R, S, T, U, V, W, X, Y, Z,
Now I know my ABC's,

tell me what you think of me.
And there are so many different
ways of learning your own language,
your own songs.

I remember Henning teaching me the
rhyme:

Schlapp, schlapp, schlapp,
die Milch ist gut.

Guten Morgen liebes Kätzchen

And you learn
in terms of values.

Some cats are your companions, and
some cats you don't want to
pet. You learn to differentiate and you
can learn to find those relationships that
allow you to *be secure*.

And in a trance you can go very deeply
in your own security.
And as a child you learn, for example,
many many things
to ride a bike.
Many children learn how to swim.

You learn to ride in a car and
look out
and see: the *different scenery* is *changing*.
The images are changing,
the feeling of movement
is changing. And
feeling the *security* in a trance . . .
feeling the security in a trance
through and through.
And even move *back* in time *further* . . .
And for a nickname,
and knowing which nickname meant
which relationship,

a certain name for you, how your parents
were calling you,
when you knew you were in trouble.
A certain name, parents will call you,
knew you were well liked.

Ist hier noch ein freies Plätzchen?

Schlapp, schlapp, schlapp,
die Milch ist gut.
Schlapp, schlapp, schlapp,
wie wohl das tut!
Now you were very proud to learn
a song.

So go and take some time to remember
a certain song that you learned . . .
as a little girl, as a little boy.
Maybe she used to sing you:
Guten Abend, gute Nacht
mit Rosen bedacht
mit Nelken geschmückt
schlüpf unter die Deck.

Morgen früh, wenn Gott will
wirst du wieder geweckt,

Morgen früh, wenn Gott will,
wirst du wieder geweckt.
And as a young baby

you understand *feeling*
and you *hear a voice*
and you don't need to hear the words,
you can just *understand the feeling,*

when you hear an angry voice,
you feel that anger.
You don't need to know what that
voice is saying
you just know the anger.

And when you hear a loving voice.

And different names and different
values
and different associations.

And different roles in the classroom.

Some of which you learned how to stand
out
as the one with the good song,
as the one with the jokes,
as the one with that special part,
as the one with that special ability,
as one with a certain value,
belonging to a certain family,
belonging to a certain culture,
belonging to a certain set of
understandings.
And in trance you can *review those
understandings.*
You can *shift* through those
understandings
with the feeling of *security,*
with the respect for all the learnings,
with an appreciation of the
developmental ability
to learn *new values*
appropriate for the present self,
new values . . .
and that's very difficult to hear
sometimes
name changes . . .
you hear sadness.

You can hear voices through walls

and you learn about relationships.

you know that feeling
and you don't need to know
what she's saying, what he's saying.

You just know that feeling of love in the voice.
And as a baby
you can hear the feeling
and you can understand
the experience full and completely.
As a child you learn to explore
with your mouth.
As a baby everything goes to
your mouth.
You see a rock
and you want to know how it feels
in your mouth.
You see your father's shoe.
You want to know how it feels
in your mouth. You see a spoon,
you want to feel it in your mouth
and taste that spoon.
And it's nice to put your fingers into
your mouth, your thumb.
And it's a good feeling as a baby
to have a thumb
or a couple of different fingers
in your mouth and enjoy the taste

and *feel security* of that *thumb*

in your mouth.

And you *enjoy* a *simple movement* as
a baby.

And how many of you may remember
the *gentle rocking*

And in trance you can be able,
*with the security*

*of the Deeper Self,*

to review those experiences

with a sense of knowing the values
for the present self. As a child I had a
windbreaker jacket.
I really enjoyed that windbreaker jacket.
And then one day
there was a loss . . .

a loss of that windbreaker jacket.
There was a sense of attachment
to something very special . . .
the jacket wasn't there. I thought . . .
*Look over and find it.*
But the loss couldn't be denied.

I didn't know what to do . . .
what to say . . .
*Go to a different state*

go to a different place

go to a different state of security

a state in which you can be all alone

with your own *sense of safety.*
You may not know
how you get there,

*back* and *forth*
*back* and *forth*, *back* and *forth*.

And you can feel that rocking now,
that gentle movement
*back* and *forth*
a *loving* movement
a *loving* pose in your *body*.

And you might feel very *secure*,
when someone rocks you back and forth,

back and forth
it's so nice to feel that *good sensation* again inside your depth.

And there are so many memories within you . . .
so many experiences of the self

and at this time

we would like to ask you to allow an image

to *allow an image*
*of a small child to develop*.

And you may recognize this child
or you may not
you don't need to.
Just allow yourself to see

or to sense, to feel
a young child near you.

may not know where you are,
may not know how the solution will develop,

how the reorganization will develop
how those new learnings
are developing,
how you learn to move your hands differently.
*One* little hand

*one* little finger. This little piggy went to the market,
this little piggy goes to the store,
and where does this little piggy go?

And you have a sense of your hand
*changing inside* . . .

of the different values of self . . .

reorganizing . . .

in accord with your *present needs* . . .

so much to review and reframe . . .
different grades . . .

different subjects . . .
geography . . .
history . . .

mathematics . . .

language . . .

reading . . .

Maybe one year old . . .
maybe two years . . .
maybe four years old . . .
maybe five . . .

some young child . . .

Allow yourself to begin to develop
a sense of that young child.
Is it a boy or a girl?
How old is that child?
What's he or she look like?
What is he or she wearing?

How big is that child?

15cm, 20cm, 25cm?
50cm? A full meter?
How big is that child?

And as you begin to get acquainted
with this child,
notice that that child is beginning
to move closer to you.

And just observe that child . . .
observe how he or she moves
get a sense of him
the expression of his face

and let her, let him
come closer to you
and let that child take your hand . . .

take you by the hand
and feel that small child's hand
in your hand.

the reading, the learning . . .

the patterning . . .

*You can feel it!*
*You can feel it!*
*You can feel it!*
And that sense
of knowing where it is: the center
*Here you are:* . . . the *center*

Here you are: . . . the center
The child is getting bigger.

Here you allow yourself to appreciate

varieties of ways that you can become

experientially intimate.

And you can really enjoy
developing further
that which is there . . .
that which is there . . .
yourself *over there* . . .
yourself *over there* . . .

moving *closer* now . . .
it is *coming closer now*, little bit more . . .
moving . . .

a child moving

Feel the softness
and you can feel very secure
being with yourself.
How you don't need to hear me,
you don't need to hear Stephen
and you can let yourself
simply be in your own world
alone with the child.
And you can be very secure
alone with the child

and feel the softness of that hand,
the littleness of that hand
and let yourself enjoy
the experience with a tear
with a sense of feeling
with an awe of that little hand.

And in a moment
when next we say the word "now"
to take a couple of minutes of
clocktime

unconscious to *let that child take you*
*on a journey*

And that child can take you by the
hand and lead you
and that child's hand in your hand
leading you, guiding you somewhere
in particular.
And you can let your unconscious help
you going along
go along

And you can let go, and you don't
need to hold on to.
You simply enjoy a journey

a child feeling
a child feeling

Hear the other sounds . . .
and that beautiful sense of music
of integration, of intimacy
. . . the sense of being alone together now.
Where two selves become
one with the other . . .
with the other . . .
for the other . . .
You can experience various emotions

right in the inside.
You know when it's time

and know that you are here
and there.
You can be able . . .

All the time in the world for you

to let that child share with you something
the child knows

and you have forgotten about.

And you really can enjoy
letting that child show you

in a fresh fashion
a very very fresh fashion
in a new fashion, a very very precious . . .

And observe your feeling
your vision
what you hear and see and feel

as that child takes you on a journey

and the journey beginning

in time

second time, foreign time, here back,
the journey
with that child

Now . . .
And you can let go my voice and
go all the way
And sometimes the child will show
you a very special place.

And you can stay there for a
while and just observe
*feel* and *sense*
at that place.
And sometimes
the child will show you *something*,

something that you need.

To pay attention to in order to *heal*
your own self-image

in order to *heal* your own
self-awareness
in order to heal your own self home
in order to make whole

very very valuable

learning . . .

nourish the self

many years of clock time

through the years

1975
68, 67
where will it be?

who knows?
*Nowwwww!*

In a very very *tender* fashion

in a very very *gentle* way

in the middle of nowhere.
An opportunity to review
*here* and *there*
*simultaneously*.

And to know of the reformulation
the value
to respect then
to respect now

the needs of the child
the needs of the adult

your own being again

our being that is soft and hard

big and small.

You can feel free to get a sense
of anything you might need
at this moment
perhaps a hand
a *gentle touch*

perhaps some time
to be with yourself and feel
and see and listen

perhaps the chance to say something
that you need to say

say it
and begin the process
of making yourself whole again
speaking a word

expressing a feeling

*redeem the time*
asking
a man

moving your body.

And when you are ready, feel free
to take a moment
to simply appreciate
and find a place for this child in you
a simultaneous self

the needs of then, the needs of now

two hands
two shoulders
one neck . . .

two hips, two ears, one spine . . .
two eyes
two hands
one self

two understandings
then and now
one unified vision . . .

the middle third
the middle third.
*A Trance Parent self*

to guide the child

to guide the child
a sense of letting go

hearing

*redeem the time*

and the unread vision

of the bigger dream.
Why should we celebrate the dead men
more than the dying?

a sense of *growing*
. . . the sense of *knowing*

find a place in your own being
for this child
and you may be aware of the need
to spend more time with the child

you may be aware of the need to cry
the need to laugh
you may be aware of the need to
move . . .

And for that reason
find a place
to keep this child near you.
And in your unconscious you can
find that place
a place which is appropriate
and comfortable for you . . .
in your heart?
in your mind?
in your need?

in the back of your head?

Find some place to keep that child
so that you know you can return

and dream again, play again
with the child.

And yet for now allow yourself

to *let go*

to absorb the journey and its memory
in you
the memory of the soft feeling.
And bring back with you
what you want to continue

a life of learning

a simple self

finding new relationships
And you really can't
predict how

that movie
that past with the heart
That path with a heart
that past with a heart.
that path with a heart

Take steps from your path.

Take steps

little baby steps

little baby feet

little baby's
shoes
little baby's nose
little baby's toys

little baby's love

the love of the little baby

for the self

the little baby's eyes
to tell you
*Grow . . .*
*know . . .*

to think about and leave
with the child what you prefer
to leave with the child for now.

And when you first begin to walk
it is quite a thrill
just to be able to take one step
and then another
and still stand up

First it was easier to run than to walk

It was sort of like falling forward
and letting your legs follow along as
fast as they could. But after not so long
you mastered walking and it became so
natural that you didn't even think
twice about it. You were already
learning to skip, to jump, to hop, to
walk on one leg, to walk backwards.
When you have mastered one skill you
move on to another. And each new one
again as you learn to experience
it more and more completely in yourself.
And when you get stuck, it's nice to
return to some of the earliest skills,
so that you can remember what it's like
to learn. And sometimes you'll be very
stuck, because you are working on a
task too complex for you at this time.
And so it's good to let go a bit for
a while.

Return to something of a more simple
form, something more basic

Yes . . .
*Grow* . . .

And your unconscious can organize the
best variety of different ways to learn to
be able to develop mental strategies
that fit . . .
organizations that reflect
inward and outward
the depth of

your own being.
You have that voice

and baby is there too.

And be able to return . . .

like the movement of taking a sweater
off, like breathing . . .
like the experience of opening and
closing your eyes . . .
like the feeling of the first time you
lifted your hand and found your face.

And remember whether your tears are
crying or your tears are laughing.
The tears are water
and they are the same

tears.

And both are water of your heart

or water that is nourishing for both
your eyes and your inner being.

So when you are ready, feel free to
allow yourself to come out
and reorient
to the room again
and appreciate your ability to do what
you have done. To let go as much as
you did let go, to hold on as much as
you did hold on, and know that both
are important to your growing power.
To appreciate your ability to remember
what you did remember

Have the experience to be able to
let yourself know there is a lot more
where that came from. So take a few
moments and give yourself some messages
of self-appreciation

and thank yourself
for that degree of movement

in that style

in that way that suited the needs
of the entire self.
And going to a light trance,
*come out: gently.*
You may go into a deep trance,
*come out: gently.*
going to a medium then, *deeper trance,*
light trance; come out, gently . . .
Go into medium and deep and light and
deep and light
and a deeper trance; come out, gently . . .

and give yourself that sense
of knowing *both sides now.*

| | |
|---|---|
| and did not remember what you didn't remember. And appreciate your ability to begin to develop the feelings and sensations in a trance state and to let them go again also. | That's it! |
| And then, when you are ready let yourself awaken. | |
| | Reorient back to the community of big people in your own rate and pace! |
| And you don't need to come all the way out of the trance, when you reorient back to the room. I remember, when Erickson regressed with me, took me on a trip in the Grand Canyon back, ate breakfast with me went to the swimming pool and then asked me to come all the way back to 1978, 77 or whenever it was, come all the way back | |
| | at a very very gradual grade |
| I opened my eyes and smiled at him | |
| | and very very gently |
| and he said: You haven't come all the way back, have you? | |
| | Let that breath |
| I said: no | |
| | be able to shift! |
| and he said: You really don't need to, do you? Because you really can learn | |
| | time to come out. |
| and better in a trance. | |
| I was there to learn. | And need go back here. Come out very very gradually at time feeling your hands feeling you hear now as you are here now! |
| Now for the completion of a trance it's often-times useful to take as much time as you need. *Hello!* | *Hello!* |

## COMMENTS
*by Hildegard Klippstein*

This Dual Induction by Paul Carter and Stephen Gilligan gives a theoretical and practical course on how to do a group induction at the beginning, especially focusing on the aspect of getting a response from the group, "utilizing" what is in the situation. Meanwhile, when the official group induction begins, the group has already oriented to trance and a task can be given. This writing task is especially good for eliciting regression.

When the authors find their particular rhythm, I always think of their way of doing a double induction as creating spoken songs. Here they play together like children, their voices first alternating, then slowly tuning in together in harmony. As with all of these powerful confusion techniques, they create a frame for letting go, because we cannot follow consciously any longer. Paul Carter and Stephen Gilligan have found a perfect balance with each other, and although it has a somewhat shocking aspect with both voices speaking at the same time, this induction allows extreme relaxation and regression, once we let go. After letting us regress before school, Paul Carter sings us songs in German, language "little children like," while Stephen Gilligan utilizes the time to give us subtly imperceptible therapeutic suggestions. What a wonderful form of therapy, caring for us competently like parents with touching songs, constructive words, and full awareness of our process of growing and developing! Notice how they create a balance, for example, when Stephen Gilligan talks about a loss, Paul Carter juxtaposes humor and spreads the idea of how a little baby wants to put its father's shoe into its mouth.

There is the simple idea of returning in time to the state of a baby and letting us grow and gain more, again, letting us develop a picture of the young self and meet it for integration with the present self. It is really a touching atmosphere where this giving hands can happen and new self-appreciation can grow. Notice also the gentle way they lead us back to our grown-up state and the present. Connecting us with our resources can be done in a loving, respectful way.

# Chapter 10

# THERAPEUTIC RITUALS: PASSAGES INTO NEW IDENTITIES[1]

Not too long ago, my father died. Resting and reading in the afternoon, he was felled by a massive heart attack. Upon hearing the news several hours later, I burst into a torrent of tears followed by wave after wave of overwhelming emotions and images. Emotional riptides carried me over great distances, bringing to the surface a multitude of feelings, images, memories, and conversations.

Luckily, this journey was navigated with a special context. For three days, family and friends gathered for the ritual process of honoring my dad and saying goodbye to him. With his body as a focal point, ceremonies were performed, a large wake where people gave moving testimonies, a funeral mass, a party and the burial.

In retrospect, this process was a conversation of the deepest sort, a conversation that midwifed within me (and presumably others) a significant new self-identity. Immersed in the multi-level, multi-participant, multi-modality conversation, yet buoyed by the support of friends and the ritual structures, I found myself saying good-bye to an old self-identity and allowing a new one to be born.

---

[1] This chapter is dedicated to the memory of my father, John Gilligan, Jr. I am proud to be his son.

This essay appeared previously in S. Gilligan and R. Price (Eds.). 1993. *Therapeutic conversations*. New York: W. W. Norton.

Such crises are inescapable in each of our lives, cutting to the core of our basic identities and demanding the creation of new ones. These crises may be planned or expected — as in a birth or a marriage, a retirement or a diploma — or they may be quite sudden and shocking — as in a rape, the loss of a child, a brutal assault or a major illness. Regardless, they all provoke a challenge to redefine one's world in significant ways.

When these challenges are successfully navigated, people grow stronger, more confident and perhaps a bit wiser. Unsuccessful attempts may leave one stranded on an isolated island of despair, subsiding on the bitter shadow fruit of depression, guilt, fear, and shame. Such a diet gives rise to strange and undesirable behaviors, from self-abuse via food, drugs or sex to self-focus on weaknesses, failures, and doubts. A life of quiet or not so quiet desperation develops, with the greatest passion devoted to self-devaluing acts.

When individuals become mired in these struggles, they sometimes see a therapist in hopes of changing things. Our challenge, of course, is to help them. Our cultural histories are rich with traditions for doing this, for such problems existed (and were solved) long before the advent of modern psychotherapy.

This chapter explores how one such tradition, that of healing rituals, may be used in psychotherapy. Some basic distinctions regarding rituals are first outlined. A four-step model for using rituals is then developed. These four steps include: (1) suggesting a ritual as a possible solution, (2) planning the ritual, (3) enacting the ritual, and (4) post-ritual activities. A case history illustrates each step.

## WHAT ARE RITUALS?

Rituals are perhaps the oldest form of therapy.[2] Virtually every culture has developed rituals for major social-psychological functions. Transitional rituals such as baptisms or brisses, weddings and funerals have been used as bridges from one stage of life into another — at birth, graduations, promotions, rites

---

[2] My understanding of rituals has been helped by many authors, especially van der Hart (1983) and Turner (1977). Others include Campbell (1984), Haley (1984), Imber-Black, Roberts, and Whiting (1989), Madanes (1990), and Palazzoli, Boscolo, Cecchin, and Prata (1978). My biggest influence, however, is Milton Erickson (1980 a, b, c, d) and his contributions to working with "the unconscious" with an awareness of social context.

of passage into adulthood, marriages, retirements, deaths and so on. Continuity rituals such as anniversaries and holidays affirm and regenerate the values and identity of a system. Healing rituals provide recovery from trauma and reincorporation of the dissociated person into the social-psychological community. And atonement rituals provide vehicles for apology and redress of damages done.

In the present view, a ritual may be regarded as an intense, experiential-symbolic structure that recreates or transforms identity. It is intense in that participants develop heightened absorption that excludes all other frames of reference. It is experiential in that analytical and other "one-step removed" processes are depotentiated, leaving participants deeply immersed in primary processes such as bodily feelings, inner imagery and automatic (spontaneous) process. It is symbolic in that the thoughts, feelings, and behaviors stand for other meanings. (For example, the flag placed on the funeral coffin stands for the deceased's contribution to his or her country; the marriage ring stands for a sacred union.) And lastly, rituals perform meaning at the meta level of identity; they affirm or transform in a deep cultural language a person's place in a community. In other words, they constitute a meta conversation between individual(s) and community.

Rituals are more than ceremonies and distinct from behavioral tasks. A ceremony becomes a ritual only when participants become fully immersed in nonrational, archaic language; until then, it is merely a traditional behavior sequence having little therapeutic value. (For example, as a child growing up in an Irish Catholic family, I most definitely did not enter ritual space during the nightly ceremony in which the entire family knelt down through five decades of the rosary!)

Similar characteristics separate rituals from behavioral tasks. Rituals involve a pre-determined behavioral sequence, such that little cognitive decision making is needed during its enactment. No *meta commentary* (such as self-talk or evaluations) is permitted, such that no part of the system is split off in an "outside observer" role, thus allowing holistic properties of the system to be expressed (see Bateson and Bateson, 1987). *Special symbols* mark ritual space: The place where it occurs, the clothes worn, the words expressed, the behaviors enacted, and the artifact used all indicate a special, unique situation. Pre- and post- phases are used as inductions into, and exits out of, ritual space. Binding commitments are secured to promote commitment and heighten the drama and significance of the event.

Rituals occur simultaneously and equally in private and public realities.

The inner world is amplified and reorganized, as in a hypnotherapeutic trance (Gilligan, 1987). At the same time, outer behaviors signifying crucial relationship changes are performed and witnessed by significant others in the social community. This co-occurrence of inner and outer changes makes rituals especially powerful and relevant to psychotherapy.

In fact, this feature of rituals is what led me to become interested in them. I had been working a great deal with clients recovering from sexual abuse. The hypnotic tradition (with its orientation to "going inside," relaxing and "just letting things happen," and "going deeper") proved markedly unsettling to a number of these individuals in many cases, especially in its parallels to the traumatic event(s). Cognitive talk also seemed inappropriate, especially in its inability to handle the emotional intensity and dissociational nature of many of the processes. The question thus arose as to what method might make room for what clients were bringing into the conversation while supporting them in reclaiming their connections to themselves and to the rest of the community. Rituals was one of the emerging answers.

Of course, not all rituals are therapeutic. In fact, many symptoms presented by therapy clients may be expressions of dysfunctional rituals in which individuals recreate a negative self-identity characterized by self-abuse and helplessness. For example, sexual abuse may be viewed as a traumatic ritual in which a person's biological and psychological boundaries are invaded and desolated. This triggers an automatic and immediate "break in belonging" with the rest of the world, engendering a sort of negative trance characterized by hypnotic phenomena such as time distortion, body dissociation, regression, amnesia, and so forth (Gilligan, 1988). This dissociated state can last indefinitely (years and even generations), leading to a disidentification with the rest of the world and a misidentification of the self as "being" the traumatic event. This misidentification includes a constellation of distinctions — e.g., "my body is to be abused," "I have no boundaries," "My own needs are non-existent" — that when operating elicit further self-abusive behaviors (involving food, drugs, relationships, etc.).

Viewing such traumatic processes in ritual terms suggests possible therapeutic interventions. Following Erickson's (1980a, 1980d) principle of utilization, the problematic pattern may be used as the solution pattern. That is, if a person's complaint may be framed in terms of a recurrent ritual, then another ritual may be used as a solution. The remainder of the chapter describes how this might be done in a 4-step method.

The method usually takes four to six weeks, and can be done with individuals, couples, families, or groups. It assumes that certain long-standing, somatically-based complaints may be advantageously described as symptoms of a negative self-identity generated from invasive traumatic experiences. It works to experientially activate and externalize the verbal, visual, and kinesthetic symbols of such "identity events" so that a person may perform a ritual act of casting away the "old identity," and taking on a new one.

The model further assumes that conversations involving "identity shifts" cannot occur within normal analytical processes, since such processes generally function to conserve one's existing frame of reference. Thus, the therapist uses hypnotic or similar processes to develop a conversation that utilizes a more experiential-symbolic emotional language. (This use of a different, more archaic language can be found in many traditional rituals, such as religious ceremonies.) The use of hypnosis occurs within the tradition pioneered by Milton Erickson, featuring a cooperative relationship organized around client values, styles and resources (see Gilligan, 1987).

## STEP 1: FRAME SYMPTOM IN RITUAL TERMS

Table 10.1 lists the components of the first step. The therapist first elicits a description of the symptom the client wishes to change. This description should include both a specific behavioral sequence and any inner experiences occurring during the sequence. For example, Joseph was a 32-year-old computer scientist who sought relief from "an uncontrollable facial grimace" that occurred especially in the presence of his superiors at work. In a typical instance, Joseph would go to present his research at an in-house meeting and find himself tremendously anxious and self-conscious as his face contracted into frightened grimaces when he began his presentation. This usually severely compromised his presentation to the point where his projects were not being supported and his job advancement retarded. Joseph further reported that he usually sank into the gloom of depression each time the pattern occurred, and added that depression was experienced by many people in his family.

Joseph was the second of three boys in his family. He described his father as a "brilliant inventor" who was "extremely brutal" with his sons. Joseph emphasized that he had little contact at present with his family (they lived 3,000 miles away) and that he wished to move on with his life without them. He specifically requested hypnosis for symptom relief of his facial grimaces.

1. Identify repetitive symptom, chronic-body symptoms, low cognitive insight, non-rational expression.
2. If needed, use hypnotic methods (ideomotor questions, art work, trance work) to identify emotional trauma or developmental challenge underlying symptom.
3. Frame symptom positively as incomplete attempt at developmental change or healing process.
4. Elicit full experiential cooperation and motivation to perform ritual.

Table 10.1.
Suggesting a ritual as a possible solution.

The complaint of facial grimaces had several characteristics suggestive of a ritual intervention. Specifically, it was (a) long-standing, (b) somatically focused, and (c) non-rational and non-cognitively based. In the domain of hypnosis, which is an intimate cousin to rituals, these are characteristics of trance phenomena. In other words, such symptoms may be viewed as the spontaneous occurrence of a "negative trance," a sort of ritual enactment of some traumatic experience. Of course, not all such symptoms are best resolved via rituals. Many can be handled by more simple and less time-consuming procedures. (In fact, I usually try such procedures before considering rituals.) To determine the appropriateness of a ritual, a next step is to explore whether the symptom is strongly connected to some emotional trauma or developmental challenge. With Joseph, I initially took his complaint at face value — that is, as simply an undesired behavioral expression that might be modified via some straightforward hypnotic processes. I therefore guided Joseph into a hypnotic trance with a general hypnotic induction centered around suggestions of relaxation and ideomotor finger signaling (Gilligan, 1987). Joseph initially seemed to develop a comfortable trance state, but then suddenly the unexpected occurred. Joseph rapidly dissociated into what appeared a terribly unpleasant state: His body and breathing froze and his face blanched and grimaced. Completely unresponsive to my requests for a verbal report, he seemed to be tailspinning into some otherworldly nightmare. Further suggestions to reorient were also unsuccessful, so I tried to simply join him in his state, saying with soft intensity something like the following:

> Joseph, I don't know where you are. Joseph, I don't know why you had to go there. But I do know that you are also *here* with me. I do know that you can *hear me* and *listen* to me. Joseph, I don't know how far away you had to go. I don't know if you need to go even further away in order to comfortably listen to me. But I do know you *can hear me* and respond to me in ways that are appropriate and helpful for you.

Using this sort of talk I was able to develop a link with Joseph. Over the next 10 minutes, I extended this connection to include holding his hand and developing finger signals to communicate with his unconscious mind.

Gradually he reoriented, but upon opening his eyes he froze again in wide-eyed terror, apparently "seeing" someone or something in front of him. I asked if it was his father he saw and his head nodded. Taking hold of his hand and encouraging him to breathe, I gently coached him to expand his attentional field to include me on his right side and to hallucinate a friend on his left side. Gathering strength from these additional relationships, he shouted at his "father" to "get the hell away." The terrifying image receded and Joseph collapsed in a paroxysm of tears. To reorient him, I walked him around my office for awhile. When we sat back down I sought to ease the seriousness by asking him in a soft humorous tone what he thought of his "standard hypnotic experience." We chuckled a bit, then rode the release to a serious but more relaxed connection. I suggested that perhaps his unconscious mind had decided it was time to say goodbye to some relationship and that this might be the meaning of his recurrent symptom. He was curious about this hypothesis, so we used ideomotor finger signals to ask his unconscious mind: (a) whether his symptom of facial grimaces was connected to experiences with his father; (b) whether the preceding hypnotic dissociation was connected to some past emotional event with his father; and (c) whether it was time to say goodbye to that abusive relationship.

His "yes" finger signaled to each of these questions, as it did to the inquiry of whether a specific memory had been accessed. It turned out that the remembered event occurred when Joseph was six years old. He had received a toy train on Christmas morning and later that day was playing with it and his brother in the basement. Joseph somehow broke the train and its tiny ball bearings scattered across the basement floor. His brother ran and reported the incident to his father, who came roaring down stairs to unleash a brutal physical assault on Joseph. The boy spent the rest of the day in the basement trying to pick up every last ball bearing while his father periodically returned to beat him again.

This event became the symbolic representation of the "old self" under the influence of his abusive father. (In rituals, like in hypnosis and any form of artistic expression, it is very important to deal with concrete symbols — i.e., specific stories rather than general identities. This event is not seen as the original or singular "cause" of present experience, but rather as a representation of a relationship around which one's identity is organized. Working with more general descriptions such as "wounded child" or "low self-esteem" does not seem to provide the requisite experiential ground needed for a ritual act to work.)

Joseph was extremely impressed at the responses generated by his unconscious. He voiced an interest in doing something to change his relationship to the memory, and inquired about how this might be done. I introduced the possibility of performing a ritual, suggesting that sometimes terribly invasive experiences led people to self-identify with voices, images, and behaviors that really belonged to someone else. It was further noted how such a self-misidentification could give rise to various uncontrollable expressions such as Joseph's grimacing and depression. Healing rituals were described as processes wherein one first externalized (through letters, paintings, and other experiential processes) these voices, images, and body feelings, then planned and enacted a ritual to once and for all say goodbye to the external influences and hello to one's own voice, images, and feelings. A few simple examples were offered to emphasize how rituals were co-created by therapist and client, with the therapist providing expertise on structures and the client generating the specific materials, making the decisions and enacting the ritual. It was also noted that individuals really needed to sense that the time was right to do the ritual, for it required their full commitment and participation. To stress this point, Joseph was asked to take the next week to decide whether to commit to such a process. He returned the following week and said he was definitely interested in doing the ritual. (If a full commitment is not possible, the therapist should abandon the possibility of a ritual and explore other interventions.)

The above description indicates the importance of connecting the complaint to an emotional trauma or developmental challenge, framing the symptom as an incomplete or unsuccessful attempt to change one's identity in relation to the event or challenge, and then suggesting therapeutic rituals as an effective means for transforming one's identity and dissolving the symptom. The success of the ritual requires the client's full motivation and participation.

The case also illustrates how the connection of the symptom with a trauma must occur experientially. An intellectual hypothesis that symptom X is connected to event Y is wholly inadequate, for it leaves the therapeutic conversation at a cognitive level. (To reiterate, it is precisely those cases where cognitive understanding is of little or no value that rituals may be indicated.) The language of ritual operates at a more primary, experiential level, in much the same way as symptoms and hypnotic phenomena (Gilligan, 1988). Thus, the therapist should make use of such language to lead into the possibility of a ritual.

There are, of course, other methods for conducting this experiential inquiry. With some clients I suggest that they develop a light "centering" trance, contemplate the question, "What is this (symptomatic) experience connected to?" and then use crayons or paints on art paper to let their "unconscious mind" express a response. This can be done in the office with me or at home during the week. In the latter case, therapists should ensure clients have adequate resources for example, the presence of a friend or a physical symbol (see Dolan, 1991) — to stay centered if the process recalls difficult material.

Another possibility is to use other hypnotic explorations — for example, general "searches" for relevant material (Gilligan, 1987; Lankton and Lankton, 1983), or ideomotor questions. Whatever the method used, the therapist seeks to frame a chronic symptom over which the client feels no control as an "identity event" that may be transformed via ritual.

## STEP 2: PLANNING THE RITUAL

This second step typically takes 3–6 weeks. As Table 10.2 indicates, it involves generating and externalizing the experiential symbols of both the old and new selves and then evolving a ritual which allows the transition from the former to the latter. Time and care is taken to ensure that this process is generated, guided, and ratified each step of the way by the client's inner self ("the unconscious") rather than their normal, intellectual process.

The first two parts of the planning are usually done concurrently. First, the verbal conversations that the person has internalized are experientially activated and externalized in physical form. This is often done via letter writing. In the case of Joseph, I suggested (and he ratified via finger signals) that he take 40

1. Have client select/generate/elaborate physical symbols of old self-identity (letters, photographs, art work, artifacts, jewelry, etc.)
2. Have client select/generate/elaborate physical symbols of new identity (same as above, but perhaps including living symbol such as plant or pet).
3. Identify basic ritual act (burning, burying, declarations, etc.)
4. Plan actual ritual (where, with whom, when, what specifications).
5. Have client emotionally/spiritually prepare (prayer, meditation, diary writing, etc.) for ritual.

Table 10.2.
Planning the ritual.

minutes each day to write two letters. Following the more structured approaches inherent in ritual, we decided upon a specific time of day (8 p.m.) and place (his study) to write these letters. After a brief centering process, he would spend 20 minutes writing a first letter to someone involved in the "old self" event of the broken train. On different nights, this person was (six-year-old) Joseph, his brother, his father, and his mother. The letter was to describe what happened, how he felt then, how the event had influenced his subsequent self image, and what he wanted to do about it now. The second letter (also 20 minutes) was to his "future self" and specified the life he was interested in living and differences in his behavior. (Sometimes in this letter a person finds it more helpful to write as their future self back to their present self or to a childhood, younger self.)

Before this task is carried out, hypnotic questioning is used to ensure that it is appropriate and that sufficient resources are available. Often, some modifications are needed — e.g., a person or other resource may need to be present with the client while letter writing (Dolan, 1991). Hypnotic questioning is also used in the next session to determine whether any more letters need to be written. The therapist might read the letters to ensure the client is centered and connected to the process. (For example, I discontinued the ritual process with a client who wrote letters to his younger self in a nasty, caustic manner, sensing that it was premature to develop a healing ritual.) Each of these ongoing "checks" indicate how the ritual planning is shaped and modified by an ongoing collaborative process between therapist and client(s).

The next externalization process involves images. As in the letter writing, it is suggested that the client take 40 minutes daily (over a week or so) to paint, draw (with color), collage, or otherwise visually display first the "old self" event and then some version of the "new self." Clients concerned about any lack of artistic talent ("I can't draw") are encouraged to just let happen whatever happens, from actual depictions to just intense colors. They are encouraged to let these expressions come from their own inner selves while focusing on the questions, "What did the traumatic event look or feel like?" (for the first drawing) and "What will things look or feel like after the symptom (or problem) is resolved?" Again, the therapist takes steps to check (a) that the process is appropriate; (b) that sufficient processes are available; (c) that the person is emotionally connected and centered in the process; and (d) whether any further work needs to be done after the person returns in the next session with the externalized images.

The client is then asked to take the following week selecting physical symbols of the new and old selves. Self-hypnosis, meditation, and open curiosity might be used in this regard. The person need not cognitively understand or explain why they selected a symbol. Examples of "old self" symbols include the baby clothes knitted by a woman who had lost her baby daughter; the photograph another woman found of the uncle who sexually molested her; and the toy train (resembling the old train) that Joseph bought. Examples of the "new self" symbols include Japanese bonsai trees purchased by the woman grieving her daughter; African shields and spears chosen by the sexually abused woman; and a ring by Joseph. Again, the therapist works to ensure that each of these selections are appropriate and complete.

The client has now concretized, physicalized, and externalized symbols of the old and new self. The next step is to select the basic ritual acts for saying goodbye to the old self and welcoming the new self. The therapist might outline "menu selections" — e.g., burning or burying — and then support clients (e.g., via hypnotic process) in making their own choice. Hypnosis helped Joseph to generate the ritual acts of (a) dumping ball bearings of a toy train over actual train tracks and then (b) crossing the tracks to "the other side" to declare his new self. These choices were ratified by his ideomotor finger signals.

The next session involves planning the details of where, when, how, and with whom the ritual will occur. Each should be considered carefully, and all discussions should be ratified in some significant way by the person. With Joseph, the plan was to go to the train tracks a mile or so from my office. He would bring the train along with the letters and drawings. The "saying goodbye" part of the ritual would involve reading aloud the "old self" letters and showing the pictures before dumping the toy train's ball bearings over the train tracks as a way of declaring his letting go of these symbols. He would then cross the tracks and do several ceremonial declarations of the new self.

The issue of who else to include is especially important since, to reiterate, a ritual takes place at the intersection between two worlds: the public and private, or the inner and outer. Persons performing a ritual act are not only reorganizing their inner world, they are also declaring to others a new social self. Witnesses not only observe a person's declarations, they participate in and validate the creation of a new social and psychological identity. This extraordinary complementarity is a major reason for the effectiveness of healing rituals.

With Joseph, this issue proved to be painful. After much deliberation he decided that he didn't feel sufficiently close to anyone to invite them to participate. (Developing friendships and community became a major focus of his post-ritual activities.) He asked me to participate, and I reiterated that I would, though primarily in the role of the "ritual specialist" guiding the process and providing minimal coaching if needed. He also accepted my suggestion to consider communicating the effects of the ritual to family members (all of whom lived 3,000 miles away).

As a last preparation step, the client is asked to take the week before the ritual to orient inwardly and emotionally prepare for the event. Depending on a person's practices and values, this might include solitary walks, diary writing, self-hypnosis or meditation, light fasting, prayer, etc. This is a crucial step in most traditional rituals (as well as other important performances), since it shifts attention away from normal "business as usual" process toward a more dramatically heightened inner focus.

## STEP 3: ENACTING THE RITUAL

As Table 10.3 illustrates, the performance of the ritual has three parts: The pre-ritual induction that develops the liminal consciousness of ritual space (Turner, 1969); the ritual itself; and the post-ritual process that incorporates a person back into the normal social space. The pre-ritual induction is similar to

1. Pre-ritual induction.
2. The ritual itself.
3. Post-ritual processes: celebration, vacation, outing, etc.

Table 10.3.
Enact the ritual.

a hypnotic induction, involving the use of attentional narrowing, repetition and rhythm, and symbolic activities that shift the person into a heightened state of experiential-symbolic consciousness (Gilligan, 1987). This may involve convocational speeches, chants, prayers, inward meditations, ceremonial acts, etc. The induced mood is generally serious and intense, with a sense that something very important is about to happen.

In the case of Joseph, he arrived at my office on the appointed day, bringing with him his ritual symbols (the letters, drawings, train, etc.). In a soft and focused conversation we reviewed all that had happened over the past month and he reaffirmed his commitment to performing the ritual. We drove in separate cars to the ritual site (the railroad crossroads), got out, and marked out the ritual space with rocks and sticks. Joseph faced the tracks, laid out the ritual symbols of the old self, oriented inwardly for several minutes, then turned to me and indicated his readiness.

When I nodded solemnly for him to "go for it," he again closed his eyes to deepen his involvement. When he opened them several minutes later, he appeared intensely focused and in an emotionally heightened, altered state of consciousness. Fighting back tears, he visualized all around him the members of his family. His strong, vulnerable voice cracked with emotion as he greeted each person and declared his purpose in summoning them to the event. He picked up the "old self" letters and read them one by one, declaring after each that he was finished with those words and then proceeded to tear up the letter. His emotions appeared ready to overwhelm him periodically but each time he paused to compose and center himself before continuing. (Some clients may benefit from some gentle support and encouragement during such times.)

He next displayed each "old self" drawing, describing what had happened, how he felt then, how his identity had been influenced, and how he was ready now to let go of this self-image. He would then rip up the images and place the torn tatters into a box (that was later burned). A variety of emotions — grief, anger, sadness — surged through him during this process.

The final "goodbye" process involved the toy train. He had removed its bottom to expose the ball bearings, which were now held in place by a single piece of tape. As he focused his attention on the train in his hand, he lapsed into convulsive sobs. After a minute or so, I moved in, whispered for him to breathe and allow the feelings to just "move through," and gently encouraged him to continue. This helped him to center and refocus his attention on the ritual task. Looking at this imagined family, he declared that the time had come for him to move on. He recounted the "train incident" in slow, emotional measures, then announced that he was ready to reclaim that event for his own development. In ceremonial declaration he held the toy train over the train tracks, removed the tape, and let the ball bearings pour out all over the tracks. (I had not appreciated until then how small these ball bearings were, or how many of them there were.) Many emotions were also released, but Joseph seemed to grow in strength and stature as they did. Finally he turned to me and said he was ready to "move on."

With Joseph in the lead, we walked over the crossroads. He then performed the "new self" ritual by reading the letters written to his future self, showing the drawings, and ceremoniously donning the ring he had selected to symbolize his new commitment. This part of the ritual seemed much easier for him, as if he was guided by some newfound strength and spirit.

One final piece of the ritual remained. Joseph had decided during self-hypnotic explorations several weeks earlier to send the toy train back East to his brother (who had "turned him in"), along with a letter. In this poignant letter, Joseph mentioned the horrible childhoods they had shared together, and how it made apparently both of them depressed and unhappy during their adult lives. (His brother struggled under the clinical diagnosis of depression.) Joseph expressed his commitment to free himself from such unhappiness, and then recounted the train incident from childhood. He described the ritual process in which he had been immersed over the previous six weeks, and noted that during his self-explorations he had developed the strong sense that he should send the train to his brother after the ritual, for Joseph was finished with it. He confessed that he was not entirely sure why this was important or what his brother should do with it (he suggested donating it to charity), but felt strongly that he was finished with it and that it should be given to his brother. (At several points during the weeks of ritual preparation, Joseph confirmed to me through ideomotor signaling that this was indeed a proper course of action.) He concluded the letter by stating that he loved his brother deeply, and he wanted their relationship to deepen and grow stronger. Joseph placed this letter along with the train in a package he had addressed to his brother. We drove in our respective cars to the post office, and he went in and mailed it. Upon returning he reported that during the ritual an incredible weight that "had been there for so long I was no longer aware it was there" had lifted and dissolved. He looked and sounded remarkably calm, centered, and confident. I complimented him on the incredible courage and commitment he had shown during the ritual (and throughout the entire preparation process) and told him he had done a great job.

He had arranged (at my suggestion) to take the rest of the day off, so I encouraged him to go home to relax and savor his achievements. I also suggested that he use letter writing anytime over the next couple of weeks that he felt any "old voices" revisiting him, since it was a good way to externalize and let go of occasional residual processes that were "looking to leave and go back to where they belong." (Many clients find this process very helpful.) I also reminded him he could review any of the "new self" letters, images, or symbols that he was taking home with him, especially anytime he needed to recenter himself. (Most clients leave behind — indeed, burn, bury, or otherwise trash — the "old self" symbols and find a special place at home for the "new self" symbols.)

### STEP 4: REINCORPORATING INTO COMMUNITY

Planning and performing a therapeutic ritual is an especially intense process. Participants withdraw from everyday life — emotionally, psychologically and behaviorally — for a prolonged time and become deeply immersed in alternate, inner realities. It is therefore crucial that the person be reincorporated back into the social community following a ritual. Any further "inner work" explorations are generally curtailed and attention oriented to practical challenges and responsibilities such as friends, jobs, families, social skills, etc. Therapy ends after another session or two, unless short-term concrete goals are negotiated. Rituals generally work as an "all or none" phenomenon with transformation occurring during the ritual act itself. Thus, additional "inner" work on the issue is often counter-productive.

When Joseph returned the following week, he looked great. He said that after the ritual he celebrated by going shopping for a new wardrobe. He felt

1. Give structure for expressing remnants of old identity (letters, physical activities, simple exercises).
2. Develop structures for expressing new identity (social activities, new symbol, imaginal guides, new clothes/artifacts, new relationship with unconscious, etc.).

Table 10.4.
Reincorporating self into community.

alive and "open," and proudly reported making a presentation at work without any grimaces. (He reported feeling very aware of the new ring on his finger during the presentation.) He felt confident about continuing these new behaviors, and we mutually agreed after a little further talk that the therapeutic goals had been achieved and that therefore we could stop meeting.

About a year later, Joseph called me on the phone. He reported a continuing absence of facial grimaces, and requested some hypnosis to help him in his new hobby of kick-boxing. We spent several sessions on this project, during which time he reported having a great time at his job.

## DISCUSSION

The case of Joseph illustrates how rituals may be powerful mediums for therapeutic change. They allow the transformation of identity and the dissolution of undesired symptoms. Rituals are decidedly nonrational events in which individuals tap into deep inner resources and engage in profound experiential-symbolic conversations. Most important, they empower individuals to externalize self-negating images, voices, and behaviors and rediscover and claim their own voices, visions, and bodies.

While the case example involved an individual, rituals may also be used with couples, families, and groups. They may be helpful with many different types of complaints. I have used rituals with individuals, couples, or families dealing with sexual abuse (e.g., incest or rape), and also with groups of incest survivors. Divorce ceremonies (with one or both people) including friends and family can be helpful. Purification and atonement rituals may work in cases of infidelity. Rituals marking deaths (including abortions) have been profoundly moving. Other rituals may be co-created for rites of passage, eating disorders, substance abuse, and leaving abusive communities (e.g. cults, ritual abuse).

In each of these cases, the therapist respects and empowers the inner uniqueness and intelligence of clients so that the actual symbols and acts of the ritual emanate from them, not from the therapist. The therapist acts as a "ritual specialist" who provides possible structures, supports clients in staying in relationship with their primary processes and witnesses and occasionally guides the process. When clients and therapists are both fully participating and contributing, each in their own way, the ritual can indeed be a therapeutic event.

# Part III:

# Moving Beyond Erickson

Chapter 11

# Living in a Post-Ericksonian World[1]

The deep parts of my life pour onward,
as if the river shores were opening out.
It seems that things are more like me now,
that I can see farther into paintings.
I feel closer to what language can't reach.
— Rainer Maria Rilke, "Moving Forward"

It was twenty years ago today
Sgt. Pepper taught the band to play.
— John Lennon and Paul McCartney

Before his death, Rabbi Zusya said, "In the coming world, they will not ask me: 'Why were you not more like Moses?" They will ask me, 'Why were you not more like Zusya?' "
— Martin Buber, *Tales of the Hasidim*

For many years I tried to be more like Milton Erickson. This paper is about the more difficult challenge of trying to be more like Stephen Gilligan. It is based on 22 years of teaching, practicing, and writing about hypnotic psycho-

[1] This chapter originally appeared in W. J. Matthews & J. Edgette (Eds.). 1997. *Current thinking and research in brief therapy: Solutions, strategies, and narratives, Volume I.* New York: Brunner/Mazel.

therapy. It indicates how my path has diverged from Ericksonian thinking. I hope it encourages others on their own paths.

The thing that was really astonishing about Erickson was his willingness to be himself, to accept his "deviancies" from the norm, as I like to say. This courage translated directly, I believe, into compassion and acceptance of others. To follow a similar path is remarkably challenging. But this is what we stand for as therapists.

In describing where this post-Ericksonian path has led me, I'll start by honoring a few core ideas from Erickson's legacy that still light my way. I'll then raise questions about how these ideas are put into practice. The main intent is to stimulate thinking, rather than arguing about truth.

## THE HEART OF ERICKSON'S LEGACY

Milton Erickson contributed to psychotherapy a handful of radical and enduring ideas. These ideas are deceptively simple, slowly revealing their extraordinary value over years of practice. The first has to do with the uniqueness of each person. In these days of corporate domination of mental health, where diagnostic labels loom larger and therapy freezes into more standardized forms, the idea that each person is unlike anybody else is increasingly disregarded. One-size-fits-all methods proliferate, and an alternative model based on each case being unique is even seen as unethical in some quarters.

But in many ways, problems arise when individuals lose a felt sense of their unique goodness and gifts. To me, Erickson emphasized that the therapist begins by sensing that goodness and those gifts, and that all effective technique arises from that relational connection. We in the Ericksonian community have been surprisingly silent about how to experientially — especially nonverbally — make and sustain this connection. Without specific traditions from which to draw, seeing and sensing the unique consciousness that is each person may exist only as platitude or concept, not practice or experience.

A second extraordinary idea offered by Erickson is that the therapist accepts and utilizes whatever the client presents, no matter how strange, unusual, or aesthetically repugnant it might seem. This includes behaviors, experiences, cognitions, idiosyncrasies, and so forth. Since the potential value of a given aspect of a person's experience is often not immediately clear — indeed, in symptoms it seems to have a distinctly negative value — this simple idea is immensely challenging to consistently translate into practice. It requires that before "doing," the therapist must find a way to "be with" a person's experience. This experiential relationship is, of course, central to the hypnotic relationship, where a person can fully "be with" an experience without a "fight" (domination or control) or "flight" (dissociation, denial) response. Moving beyond the inner world of traditional hypnosis, Erickson applied this principle in a dynamic way to ongoing relationships with patients. He was like an aikido master, blending and harmonizing with whatever was presented, neutralizing the violence and reconciling the conflicts inherent in a symptomatic behavior.

This idea of acceptance and cooperation puts the idea of deliberately trying to change a person in a different light. It means that life is moving through the person, distinct in each moment, and therefore change is already in motion. Rather than imposing something on clients, you sense and blend with their immediate processes. This is an active and dynamic responsiveness, not a passive and purposeless one. It is an art that requires enormous devotion and study. How does the therapist center his or her attention, be attentive yet flexible, expecting nothing but ready for anything, soft yet effective? We need practitioners to talk more about how this might be done.

A third key idea in Erickson's legacy involves therapy as a restoration of balance in a person's life. To me, one of Erickson's great talents was moving effortlessly between the interior worlds of experience and personal meaning and the exterior worlds of behavior and social community. In reading Ernie Rossi (Erickson & Rossi, 1977; 1979; 1981), one sees transcript after transcript in which patients are hypnotized and their inner worlds of experience are activated and transformed. One gets the impression that Erickson's primary interest was to activate inner resources and "spontaneous creativity" in others. But in reading Jay Haley (1967; 1973; 1985a, 1985b, 1985c), more emphasis is placed on how Erickson manipulated patients to behave differently in their outer worlds. Here one gets the impression that Erickson's primary interest was in directing behavioral changes.

Which version of Erickson is the "true" one?[2] The answer seems to be

[2] It should be noted that Haley studied with Erickson in the latter part of the 1950s into the early 1970s, when Erickson's health was much better. Rossi was a student during the 1970s, when age and illness took its increasing toll on Erickson. It may be that Erickson was a different type of therapist during these two eras, contributing to some of the differences in the two authors' versions of Erickson. A counterpoint to this argument, however, can be found in Erickson and Rossi's (1989) publication of the February Man case

both: Erickson went both ways. Sometimes he focused on the outer world, sometimes on the inner, but at all times the importance of both seemed to be held. I believe this skill reflected an enormous appreciation of a principle of balance.[3] This balance might be between doing and not doing, between experience and behavior, between self and other — indeed, virtually any distinction to be made has its important complement. Erickson seemed to operate with what Jung (1916/1917) called the "transcendent function" or what the Eastern traditions call "the way between the opposites", where a course including and often integrating opposite or complementary values is navigated. This might translate into a hypnotic induction where a person is encouraged to both withhold or resist *and* let go and disclose. Or it might translate into a therapy where strategic directives to do something different in the social environment are interlaced with hypnotic trances for self-identity reorganization. Erickson was remarkable in his capacity to know when to use one and how to combine both approaches. None of us, it seems to me, has remotely approached this skill. A deeper understanding of the balance principle might be helpful in this regard.

A fourth idea central to Erickson's legacy is that life is to be experienced and enjoyed. For Erickson, therapy was not primarily about analyzing the past or teaching a new conceptual approach, but about helping people to enjoy the "here and now" of life. There was a preference for curiosity over control, acceptance over rejection, experience over intellectual understanding, and flow over fixity. Erickson was a beautiful example of living life on life's terms, and accepting and working with whatever life has to give.

## DEPARTURES FROM ERICKSONIAN TRADITIONS

Erickson and his students have detailed some of the many ways his simple yet generative ideas can be applied in therapy (Zeig, 1982, 1985a, 1985b, 1994;

---

that occurred in 1945. Here, as in most other cases reported by Rossi, the primary emphasis is on hypnotic work. So while Erickson may have changed some, the differences between Haley and Rossi may reflect more of their own biases. That Erickson's work could support such differences is perhaps the most interesting point.

[3] A good example of this commitment to balance is found in Erickson's dedication to Erickson, Rossi, and Rossi (1977): "Dedicated to an ever progressing understanding of the total functioning of the individual person within the self separately and simultaneously in relation to fellow beings and the total environment."

Zeig & Lankton, 1988). The appreciation of his work has led, inevitably, to some reified version of "Ericksonian psychotherapy" which, just as inevitably, seems more limited and less creative than the original version. Jung used to say, "I'm certainly glad I'm not a Jungian." Erickson would no doubt echo such sentiments, and I hope most of us would ultimately concur.

Letting go of defining one's self as an "Ericksonian" allows new understandings and approaches to emerge. In my own case, this process has raised questions about premises that seem to be implicit in the Ericksonian community. I raise these questions here with the intention of nurturing the "beginner's mind" so crucial to therapists. As in hypnosis, the holding of a question is usually far more important and productive than the seizing upon any specific answer.

**1. What do we call these "other than conscious" presences?**

A cornerstone of the Ericksonian approach is that an intelligence exists within a person that is beyond the normal egoic self. Erickson talked about this in terms of "the unconscious mind," and demonstrated beautiful ways to work with it (Erickson & Rossi, 1981; 1989). In my own explorations, it has become increasingly clear that to singularly refer to this "other than conscious" process as "the unconscious mind" is too limiting and sometimes misleading. The possibility for reification is too great and the connotations of the term are too limited for therapeutic flexibility. Alternative references include "the inner self," one's center, heart, soul, or what Chogyam Trungpa (1988) has called the indestructible "tender soft spot" that each of us is born with.

We use such terms primarily for practical reasons. We approach therapy assuming that a client has become stuck in a narrow understanding of, or limited connection to, their potentialities. Identifying and activating resources is seen as central to helping the client. The idea of the unconscious is used poetically, not literally, to access an intelligence greater than, and different from, what a person is doing. As a poetic term, it invites and evokes a different, hopefully more productive way of being. The term is not used within an intellectual exchange as much as an experiential-symbolic one intended to produce a felt sense of nonintellectual intelligence. In short, a major purpose is to open the language of the heart to complement the dominance of the language of the head.

If we appreciate "the unconscious" as poetic language, then we can become curious about other poetic terms as well. Each will carry different nuances for the client, and each is associated with a different tradition of acting and understanding. From this perspective, a good therapist will be skilled in finding and using those poetic terms that are most helpful in a given situation.

For example, consider the Japanese martial art of aikido. In this situation, one is faced with physical attacks from all directions. The challenge is how to neutralize violence by receiving, harmonizing, and redirecting the attack. Nothing is ever resisted or opposed; all behavior is blended with and utilized. (As I said earlier, Erickson was quite the aikido master.) To perform aikido, one does not talk about going into trance and trusting the unconscious, but instead emphasizes finding one's center. This mind/body center is not an esoteric or theoretical term, it is a felt sense of an intelligence that allows relational creativity and calmness. Without it, one can only "fight" (dominate) or "flee" (submit); with it, the third choice of "flow" is possible (see Leonard, 1991).

Is the notion of a center relevant to therapy? I think so. For example, consider a therapy problem where a person is experiencing anxiety when criticized. Will it be more helpful to appeal to the client's "unconscious" in a trance, or to help the person find his or her center? Each tradition would share an interest in relaxing the grip of muscle-bound, head-oriented, control-based thinking. But they would go about it in different ways. The tradition of talking with the "unconscious" is associated with trance and related behaviors such as eye closure, relaxed muscles, inward orientation, and resource images and stories. The tradition of working with one's center includes learning to "drop" attention below the navel as a primary focus, and then gently "open" attention to a field-based perception without grasping on any fixed points (Palmer, 1994). The therapist being skilled in both traditions will likely be more effective in finding what works best for a given client.

Other terms may also be helpful. For example, the idea of soulfulness may be quite relevant in various performance arts, such as music, poetry, oratory, and therapy. Yeats (in Jeffares, 1974, p. 104) could have been talking about Erickson when he observed:

> An aged man is but a paltry thing
> A tattered coat upon a stick, unless
> Soul clap its hands and sing, and louder sing
> For every tatter in its mortal dress.

If Yeats had used the term "unconscious mind" rather than "soul," the poem would have suffered terribly! The point is that the unconscious mind belongs to a family of poetic terms referring to something quite knowable yet ineffable; other terms might be superior or complementary in various circumstances. My suggestion is that a therapist with a felt sense of the nuances of each of these poetic terms will be more effective than one stuck with a reified understanding of just one of them.

Thinking of this other-than-conscious self simply as "the unconscious mind" may lead us to ignore what Erickson (1980b) referred to as "that vital sense of the beingness of the self (that) is often overlooked" (p. 345). It may suggest a mechanical or impersonal "thing" to be manipulated or programmed, rather than an integral human presence to be felt, honored and cultivated.

Some may say that words like "heart" and "soul" are too vague or too poetic, or that therapy should just deal "scientifically" with the mind or behavior. But of course the notion of the "unconscious mind" is even vaguer, and no loving parent or devoted artist would say that nurturing human life is done singularly via the "unconscious mind." As a human encounter, therapy includes elements of both science and art, but must also go beyond them into the areas of love and psychological struggle. Language here must help the person go beyond language, touching upon the soft, tender spots of being and interbeing. Access to multiple poetic terms can be helpful in this regard. Of course, it also carries the risk of making mush of things, so the therapist must be skillful in activating their felt senses within the client. How to do this is, I believe, one of the great contributions of the Erickson legacy to therapy.

**2. Is intelligence "in" the unconscious?**

Erickson used the metaphor that the unconscious is intelligent. He failed, however, to explain why the patient was doing so poorly before meeting with him. After all, if this intelligence were so magnificent, how did the person end up in such a mess? It seems apparent that the "intelligence of the unconscious," if we might call it that, began to manifest only after Erickson started talking with the person. So we might say that the creative intelligence was in the conversation or relationship between Erickson and the client's "unconscious."

In this regard, we might say that intelligence is a relational or field-based principle. To use Bateson's (1979) metaphor, it is the "pattern that connects," or the willingness to hold different views, descriptions, or truths within a deeper field. This echoes the Buddhist notion of interbeing (see Thich Nhat Hanh, 1975), a non-dualistic view that posits the interconnectedness and inseparability of each aspect of life.

This relational view challenges the traditional Western approach that separates and isolates mental process from their larger contexts, thereby making mind a "thing" inside somebody's head rather than a process within relational space. In the relational view, mind is a sort of Great Internet, a web of patterns that flows through each of us, connecting all of us. It is not inside of us, we are inside of it. Each of us has our own distinct place in the field, an ever-changing ecological niche with unique perspectives and specific knowledges, but the mental circuitry that moves through these vantage points is of a deeper, communal nature. We are individual, but not separate. When a person feels disconnected or separate — whether in inflated (grandiose, power-deluded) or deflated (depressed, frightened) ways — direct experience and creative responsiveness is lost. In the existentialist sense, pathology is precisely the study of loneliness (or the isolation of a process, truth, person, or experience from others). Thus, I believe a central goal of therapy is to reconnect experience and behavior to larger relational fields, rather than trying to fix something inside a person.

**3. Is the therapist really in charge of changing the client?**

This Ericksonian view, especially espoused by Haley (1967, 1973), encourages therapists to be "in control of" the therapy and responsible for its outcomes, and to think in terms of manipulating the client. This view has ultimately been unhelpful to me. It reflects an exclusively hierarchical position that egoic intelligence, particularly that of the therapist, is the only game in town. It encourages therapists to be immersed in the principle of power rather than a principle of cooperation with clients. Therapists are then faced with the problematic belief that they can and should "cure" clients.

These concerns about ideas of control were voiced by Bateson, who sent many students (including me) Erickson's way.[4] He repeatedly warned of what he called the pathological "effects of conscious purpose on adaptation" (Bateson, 1972), emphasizing that the "myth of power" is especially corruptive (Bateson, 1979). His concerns about Erickson's students were expressed in an interview with Brad Keeney (1977):

KEENEY: You're saying that people who go see Erickson come away with a craving for power?

[4] The shortcomings of the ideas of power and control have been addressed by others, including Keeney (1983) and Hoffman (1985).

BATESON: Yes! They all want power.

KEENEY: Is there something about seeing (Erickson) that induces this power hungriness?

BATESON: Well, it's the skill which he has of manipulating the other person which really in the long run does not separate him as an ego dominant to the other person. He works in the weave of the total complex and they come away with a trick which is separate from the total complex, therefore goeth counter to it, and becomes a sort of power. I think it's something like that. [p. 49]

These lucid comments encourage an alternative to the "power principle" that traditionally underlies our thinking (see Woodman, 1993). The power principle emphasizes intellect, unilateral manipulation, control, singular truth, and subjugation of nature. Addiction to this principle reduces relationship to stark contrasts: You either dominate or submit, are right or wrong, win or lose. In this either/or frame, the other-than-conscious self — whether it be "the unconscious" or another person or group — is seen as an "it" that needs to controlled, rather than a "thou" to be accepted and listened to.

A symptom is in part the breakdown of this power principle: It signals that a person can no longer maintain some ideological position, or isolated intellectual control over the "other(s)" and the rest of his or her world. It suggests that a more integrated, less mechanical understanding of self and world be developed. From this perspective, the idea of power — whether it is the client trying to control the problem or the therapist trying to control and change the client — is part of the problem, not the solution.

Our images and understandings of cooperation are often undeveloped and limited, so it is easy to underestimate the value of this principle. We need to be clear that in rejecting the idea of power and the accompanying idea of the therapist being "in control," we are not left simply with the alternative of passive acceptance of the status quo. Gandhi used to say that if the choice was merely between passive submission to injustice or violent resistance, he would choose and encourage violence. But he articulated and walked a third path of nonviolent resistance.

Similarly, if the choice is only between passive acceptance of a person's suffering and deliberate manipulation to change the person, the latter would often be a better choice. But a third path, originated but not completely developed by Erickson, involves actively accepting and cooperating with a person's ongoing process to reconnect with the natural process of change and healing that flows through each living system.[5]

This view is related to the Palo Alto (MRI) group's notion that the attempted solution is often the problem (see Watzlawick, Weakland, & Fisch, 1974). The Milwaukee group, led by Steve de Shazer (1985, 1988), further developed this idea by encouraging attentiveness to already occurring (but non-articulated) differences in the person's world as the basis for therapeutic change. For example, if the client complains of depression, the therapist might focus on exceptions (when the person isn't depressed or feels less depressed) or the "miracle question" (what the person would do differently if, by some miracle, he or she woke up the next morning to discover that the problem had disappeared). The client is then directed to do more of the different-from-symptom behaviors. In this view, the therapist doesn't create change; Life does! It is more a matter of "being with" life, a fresh attentiveness to each moment, that allows new experiences (including desired changes) to emerge.

My approach of self-relations psychotherapy differs from these approaches in its strong emphasis on felt experience as well as behavior (see Gilligan, 1996). I am especially interested in what happens when the social/behavioral mind (the "conscious mind") and the natural/experiential mind ("the unconscious") are seen as different sides of the same coin. (I want to know the name of this coin!) Self-relations suggests that since every moment in life is different, experiencing the "same damn thing over and over" means a person's conscious self is not "in life" at those times; it has dissociated from the experience of the present moment and is trying (with increasingly dismal failure) to control behavior from some satellite orbit. The social mind has split off from the natural world (including the body, its feelings and emotions) and is operating under the delusion that it is separate from it and can and should dominate it. The "out of control" nature of symptoms can thus be seen as an error-correction process that reveals the illusion of power as it attempts to establish a new mind/nature relationship based on cooperation.

---

[5] My personal view is that an admirable struggle existed within Erickson between the power principle, which reigned supreme and unchallenged during Erickson's time, and the cooperation principle, of which Erickson was a major originator. The struggle is similar to that of Morehei Ueshiba, the founder of the martial art of aikido, and also known as the greatest martial artist in Japan's history. Ueshiba, like Erickson, gave birth to a vision of how to non-violently join with an attacker to reconcile violence. Aikido is one of the traditions that has helped me to see symptoms as acts of violence against self and/or others.

Of course, the transition from control over to cooperation with the natural mind requires some workable practices of "controlled surrender" (Leonard, 1991). A first step is to "be with" experience as it is. For example, mental processes can harmonize with and bring attentiveness to natural processes such as ongoing breathing, heartbeat, physical behaviors, etc. This method is similar to the "pacing" techniques of Ericksonian hypnosis (see Gilligan, 1987), but the intent is not so much to manipulate the behavior as to touch it with human awareness. It is like playing with young children, where relatedness and curiosity are crucial to developmental process. The therapist lets go of trying to reframe or change something in favor of properly naming and attentively "being with" what is present in a person's experience.

This is a piece of what the Buddhist mindfulness tradition calls the "skillful means" of love. The idea is that when human consciousness touches an experience or behavior with loving awareness, it is affirmed and grows, to paraphrase Rilke, a little bit more like itself. It is like helping a child learn to recognize, properly name, and respond to different natural states such as hunger, sleep, and emotional needs. If these states are not properly named and attended to, suffering and "acting out" will occur.[6] Similarly, the distressed "acting out" of a symptom suggests a recurring natural state that has no mature human presence to be with it. This natural state might be the need to be seen, to have privacy, the interest in relatedness, fear, and so on. The idea is that these natural states are not complete within themselves: without a mature human presence to "give them space," they will likely be experienced and expressed as negative forms with little redeeming value.

Mindfulness is in part a training of how to listen, "be with," and allow the human nature of each of these states to unfold. It is a skill that offers a third choice of what might be called "human sponsorship" to the existing extremes of (1) repression of or (2) identification with an experience. Sponsorship, distinct from ownership, recognizes the autonomy of the "other" — whether it is a person or an emotional state or a symptomatic behavior — while also realizing the need for guidance, discipline, human social traditions, love, and relatedness. Since the experience or behavior of the other is unique and different in each moment, sponsorship is a considerable skill to practice. It requires the

---

[6] Interestingly, a major tool in 12-step recovery programs is the acronym HALT, standing for Hungry–Angry–Lonely–Tired. The idea is that these states, if active yet unattended to, are triggers to addictive behaviors.

cultivation of listening deeply, opening fully, concentrating, tolerating, being flexible, understanding from the heart, challenging, naming, guiding, and most of all, loving.

We generally accept the need for sponsorship as a given with children: Without a human presence to love, accept and guide them, they will not develop in positive ways. As we mature, we develop the capacity to provide this sort of sponsorship for our own experiences, in addition to the continuing need to experience it from significant others in our community. A repeating negative expression suggests that some natural experience is occurring without human sponsorship; for it to change, it must first be sponsored. The skill of sponsorship is not simply behavioral, as in the Ericksonian concept of matching behavior; nor is it simply empathic, like the Rogerian concept of mirroring. It combines both skills into a third way of artfully "being with" a person. As it develops, change occurs on its own. The therapist then shepherds that change to fruition.

For example, imagine a four-year-old with her parents. Her normally charming self is replaced by a whining, unremitting, and unresponsive crankiness. Everybody in the vicinity feels affected by the kid's mood, and the parents try nicely, then sternly to get the kid to change. These tactics, which usually work, seem to be ineffectual. So the parents finally come around to listening and wondering what's going on with this kid. In this instance, knowing the child's world a bit, the parents realize the child may be sad about her nanny leaving and her best friends next door moving. So the question becomes how to acknowledge that while also not letting the kid act out too much or for too long. Again, a key idea is that the persistent negative behavior suggests a natural state (sadness and fear about people leaving) that has not been properly named and responded to.

Let's now compare this to an adult in a psychotherapy office, whining about childhood experiences or depressed about current relationships. The same feeling pervades the social context, and the same tendency to want to shut the person down prevails. But in the idea of sponsorship, the therapist begins to listen for an underlying natural state that is active but unnamed. This might involve simply listening, or asking questions about present and past social history. The proper naming of the experience is not a scientific classification process, but a touching of an experience with human consciousness. When the naming is accurate, the person will usually soften and become more responsive. The therapist then skillfully stays with the named experience, using language to "bless it" and bring it into the sphere of the person's normal competencies.

**4. Is trance really so common?**

In the Ericksonian community, there is a view that trance is an everyday naturalistic state that is exceedingly common. In the extreme version of this idea, trance is everywhere, all the time. Formal or even informal testing of trance may be seen as irrelevant, and client reports of not feeling trance may be disregarded, as the all-knowing "Ericksonian wizard" somehow knows the person is in a trance. In this view, powerful yet subtle indirect techniques can access a trance of which only the therapist is "consciously" aware.

The more traditional view is that hypnosis is a socially constructed state or relationship resulting from formal hypnotic induction. In this view, trance is not so common. It requires a situation defined as hypnosis and direct suggestions from a hypnotist. Even then, hypnosis "tests" indicate that only a percentage of persons can experience hypnosis.

While there are merits to both views, I would like to suggest a somewhat different approach. In its present form, this view is not so much a scientific "fact" as a clinical suggestion. It sees trance as part of the language of the natural mind, and hypnosis as one of the social rituals for naming, shaping, and giving meaning to its form and expression. This relationship is similar to the idea of sponsorship of other natural experiences: Trance is going to occur, like it or not. Without social traditions (such as hypnosis, art, religion, or ritual) to guide and artfully contain its expression, it will manifest as symptom(s) and be experienced as suffering.

So what kind of natural state is trance? *One that occurs when identity needs to be preserved, transformed, or recreated.* Identity is organic and impermanent, and undergoes major changes at certain times — for example, family events such as births, deaths, marriages, illnesses, job changes, graduations, traumas, divorces, leaving home, and so forth. At such times, the old way of knowing one's self and one's world "dies" and a new identity must be born. This is a second-order, and occasionally a third-order, level of change (see Bateson, 1972). Since the normal conscious processes are designed to maintain the present order — they are conservative in nature — they must be relinquished for a different type of mental process.

Trance is precisely this type of process. In the experience of trance, time is suspended, logic is more flexible, focus is intensified, frames loosen, receptivity is deepened, and primary process is prominent (see Gilligan, 1987, 1988b). This makes control secondary and change of perspective primary.

Thus, when a person or system is undergoing an identity change, trance will tend to spontaneously show up. Trance and trance rituals are present in virtually every culture, especially at transitional points. Symptoms also tend to occur around these transitional points; that is, a person is most likely to develop a symptom following significant life changes (Lazarus, 1965). This suggests that symptoms are spontaneous trances without good social rituals and human presence to sponsor and guide them. Thus, in therapy the point is not so much to introduce trance but to introduce hypnotic forms that allow the trance that is naturally occurring to be socially sanctioned and worked with.

From this perspective, it doesn't make much sense to think of trance merely as behavioral or simply as a social interaction between hypnotist and subject. This is like reducing love to the exchange of words, or the experience of art to the commentary of critics. It makes trance too much about the therapist, and not enough about the client's natural experience of growth and change. A minimal understanding of trance requires an appreciation of the inner and outer worlds, of natural mind and social mind, and especially an appreciation of how the altered states in a person's life are always occurring within a life stream of specific events. By seeing the symptom as a trance indicating an identity shift, hypnosis becomes a social ritual that provides a skillful means for connecting the change process to healing resources.

While this naturalistic view of trance is somewhat different from the artificial or purely social view traditionally held, it is also different from the Ericksonian view that sees trance as exceedingly common.[7] To confuse trance with mental "spacing out" that occurs throughout the day is to miss its deeper clinical significance and potential.

### 5. Is trance always such a good thing?

We in the Ericksonian community have sometimes naively approached hypnosis as the panacea for all that ails you. In its extreme version, the idea is that if we could only go into trance and stay there, happiness would be ours forever. This dangerous and seductive view makes certain things more difficult — like being present as a spouse or parent, or participating as a citizen in the community. Further, it assumes that trance is always a good thing. My personal view is that hypnosis, used wisely and in moderation, can be a wonderful

---

[7] There are of course other views on the nature of hypnosis. Lynn and Rhue (1991) provide an excellent summary of the current controversies. I do believe that the present view stands up well as a clinically helpful way to join and transform the client's suffering.

and helpful experience. But it can be, and sometimes is, used as a narcotic, a drug-like state to numb or turn one away from participation in life.

Trance is especially likely to be used as a dissociative tool among trauma survivors, to protect one's self from further harm (Terr, 1994). But this dissociative skill may continue to be used long after threatening conditions have passed, thereby turning one away from the call to re-enter the life of the community. For example, a person growing up in an alcoholic family may have learned to "trance out" when a parent was abusive or intoxicated, but now automatically uses the same strategies to avoid dealing with the fear of intimacy with a spouse. Then, what had been an ally becomes a hindrance to growth.

The value of trance is in the way it is used. You can be in trance and not "be with" your self or "in" life. Erickson had a wonderful capacity to "sponsor" trance and other psychological states; that is, he really connected the natural experience of trance to the person's well-being and learning. Whereas patients had previously learned to use trance to get away from the world, Erickson joined with where they were to help them use trance to come back into the community. This skill of "being with" a person's ongoing experience — what the Buddhists call "mindfulness" — is simple but elusive. It is far more important than whether a trance is present. In fact, when more attention is spent on mindfulness, I believe trance will be used more effectively in therapy. It will be seen as a natural state that can be misused, and thus something to approach with sensitivity and awareness. Very importantly, it will not be seen as a panacea or a lifestyle, but as a resource available at various points in one's path. In this view, hypnosis is one member of a family of approaches that can promote peace of mind, relieve suffering, expand heartfelt understanding, and allow self-transformation.

### 6. Is indirect communication such a good thing?

A hallmark of the Ericksonian approach is the use of indirect communication, ostensibly to enhance therapeutic responsiveness. To me, this is one of the most misunderstood and potentially harmful aspects of the Erickson legacy. Such misunderstandings arise partly, I believe, from a confusion of signs with symbols. Signs are context-invariant descriptions: that is, they mean roughly the same thing in any situation; while symbols are context-variant: their meaning is contextually constructed (see Pribram, 1971).[8]

---

[8] As Pribram (1971) notes, signs can sometimes be used symbolically and symbols can

Signs and symbols may be seen as two poles on a dialectic. I believe the Ericksonian community is making the same mistake as traditional therapy by biasing too much toward descriptions as context-invariant signals. A problematic behavior is seen more as a sign to be interpreted by the person in power, i.e., the therapist. Thus, the meaning of a headache, a dream, or a marital fight is invariant, and is listed in the code book of the therapist's system. For example, a headache might "signal" sexual repression, which the therapist then takes as the "real" underlying problem to be defeated.

In this view, the therapist's superior training and expertise gives privileged access to the deeper (problematic) meanings of the client's life. The therapist is justified, even ethically obliged, to technically operate on the client with a method — such as an indirect technique — that presumably will causally change the underlying problem. This "benevolent dictator" approach assumes that since the meaning (or "deep structure") of a problem, such as a headache, is context-invariant, the method (e.g., story or indirect technique) used to "treat" the problem is also context-invariant (cf. de Shazer, 1994). This gives rise to popular practitioner "storybooks," similar to the dream interpretation handbooks, where the therapist can look up and discover the proper story to be used to "cure" a given problem.

From a relational point of view, this is the power principle in action. The implicit premises are that (1) the therapist knows things about the client that the client doesn't and shouldn't know (presumably because he or she couldn't handle this self-knowledge); (2) the therapist can and should use this information to deliberately influence the client without her permission or awareness; and (3) this deceptive practice actually works and is helpful to both the client's and therapist's growth.

This is, I believe, a dangerous trend in the way the Ericksonian community has used the ideas and techniques of symbolic emergence of new communication. It gets away from Erickson's cornerstone emphasis on the uniqueness of each person and each situation. Such an emphasis implies that meaning is never fixed: it is different for each person and, to some extent, for each moment. If nothing is fixed, the therapist has no ground to stand on, no code book to consult, no deep structure to discern.

---

be used significantly, but this level of analysis is unnecessary for the purposes of the present discussion.

This other pole on the dialectic suggests that problems, as well as the therapist's theories and responses to them, should be read more like poems than scientific facts or entities. In poetry, as in hypnosis, the goal is to reconnect language to felt experiences or, to quote Rilke, "to feel closer to what language cannot reach." The idea is that descriptions become dysfunctional when they are no longer context-sensitive, that is, no longer connected to the pulsation of the present moment. When disconnected, descriptions function as fundamentalist texts that reject what is for what should be, thereby creating suffering (see Gilligan, 1996).

The repoetization of description is first and foremost a shift not in the content of the text, but in the relationship of the reader to the text. Thus, the magic is not in the story or its cleverly constructed details, but in the re-engagement of consciousness to a story such that new meanings and experiences are unfolding. This is the primary goal in experiential-symbolic communication: not to cleverly deceive but to experientially revive the client's consciousness.

Thus, the client with a headache complaint is seen to be rigidly attached to a frame of reference. The peculiar way that the client is holding on, no doubt in an effort to avoid further suffering, is shutting down the healing principle that permeates the present moment. The therapist is looking to reconnect with that healing principle by joining with the client's process, listening to the "reified poem" of the headache complaint, feeling his or her own poetic responses ("it reminds me of . . ."), and then using therapeutic skills to feed back a related poem (that is, a story, a paradox, an indirect technique).

Such a "poetic" exchange is not an associational free-for-all where anything goes. There is tremendous constraint and discipline involved in any art. In the art of therapy, the therapist is committed to the responses from the client, so considerable concentration is needed to stay engaged with the client at multiple levels. At the same time, the therapist realizes he or she is not "in control" or has some privileged access to deep structures; he is more trusting and curious of how this engaged poetic process can produce new meanings that are more vital and workable for the client.

The important point is that the meaning of the indirect communication is relationally derived. Just as sweetness is not a property of sugar — rather, it is an experience of the relationship between the sugar and the tongue tasting it — the therapeutic meaning derives relationally from the connection between therapist and client. This leads to a more collaborative, indeterminate, curiosity-based understanding of indirect communication.

Thus, I believe the way in which indirect communication has been talked about in the Ericksonian community is misleading and unfortunate. I think it has led therapists to become more absorbed in their clever techniques than in connecting directly with the client. But as the great dancer Isadora Duncan said when asked to explain the meaning of a particular performance, "If I could explain it, I wouldn't have to dance it!" So rather than plotting and planning to deceive clients, therapists should, like devoted artists, join the psychic field that allows the dancers to be danced by the healing principle.

**7. Are failures important to admit?**

One of the compelling aspects of Erickson's legacy is his success stories. As de Shazer (1994) has pointed out, every therapist has a persona, and Erickson (and especially his students) described his therapist persona from the point of view of "Erickson-the-Clever." Like the brilliant Sherlock Holmes, Erickson-the-Clever astounded the reader with a common-sense brilliance and remarkable creativity. Also like Holmes, Erickson seemingly never failed.

While Erickson-the-Clever makes for fascinating reading and inspirational thinking, its value as a teaching style is less clear. Therapists (and clients) must find ways to accept and work with the differences between ideal and actual outcomes, especially failures. Surely Erickson failed many times, but we know little of how he struggled to learn from them.

In my own case, this type of omission has not been helpful to my development. For too long I downplayed my weaknesses and failures, and tried to act ever confident and always in charge. My taboo against failure especially compromised the capacity for disciplined "not-knowing," that essential ingredient of curiosity and creativity.

I have come to believe that therapist failure is essential to therapy success. It is precisely when the client throws the theory back in the therapist's face or resists the therapeutic (or hypnotic) suggestion that therapy actually occurs. At that point the client is discovering his or her own way, realizing it is significantly different from the therapist's understandings. The therapeutic process that begins with the failure of the therapist's way must then be cultivated by following and gently giving human presence and structure to each successive expression of the client's way.

We see this process especially in working with hypnosis and with metaphor. Erickson used to encourage hypnotic subjects to translate his meanings, words, and images into their own meaning, words, and images. I believe the therapist should be quite concerned if the client is literally following each suggestion offered, as it suggests the person trying to be a "good boy" or "good girl" and follow the therapist's way, rather than discovering his or her own way. As clients develop openness and self-love they discover increasing differences between them and the therapist. The inadequacy of the therapist's perspectives for the client's needs is realized, and the client learns that he or she must rely increasingly on his or her own thinking and feeling. Thus, the revelation of the therapist's failures become the basis for therapeutic progress.

**8. Is love a force to be reckoned with?**

The discussion thus far has been somewhat critical of ideas of power, manipulation, and deception. It leads us to ask: Is the power of love greater than or equal to the love of power? Is "love as a skill" relevant to doing therapy? Can it be effectively used to absorb and transform the violence implicit in a symptom?

I believe the answer is yes to each of these questions. Once we move beyond our immature and rigid understanding of love as a state that "happens to you" under favorable circumstances, we can appreciate it as a cultivated skill and force available under the most adverse circumstances (see Fromm, 1956). We see examples of this in the work of Gandhi, King, Christ, and others. I think we saw it also in the work of Erickson. Love as a skill has many aspects, including opening, understanding from the heart, grounding, receiving, compassion (suffering with), protecting, being with, blessing, noticing growth, commitment, warning, flexibility, and so forth. I think therapy involves a great deal of love,[9] and that it is unfortunate that we talk so little of it.

I have been encouraged by Erickson's example to move from a place of trying to dictate, dominate and control life to learning how to cooperate with it, both in inner and outer worlds. I felt tremendous love in Erickson's work, and find it a good example to remind me of what's possible. The core importance of thinking about therapy in terms of love, rather than power or manipulation, is growing steadily clearer to me. Thus, I believe it is helpful to open discussions of what love as a skill is in therapy, and how to promote and cultivate the courage to love.

---

[9] Mother Teresa was fond of saying that there are no great acts, only small acts done with great love.

## SUMMARY

My development as a therapist has been strongly influenced by the example of Milton Erickson. His emphasis on the uniqueness of each person, accepting and cooperating with whatever the person offered, the restoration of balance, and the enjoyment of life continue to light my path and point onward. As this path has changed, my style has also changed. Some of the aspects of Ericksonian work that I leave behind include the emphasis on power and manipulation; the other-than-conscious self as a mental apparatus; intelligence being "in" or "of" the "unconscious"; trance as always a good thing or an everyday event; the value of indirect communication; and a singular emphasis on success and a taboo on failures.

I am more curious about love as a skill; cooperation as a skill; heart, soul, center, "inner self" and "original soft spot" as complementary terms to the unconscious; the intelligence in interbeing; the specialness of trance and its connection to "cousins" such as art and meditation; experiential symbolic communication that bypasses both the therapist's and client's fixed frames; and the skill of being with failures.

I realize others see Erickson's work differently. This was Erickson's enigma and strength; his work meant so many things to so many people. My major interest here is sharing how what I learned from him twenty years ago is still changing, for better or worse, in my work today. I hope that this remains true for all of us. As the Buddha said many years ago, Be a light unto yourself.

# Chapter 12

# A River Runs Through It: The Relational Self in Psychotherapy[1]

And we did what we did, made love attentively, then
Dove into the river, and our bodies joined as calmly
As the swimmer's shoulders glisten at dawn,
As the pine tree stands in the rain at the edge of the village.
The affection rose on a slope century after century.
And one day my faithfulness to you was born.
— From *The Good Silence* by Robert Bly

Self-relations psychotherapy is an approach developed by the author (Gilligan, 1994, 1996) over the past decade. Based in part on the legacies of Milton Erickson and Gregory Bateson (see Gilligan, 1987), it is also influenced by the gifts of Morehei Ueshiba (the founder of aikido), Gandhi, Groucho Marx, Jerry Garcia, T. S. Eliot, Martin Luther King, Jr., and my daughter Zoe. It seeks to repoeticize experience while encouraging a deeper sobriety of being present in life without sentimentality, self-pity, or grandiosity. It endorses a marriage between the power of love and the love of power, and thus seeks the primacy of being as well as the art of becoming. It offers an explicit way of thinking about how life becomes (and remains) a problem for people, and suggests specific principles and methods by which individuals may find their way out of recurrent suffering.

[1] This essay appeared previously in *Hypnosis International Monographs* 2, 1996: 195–209.

This paper presents some ideas of self-relations and then describes what the approach has to say about the multiple levels of therapist-client relationship. The informal principles which underly the approach are first presented. Then, five principles for "deconstructing" or "deframing" reality are presented, with comments regarding how they might be used by both therapist and client. Throughout, the emphasis will be on cultivating a consciousness that holds opposite truths: love and power, masculine and feminine, problem and solution, and therapist and client.

## SLOGANS FOR SELF-RELATIONS WORK

Every therapist is guided by ideas about how life works and doesn't work. Such principles are often implicit, weaving (and woven into) the multi-layered fabric of a therapy conversation. We will note four ideas that often guide self-relations methods. They are often introduced when a client has identified an impasse of some sort, and are typically communicated with an "Irish twinkle," with the intention of shifting the conversation from the dreary literality of fundamentalism to the artistic intrigue and fresh possibilities of life itself.

**1. Life sucks, but it's not a problem.**

This first principle is based on the Buddha's first noble truth: Suffering exists. On a daily basis, this much is clear: If it's not one thing, it's another. If you have a car, you're going to have car problems. If you have a relationship, you're going to have relationship problems. If you have a therapist, you are going to have therapist problems. And on and on it goes. But life itself is not a problem, and neither are you. When problems become an identity level statement ("I am a problem"), we become identified with (or as) suffering, and all hell breaks loose.

Self-relations assumes that a person's unwillingness or inability to stay in direct relationship with suffering is partly what brings him or her into therapy. Something keeps hurting badly, and the person is seeking a way out of the suffering by (re-enactment of) violence against self or others. This violence takes many forms: addiction, hostility, self-denigration, starving one's self, and on and on. Self-relations sees that there is no way out of suffering, but there is a way through it. It is especially interested in methods that help a person to "be with" suffering without becoming it. It decries attempts to "just be happy" or to just focus on "solutions" as much as it challenges methods that encourage regression or other "face in the place of spaghetti" approaches to experience. It looks to find a middle way between these opposite paths, one that will allow suffering as well as joy and happiness.

Like Buddhist practices, self-relations seeks to dissolve the attachment to (and hence the identification with or dissociation from) suffering. To do this, it distinguishes the experience of suffering from the narratives constructed to represent it. It observes that problems degrade into symptoms when the person relates to a problem or to suffering at an identity level — "I am a problem" rather than "a problem exists and I can explore how to be in relationship with it."

The idea of suffering evokes many different images and hence many different understandings, many unhelpful to the relief of suffering. Suffering is often seen through the mediating frames of self-pity, grandiosity, or intellectualization, which invariably results in distorted (e.g., overly complicated or narrow) views. Many people believe that to accept one's suffering is to submit to injustice or define one's self as a victim. The main purpose in acknowledging suffering as primary is to recognize the many pains, losses, traumas, heartbreaks, and failures that, if unintegrated, stall a person's development and perpetuate the cycle of violence. The point in recognizing them is not to wallow or otherwise identify with them, but to open the possibility of being with them in a way that allow them to move through us. This leads to our second principle.

**2. Life moves through you, except when it doesn't.**

We often think of mind and experience as occurring inside a person, rather than a process that flows through the organic circuitries of relatedness connecting everything. Mind is a verb. You are a receptor site in the Great Internet, a conduit through which the mystery of life flows. As I suggest (with an Irish twinkle) to many clients, life is out to get you. Or as Rilke (1981) wrote in "The man watching":

> What we choose to fight with is so tiny!
> What fights with us is so great!
> If only we would let ourselves be dominated
> As things do by some immense storm
> We would become strong too, and not need names. (p. 105)

Life relentlessly follows you, calling on you to change your point of view, to develop a deeper understanding of yourself and life. The illusion of control is tragic and costly, though the possibilities of cooperation are endless. In our models of isolated patriarchy, the power principle reigns, urging us to control and oppose that which is outside our narrow identity. The idea of surrender to a power greater than our ego (it doesn't take much!) is regarded with horror and indignance, seen as a loss of control or a submission to injustice (which it can be). We are reminded of Eliot (1963):

> Do not let me hear
> Of the wisdom of old men, but rather of their folly,
> Their fear of fear and frenzy, their fear of possession,
> Of belonging to another, or to others, or to God.
> The only wisdom we can hope to acquire
> Is the wisdom of humility: humility is endless. (p. 185)

The effort to control life, to hang on to a fixed position, inevitably fails. Symptoms represent a breakdown of the power principle, a failure of the person to maintain a static representation of self and world. In mythological terms, it signals the end of a middle stage of a journey. The first stage is living in the garden. Here life is innocent, spontaneous, complete. My four-year-old daughter Zoe still pretty much lives in the garden. At some point — it could be through violence, trauma, formal education, systemic injustice, whatever — life forces you out of the garden and into exile. This poignant tragedy befalls each of us; there seems to be no escape from it. As we walk our forty years (of mythological time) in the desert, operating from an exiled government, we are forced to learn a new language. We are challenged to rely on ourselves, to differentiate and hold differences, to develop our own understanding of things. But at some point, life begins to call us back to our selves and to our connection with others. Symptoms can be seen as a call to "return from exile," back to ourselves, to learn what Erich Fromm (1956) called the "art of loving."

If we disregard or otherwise don't properly respond to this call, symptoms and other forms of violence develop. As Fromm (1956) noted, the alternatives to learning to love include addiction, fascism, fundamentalism, indulgence (sex, drugs, rock and roll), and conformity. Such processes are attempts to regress to a pre-individual, pre-rational mode of consciousness (cf. Wilbur, 1983). They are primarily acts of violence because they require us to kill off parts of ourselves or others as "final solutions" to our pain. In psychological experience, there is a world of difference between killing and dying. We cannot kill ideas, though we can "be with" a death/rebirth cycle. Symptoms signal a death/rebirth cycle, an identity in transition. As life moves through us, it brings death to old ways and birth of new possibilities.

Symptoms are thus attempts to change that are thwarted in part by violence. As we say in self-relations, symptoms signal that the person is "up to something big." We assume that some life force keeps moving through them, over and over again. The person has tried everything to turn away from, control, or otherwise deny this force — it feels meaningless and threatening — but has failed miserably. Rather than regarding this force as bad, we see it as a life-giving presence. This is not meant flippantly, for it is a dangerous time. If a person cannot somehow be changed by the experience, he or she may be damaged significantly. As the wave rolls to shore, you may be thrown down to the bottom of the sea, caught in an undercurrent, so it is important to stay tuned. Sentimentality, intellectualization, and other false approaches must be avoided. So the challenge of therapy is how to sense the presence of this "other than ego" life force that is moving through the person, and help a person move through it without resorting to violence against self or others. (A symptom is thus a type of violence.)

In this regard, the principle of "neuromuscular lock" is central. To quote William Blake: "Satan has many names, Opacity being the most common." The easiest way to create opacity, such that you can't feel or see through things to a deeper level, is to "freeze" the muscles, prompting an excitatory/inhibitory imbalance in the nervous system (Gilligan, 1996; Shapiro, 1995). This moves the experience of life from a dynamic to a static orientation, and makes the mind/body sheathing (or boundaries) "opaque" rather than translucent. "Inside" and "outside" the self seem irreconcilable, as no common-unity ground is sensed to underlie differences.

Neuromuscular lock occurs in every threatened organism, but only humans can persist in the frozen state long after the threatening conditions are removed. Most of what we call thinking and acting are performed from this state of neuromuscular lock, and the result is that we feel alienated from ourselves and the world within and around us. Thus, the meaning of "life moves through us, except when it doesn't" is that we can (and have) shut down to the currents of life moving through everything. (As Thoreau observed, "This current allies me to the rest of the world.") While shutting down was probably unavoidable at an earlier point, the symptom is demanding that we learn to open back up to life. As long as neuromuscular lock persists, the gift of the symptom will feel alien and threatening, and thus lead to further (violent) attempts to destroy it.

The MRI group (Watzlawick, Weakland, & Fisch, 1974), in crystallizing their work with Bateson and Erickson, emphasized that the attempted solution is the problem. In trying to separate from the symptom, we co-create it as a self-destructive act. At the heart of this unwitting act is neuromuscular lock: Our bodies shut down to the energies of life and our images get locked into a fundamentalist freeze about how life should look and about what something means. To relieve a symptom, we must soften neuromuscular lock; in technical language, we must "chill out." It can help immensely to examine how agitation and neuromuscular lock underly most of our activities.

*Self-relations suggests that a cardinal feature of a mature consciousness is to think, experience, and act without neuromuscular lock.*[2] The whole idea in hypnosis and meditation is to "just let it happen," to learn to let life move through while we stick around to learn from it. In the larger sense, all of art is based on sensing and being used by energies greater than the ego. As Faust spoke through Mephistopheles (cited in Edinger, 1990):

> The stuff lies there, the problem is to win it:
> That calls for art, and who can now begin it? (p. 48)

Every artist knows the importance of learning some workable traditions for relaxing and letting go. This letting go is not a stuporous drool; it is a heightened sensitivity that allows a greater sense of control, albeit one distinct from egoic muscular contraction. It is not a trance state, though trance could be developed from it. In such a state, one can better carry out the aikido slogan of "Expect nothing, be ready for anything." The principles in the second part of the paper all have to do with this process.

**3. There are two of you.**

At some point in a therapy, usually in the first or second session, I suggest

---

[2] It is interesting in this regard to note that Milton Erickson's severe polio attack at the age of 17 left him paralzyed and without the capacity to think by squeezing his muscles. He had no felt connection to his muscles! Thus, he had to learn to think without moving or talking. A common line in his later hypnotherapy inductions was, "you don't have to move ... you don't have to talk ... you can let your unconscious mind begin to do the work for you ..." I suspect Erickson's polio forced him into learning this non-muscular type of mature thinking at a relatively early age, and that he passed his learning onto others via hypnotic processes.

to a client that once you wipe away the "booga-booga" aspects of hypnosis (which are about 95% of it), a handful of ideas remain that can be quite helpful to therapy. One of them, I say, is that there are two of you. Many clients wryly smile, responding, "Is that all?" I acknowledge that there are many faces and many forms of Self, but there are two distinct psyches through which they are known. In hypnosis, of course, they are referred to as the "conscious mind" and the "unconscious mind." I rarely use these terms any more, mostly because I lost any felt sense of what they meant. They suddenly seemed too impersonal and mechanical to describe the struggles and mysteries of human experience. Still, they have value in suggesting that you are more than simply an egoic self, that someone else lives inside of you. Robert Bly (1986) observes in his poem, "The Watcher":

> Inside us there is a listener who listens for what we say, a watcher who watches what we do. Each step we take in conversation with our friends, moving slowly, or flying among worlds, he watches, calling us into what is possible, into what is not said, into the shuckheap of ruined arrowheads, or the old man with missing fingers. (p. 135)

This idea of the "other self" is, of course, central to artistic awareness. The Chilean writer Isabelle Allende offered a beautiful description in an interview about her writing style (Toms, 1994). She described how the characters in her novels first appear as "beings in her belly." She holds these beings in a sort of pregnancy. Her process of "giving birth" to them includes falling in love with them on their own terms, accurately describing them, and listening to the story they have to tell. (How much this sounds like good parenting!) In the first stage of the process, these beings in the belly are guiding the story; in her second stage of editing, her writer's ear and craft are more active. In both stages, the Relational Self is the felt sense of connection between these two orders of being.

So the conscious/unconscious distinction of Erickson's work is modified in self-relations work to emphasize a "normal" (everyday) sense of self located in the head, and an experiential/archetypal self located in the belly (see Gilligan, 1996). If a person identifies only with the normal self, alienation from life as it "moves through the belly" will ensue, and fear and (unsuccessful) attempts to control will predominate. If the identification is with ongoing experience or with the archetypal self, a person will be lost in emotion, trauma, and fantasy, suffering what the Jungians call "inflation of the archetype." (If you look this term up, you'll see pictures of such luminaries as Michael Jackson and Marilyn Monroe.) So what self-relations looks to do is develop a felt sense of both at the same time. The approach says that you are the field that holds, and the spirit that connects, the differences. It thus encourages therapists to sense a client as a relationship between selves, rather than as a position of a given self.

The Relational Self can be noted in diverse contexts. Seymour Epstein (1994) reviewed a wide variety of research supporting a dual-processing or "double-mind" model. William James used the "rider/horse" metaphor to describe it. Good parent/child or teacher/student relationships embody it. Art raises it to a beautiful level. Milton Erickson's therapy demonstrated it, though I believe Erickson misdescribed it, committing the typical Occidental epistemological error of not including the observer — that is, himself — in the description. He would emphasize the intelligence of the person's relating with it. I believe a more complete description is that "Erickson plus Client's unconscious" was the generative unit. Of course, this raises the question of whether "Client's normal self plus Client's other self" might not be a better fit in the long run. This latter relationship is what self-relations tries to establish (see Gilligan, 1996).

One way is to move the relationship between the normal self and the "other self" from an "I-it" to an "I-thou" connection. For example, the symptomatic "it" (e.g., depression) is moved to a personal "he" or "she" that has a felt center in the body and often an age. Thus, the person is not the symptomatic experience but can be helped to "be with it" in a way that provides a container within which it can be felt and expressed. Like in mindfulness meditation, the self is not acted out via muscular behavior, but experientially held in a mind/body container.The "other self" can be named in various ways — one's center, soul, "he" or "she," the guest, the inner being, etc. This other self cannot be reduced to any given image or description, such as an inner child or wise old man. It is a center through which every psychological form moves, as in the young child who manifests in the course of a day every psychological form known to humankind at least twice. Each form moves through except when it doesn't, that is, when fear and contraction hold it in neuromuscular lock, spinning in reiterative cycles until human presence is there to "bless" it and work with it.

It is also important to remember that this other self doesn't belong to you. It is part of your larger Self, but not a part or extension of you. It has its own autonomous life, in many ways different from your own. You might regard it as a mate. In this regard it matters whether I regard Denise, my wife, as

"Denise" first and "my wife" second, or the other way around. Similarly, when we regard the "other self" as autonomous, we can begin to realize that life moves through him or her. Our mission thus is to feel the center in our body that "houses" this self, and to listen and feel each experience of life flowing through it, responding to it without identification or dissociation.

To reiterate, the notion of a relational field that underlies both selves is crucial to doing this. When "I" and "thou" are both sensed, an "us" emerges. As Figure 12.1 illustrates, the sensing of this field is crucial to holding different positions simultaneously in the field. This is a natural state known to most people. For example, if you review what you do when you need to "get back to yourself" — activities such as reading, walking, listening to music — you probably will notice that at some point you sense an expanded sense of feeling beyond your body boundaries. If you were asked where your self ends in such an experience, you would probably find it an inappropriate question, for it is sensed as a unitary field. Self-relations is especially interested in what practices or traditions a person may engage in to enter this field, and is curious as to how they may be generated and maintained under adverse circumstances (such as the problem context).

**4. You are an incurable deviant, but so is everybody else.**

One of the concerns many clients have is that they are weird and strange. I try to assure them as soon as possible (again with a sympathetic Irish twinkle) that they have understated the matter tremendously. They're a lot weirder than their deepest fears suggest, and it's only going to get worse!

One of the obvious implications is that a person will have to face the fact that he or she cannot meet other people's expectations. This signals the end of what might be called the "camel" phase of human development. I believe it was Nietzsche who suggested that for the first part of life, we are camels, trudging through the desert, accepting on our backs everybody's "shoulds" and "don'ts." Camels only know how to spit; they don't think for themselves or talk back. When the camel dies, a lion begins to emerge. Lions discover both their roar and the art of preening. It may seem a little shaky at first, so a little coaching can be helpful. But once the camel begins to die (e.g., signaled by depression), there seems to be no turning back. Symptoms occupy the space between the death of the camel and the birth of the lion. A therapist can be a good midwife during this liminal phase.

Joseph Campbell used to say that sometimes you climb the ladder to the top, only to discover that you've placed it against the wrong wall. A symptom

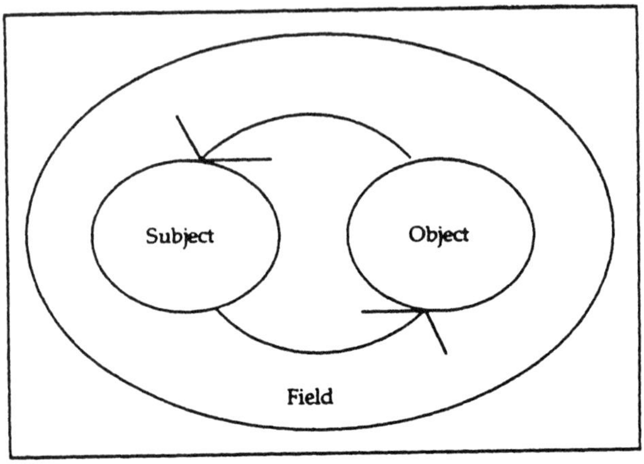


Figure 12.1.
The Relational Self as the pattern that connects differences.

can be such a message. It says the way you've directed your life no longer works. Something or somebody inside is urging you to find a new way. But first we must climb down off the ladder set against the wall of other people's expectations.

One of the values of accepting your "deviancy" (or uniqueness, if that feels better) is that you can ease the endless self-demands for change. Wanting to change is often a form of self-hatred, stemming often from the hope that "If only I was different from who I am now, then you would love me." Endless attempts to perform in hopes of love result in the horrible realization that you have failed; if you can stay with this, you will realize that it's not about you, it's the nature of the beast. Symptoms such as depression are remarkable voices of integrity at this time. They signal that "nothing will work," "it doesn't matter," and "there's no use." This signals the death of an illusory self, and if properly accepted and dealt with, can lead to enormous reconciliation between the normal and archetypal self. A need for a solid container is crucial at this point, for the dangers of acting out in violence are substantial. But the cry of a symptom is an expression in part of the need to accept some unique, unacknowledged aspect(s) of one's self.

As I suggest to clients, one of the other therapeutic nuggets that may be mined from hypnotic experience is the realization of just how weird you are. In hypnosis, everybody does it his or her own way. The therapist suggests one thing but when things are working properly, the client responds with something else. I believe that therapeutic hypnosis only begins when the client is not following what I'm saying, but doing something in parallel.[3] Without resistance or failure, therapy is invariably merely a polite social game.

Therapy is a conversation for discovering the client's unique way. Since the therapist's way is different, the success of therapy is predicated on the failure of the therapeutic theory and technique. The therapist is thus at his or her best a sort of "holy fool" who knows that his or her way is not the client's way, but must proceed with dignity nonetheless, waiting for the client to "push back" the theory and technique offered by the therapist to reveal a different perspective, one that is more true for the client. The capacity to accept and hold these differences leads to good therapy. It also leads to an increasing appreciation that the client must continue to discover their own unique "deviant" way of knowing and being in the world.

To summarize, these four slogans encourage the therapist to accept the presence of suffering in life, without sentimentality or denial. This allows a confirmation of what Trungpa Rinpoche (1984) has called the "original soft spot" (as compared to "original sin") that is the center of each human being. When the soft spot is violated, pain occurs. To avoid pain, a person spins off a persona (including a story line) that lives some distance from one's center. (Ego is founded on the denial of the original soft spot.) The mental agitation and distortion produced by this denial produces suffering, which produces further agitation and distortion, and away we go, sometimes only returning years or even generations later.

This dissociation from one's center is initially a solution. Not only does it numb the pain, it leads to the development of a separate egoic self. But as the person develops resources, the continued alienation grows into a liability, for a better way is now available. This better way involves a relational Self which connects the egoic self and the original self, as well as other self-other (Self)

---

[3] A common hypnotic suggestion Erickson used to make was: "As you listen to me, you can change my meanings into your meanings . . . my images into your images . . . my understandings into your own understandings." The idea is that therapeutic hypnosis really begins when the client is able to do this. At this point she/he is no longer following suggestions but discovering her/his own creative responses.

complementarities. This is what a symptom attempts to do for a person: It is a call to return to the original center, and an opportunity to move into a integrated relational Self. What it requires is a surrender of the power principle, a willingness to engage the other (interior or exterior) self without violence. Unfortunately, neuromuscular lock leads one to think that surrender would be a disaster, so we continue to resist the change moving through us. On this point nature seems eternally patient: It simply waits, and begins the cycle again. At some point, a person feels that control is slipping away, and they come to a therapist in desperation.

The therapist realizes that clients are well along in some process of change, but that they have been conditioned to distrust and regard their other selves as alien and threatening. A solution therefore requires a paradoxical relationship of "not resisting" (allowing experience to flow through) while "not becoming" (not identifying with the experience). Self-relations looks to develop an experience of Self as a felt field that holds two selves, one to witness and "be with" and the other to experience life moving through. From this relational Self, a middle way between repression and acting out is cultivated, and life is no longer a problem (for a while).

So the self-relations therapist enters a session with the attitude, This person is up to something big. My job is to sense it and properly name it. I need to name the suffering in a way that begins its dissolution, while keeping a connection with the part of the person who is not damaged (and doesn't need to change). To do this, remember that the client is a relationship: *Don't act until you can feel both selves simultaneously*. My job is to foster a feeling of relatedness between these two selves. What will block that relatedness is neuromuscular lock, so I need to introduce some principle of unlocking the body/mind. As that happens, I can join, bless, and harmonize with whatever is happening, knowing the solution is already in motion. Other methods (see Gilligan, 1996) can then be applied.

## STEPS IN RETURNING FROM EXILE

Influenced a great deal by the legacies of Milton Erickson and Morehei Ueshiba (aikido founder), self-relations sees symptoms as arising when a person feels "breaks" in beingness, belongingness, and relatedness. The following principles are some of the guidelines for making the reconnections. It should be emphasized that the therapist always follows these guidelines him- or herself while suggesting them to the client. They are not meant to put a person into an "altered state," but rather to "deframe" or "deconstruct" the neuromuscular fixation that is at the heart of symptomatic behavior.

**1. Sense the center.**

The basic question here is: To what (or whom) do you give first attention? A simple task for the therapist is to watch where the client's eyes project; this is where primary attention is given. Self-relations makes the observation that in stress, a person usually (without awareness) gives his or her focal point away to the stressor. This may be a physical presence — for example, another person in the room — or a remembered presence (via eye accessing cues). The problem with this is that a person is left to react, rather than respond; the stressor is the "higher power" that determines identity.

So a simple shift is to train one's self to "keep coming back," to return to one's center. In aikido, where you are faced with the prospect of people attacking you with all sorts of blunt instruments and malicious intents, this is done by softening the eyes and dropping awareness to a point several inches below the navel. In training this response, it may help to let several fingers touch that point in your body and rest gently until you can feel them harmonize with the natural in-breath/out-breath. This may take awhile and require some gentle coaching to let go, so patience and tenderness are premium qualities.

The therapist can use this process to drop into the "belly-mind" when stressed, and may also suggest it to the client. The basic idea is that when "first attention" is in your center point, you can be in a more receptive, non-reactive relationship with the "antagonistic other" (person, image, thing). Being receptive doesn't mean you allow a person to run you over. As an exercise in martial arts, lowering your center is about increasing the freedom to feel secure and to respond from a natural sense of being, rather than one foreign to you.

The underlying premise here is that your relation to your center (or what some might call their soul, or sobriety, or daemon) is your primary commitment. This is a new idea for many, so the difference between narcissistic absorption and responsible selfishness may be important to distinguish. The simple notion, testable in action, is that when you leave your center, you cannot sustain being with anything or anyone else. You make a mess of things, whatever your intention. Training attention to be centered allows one to let life move through you, and to thus allow awareness to include, but also extend beyond, egoic interests.

**2. Open awareness to peripheral fields.**

Another simple observation in Self-relations is that in symptomatic behavior, attention is fixed rigidly on the figure of the stressor, and withdrawn from the field around it. Another aikido principle relevant in this regard is, never fix your focus on the attack.

Instead, let your awareness soften and spread to the peripheral field. This is similar to advice Don Juan gave to Carlos Castaneda (1974) in *Tales of Power*, when he recommended that Carlos learn to walk with eyes spread to 180 degrees peripheral vision, watching the horizon on both sides while feeling his hands at his sides. (Don Juan added the further sobering suggestion to then sense death always stalking you over your left shoulder!) We might call this field-based (rather than the traditional figure-based) perception "juggler's consciousness": It allows one to connect with the field holding the different figures (truths, people, positions, etc.), without locking into any of them.

One simple way to do this is what I call three-point attention, which I sometimes introduce to clients as an "anti-anxiety" technique. I point out that in order to worry, you have to tense your eyes and then move them around in arrhythmic patterns. (This is why in a traditional hypnotic induction a person is asked to relax and focus on a point: It disrupts the orienting response triggered by eye movements and thereby sets hypnosis into action.) I then suggest a simple experiment, namely that they relax and allow a first point of attention to develop in their belly (or heart, or hands, whichever is most comfortable). I then suggest that they select two other points in front of them, preferably one on either side of me. We work a bit on relaxation and gently distributing attention until all three points are equally in focus. I then suggest they soften the field a bit more while remaining alert.

A nice aspect of this technique is that the therapist can easily monitor how the person is doing. If the eyes shift, gentle coaching suggestions to relax and refocus can be given. This can be a straightforward way to develop a relaxed and alert focus. (Again, the therapist can do this in parallel with the person.) Work, especially with anxiety related issues, can then be done with the person while they are in this state. It keeps a person from accessing a lot of control/fear reactions to an experience, thereby allowing the person to stay present. Also, the person may be encouraged to use this exercise before or during stressful situations as a centering method. (In public situations, one can learn to do it in non-obvious ways.)

A modification of this exercise is what might be called "orbital looping."

This is similar to a process I use in aikido, where one of the guiding principles (regarding the relationship with the attacker) is:

> "Heart to heart,
> Mind with mind,
> Center with center."

In orbital looping, the person feels gentle curved bands of energy pulsating through various channels, connecting through another person. For example, suggestions may be given that the client feel a gentle energy behind his or her eyes, a relaxing feeling that can be felt as a pulsating band. This curved band can extend through the temples of their forehead into an orbital circuit, moving through the temples and behind the eyes of the therapist. Similar orbital loops may be developed through the ears, the fingertips, and toes.

This process may sound a bit strange at first description, but it is a simple way to feel the "pattern that connects" you and another person. (I also use it as a technique with couples.) It is a process to encourage an experience of a relational mind that is a field between people rather than a position inside a person's head. The idea is that the more you can move from the isolation of being locked inside your head to the community field that holds you and others, life is no longer sensed as a problem.

**3. Soften agitation.**

Neuromuscular lock ensures that most of our experience, thinking, and acting arises from an underlying state of agitation. A simple exercise to help in the monumental task of decreasing agitation is to move through a series of gentle self-suggestions for "soft mind . . . soft body . . . soft eyes . . . soft heart . . . soft soul." (Additional suggestions for trouble spots such as the jaw, forehead, and shoulders may be included.) The idea is to simply bring awareness and then releasing to each space.

For example, in softening the mind, it may help to adopt the Buddhist view that mind is space and that space is sky. So we feel the space in which the thoughts move, feel it as a full emptiness. We then simply allow the thought of "soft mind," and wait patiently. The key is in our response to what happens. Often nothing happens at first, so we can move through the first two steps (center point, peripheral field), and gently return to the idea of soft mind. It may help to feel the most dense area, the busiest "downtown" area of your mind — for most people, this is in their head — and start there. With training, it is possible to develop a mindfulness that is full of awareness without trying to fix things. Again, this can be helpful to both therapists and clients.

If the mind is agitated, it is very hard to relax the body, and vice versa. So it is good to cycle through the different areas. The point, which is central to many martial arts, is that true resilience, strength, and courage come from softening the agitation.

**4. Erase any hypnotic phenomena.**

All of this talk about softness and relaxation is bound to encourage people to drift off into trance, so it should be emphasized that this is not the goal in following these principles. Trance states can be therapeutic and a lot of fun, but here we're exploring ways to deframe symptomatic altered states of consciousness and return from exile. A few common side effects of hypnosis are grogginess, distortion of reality, and falling out of one's chair. Since these may detract from therapeutic presence, it is helpful to have a few ways to steer away from them. A simple question may be asked in this regard: How do you know you are going into trance?

The most common answer is trance phenomena. That is, I know trance is developing because the phenomena (or appearances) of my experience change significantly. How I see things (in the exterior and interior worlds) changes; how I feel things changes; and how I hear things changes.

So an intriguing experiment is the following. Find a comfortable position and take a few moments to get into a receptive state. Tuning to your visual awareness, ask "What are the first (small) signs that trance is developing?" It could be a tunnel vision, or a certain type of imagery, or a shift in detail. As you notice whatever it is, imaginally take a "gentle, mental eraser" and tenderly erase that phenomenon, and then feel what's behind that. (Not in the sense of a hidden meaning or symbol, but the experiential space — often emptiness — that is sensed.) As you feel what's behind it, let yourself move deeper into a trance (without the trance phenomenon).

Then move your attention to the kinesthetic mode, and ask the same question: "What are the first small signs that trance is developing?" It could be a heaviness in the body, a tingling in the hands, or a dissociative feeling. Take the gentle, mental eraser and erase that distortion, feel what's behind that, and go deeper into trance as a result. Repeat the same for the auditory realm, and then recycle through each modality as many times as you'd like.

Some people have amazing experiences with this process. An experience may be developed that is neither the dictatorial control of egoic identity nor the dreaminess of hypnotic reality. It can help develop an exquisite awareness of the middle way between the extremes. In this middle way, life is not a problem — it simply "is." This can help one deal more directly with the challenges that are presented.

**5. Erase analytical phenomena.**

On the one extreme we lose ourselves to the seductiveness of trance phenomena, on the other to the thought-forms and constructs of rational consciousness. We become addicted to thinking, ruminating over images, rigidly applying rehearsed mental structures. We believe that we think thoughts, not recognizing that usually thoughts think us.

When thinking becomes unhelpful, the same "experiments in consciousness" used with hypnotic phenomena can be applied to analytical content. Thus, after the person has centered, spread to the peripheral, softened the mind/body/heart, and erased the hypnotic phenomena, he or she may wonder, What else am I aware of? As each thought, image, percept is attended to, the "gentle mental eraser" may soften it, allowing a felt sense of the tender space behind it. This is the experience of mind as a relational field. Like Erickson's "middle of nowhere," it is a space from which fresh experience can arise. It may allow relief from compulsive doing/thinking and a return to the more basic level of the consciousness of being. This is an antidote for the mind caught in the endless cycle of performance. Here one can feel the sorrow of Rilke (in Bly, 1981):

> The man who cannot quietly close his eyes
> Certain that there is vision after vision
> Inside, simply waiting until night-time
> To rise all around him in the darkness —
> He is an old man, it's all over for him.
>
> Nothing else will come; no more days will open,
> And everything that does happen will cheat him.
> Even you, my God. And you are like a stone
> That draws him daily deeper into the depths. (p. 53)

# Chapter 13

# The Relational Self: The Expanding of Love Beyond Desire[1]

The experience of Self is always a defeat for the ego.
— Carl G. Jung

Growing up in an Irish Catholic alcoholic family in San Francisco, I used to get into big trouble. Such rascality would typically earn me a face-to-face encounter with my drunken father who would demand to know, "Who the hell do you think you are, anyway?" The question arrested my attention, so it is not surprising that I have continued to ponder it over the years. How we ask and answer this question of psychological identity seems crucial to how we experience and express ourselves in the world.

Of course, much of the time the inquiry is straightforward. When I go into a store, I am in the identity of a customer, with all my understandings and associations of that role identity. At the same time, still in a rather straightforward way, I may sense the clerk as a bully, and respond by identifying myself as assertive. If the clerk speaks with a heavy foreign accent, I may additionally think of myself as a native-born American.

Although the identity question is straightforward and not so interesting in some contexts, it is of central relevance in others, especially that of psycho-

[1] This essay appeared previously in Michael F. Hoyt. 1996. *Constructive therapies, Volume II.* New York: Guilford Publications.

therapy. In fact, we might say that people become psychotherapy clients precisely because the ways they are answering identity questions don't allow a fit to the social context or a connection to an inner sense of self, and thereby generate inappropriate behavior or painful experience. For example, when a depressed person locks into the singular self-truth of "I am worthless," all other self-descriptions are functionally dissociated, and the person's response to the outside world and connection to the inside world are lost. In this sense, a goal of psychotherapy is to support the fixed identity a client may be stuck in, while expanding the field of consciousness to activate and connect additional identities.

This is what the therapeutic approach of *self-relations* seeks to do. As we will see, self-relations sees therapy problems in terms of a position, truth, or identity becoming isolated from its larger field, and sees solutions developing when relational processes are reactivated and cooperative processes developed. For example, say a client is espousing the position of "Life sucks and you can't trust anybody." (Such a person usually receives the diagnosis of adolescence.) Is this good or bad? Self-relations suggests that it is neither. It is one of the great "truths" of the world, whose value and meaning depends in large part on whether the person also has access to other, especially complementary truths, such as "Life is beautiful." In other words, *the problem is not the problem; the problem is that what is pointed to as the problem is isolated from other positions, persons, experiences, or truths.* As the existentialists used to say, the study of psychopathology is precisely the study of loneliness. The idea of a *relational self* is that every person is a conversation between positions, the holder of differences, the integrator of opposites. The person is relationship itself— figure, field, and form.

How that idea plays out in psychotherapy is the focus of this chapter. I begin by describing two different psychological approaches to experience, fundamentalism and aesthetics. I show how fundamentalism is a succinct formula for violence, and how the alternative of an aesthetic approach gives rise to the basic premises of self-relations. I next discuss how these premises suggest a psychological model of symptoms based on the alienation of a social/cognitive self from an experiential/soulful/archetypal self, and then explore a prototype structure for renewing the spirit of relatedness within the relational self.

## FUNDAMENTALISM VS. AESTHETICS

One can approach the question of identity or meaning in different ways. Some ways lead to limited answers, violence, and symptoms; others lead to growth and solutions. In the view of self-relations, the two most relevant approaches are fundamentalism and aesthetics.

Fundamentalism is the more common approach. It is not tied to a particular content or ideology. It may be used by the right wing as well as the left, in secular contexts as well as religious, in artistic domains as in scientific ones. It may be applied equally to the Bible, to the DSM-IV, to the lyrics of the Grateful Dead, to the work of Milton Erickson, to a memory, or to any other experience or view of life.

Fundamentalism starts with the premise that identity is defined according to allegiance to some single truth. This truth is revealed in a special text. I use the term text loosely here, meaning any frame of words, images, and feelings. The therapist's theory is a text; so is each memory, experience, or story of the client. In fundamentalism, a particular text is assumed to reveal *the* truth rather than a truth, and identity is based on strict adherence to that truth. The text is more important than experience itself, so in fundamentalism the primary relationship of a person is with the unchanging, single text, rather than with the organic here and now of life itself. Needless to say, this makes learning difficult if not impossible.

Fundamentalism further requires that the text be read literally; it is not to be sensed poetically, metaphorically, or with a sense of humor. (Is it not rare to hear of hilariously funny fundamentalist comics or poignant fundamentalist artists?) In fundamentalism, psychological identity is expressed by fixating on the text, rather than seeing or feeling through it to a deeper aesthetic meaning. Thus, the metaphor of an inner child, the idea of an unconscious mind, a depression, or a solution is taken literally, rather than as a process description that points beyond itself to something more ineffable, something more primary. In the words of William Blake (quoted by Yeats, 1905/1979, p. xxxii), "Satan has many names, Opacity being the most common."

In positing that one way is correct and all others are wrong, fundamentalism sees the relationship between differences as irreconcilable opposites. A person is either an insider or an outsider in relation to the truth, and the possibility of relatedness across the boundaries is forbidden. If intimacy involves the holding of two different "truths" — the "I" and the "thou," "self" and "other" — in relationship, then intimacy is disallowed. If creative activity —

whether it be humor, art, or scientific discovery — involves the holding of two different frames simultaneously, then creative activity and aesthetic experience are forbidden.[2] If altered states of consciousness such as hypnosis are developed by assuming that a person has two different selves, then trance is to be feared.

The idea that differences are irreconcilable spells trouble when opposites meet, as they have a habit of doing. (As Bateson [1972] emphasized, difference is the basic unit of mental process.) In fact, the "I-it" relationship given to one person's position and another's different position is, I suggest here, a formula for violence. The position of the "other" is deemed invalid in a way that legitimizes attempts to eliminate it, by any means necessary. The thinking is, "There's only room in this here self for one of us, so you better be destroyed." This gives rise to a series of "final solutions" that seek, in the name of freedom, purity, mental health, justice, or God, to eradicate the bad, sick, crazy, or evil "other." Our image of the "other" is degraded, as Sam Keen (1986) has brilliantly illustrated, into the archetypal face of the enemy. Once the image of the enemy is locked into neuromuscular freeze, any "freedom loving" person may feel not only justified but obligated to engage in violence to eradicate it.

In the clinical context, a client struggling with a symptom is a person struggling with, among other things, fundamentalism. For example, say a person has experienced a sexual trauma. In an almost unavoidable way, the memories or images of the trauma become imprinted as the text (or frame) by which future sexual or intimate relationships are understood. The traumatic memory becomes the fundamentalistic text that says, "All relationships are like this; you can't trust anybody." Furthermore, the text of the memory is regarded as an "it" that the person may try to keep out of his or her self, though it keeps coming back (via flashbacks, etc.).

---

[2] This idea of holding double frames simultaneously as the basis for the distinctly human experiences of humor, love, mythology, intimacy, craziness, play, and so on, has been suggested by a variety of writers. Bateson's (1979) idea of *double description* as a minimal requirement for an ecological view, stemming from his earlier work on the double bind hypothesis, was central to his later work. Jung (1916/1971) suggested the idea of the *transcendent function*, involving the capacity to hold opposite truths simultaneously, as the basic means of individuation. And Arthur Koestler (1964), in his opus *The Act of Creation*, suggested the idea of *bisociation* — involving the holding and integration of two disparate matrices — as the essential mechanism of creative activity.

As therapists, we need to have compassionate understanding for how fundamentalism develops. *The "break in relatedness" between self and other occurs via violence, and requires violence (against self and/or others) to maintain.* We need to appreciate how the consequent reduction of identity to an image or an "–ism," rather than to the consciousness of being, is a recipe for suffering and violence. At the same time, we are committed to exploring how the chain of violence may be ended rather than perpetuated. Thus, we engage in what T. S. Eliot (1963) in *Four Quartets* has called the "expanding/Of love beyond desire" (p. 205), or the expanding of identity beyond the fixed frame of a single text. We may be helped in this process by the epistemological approach of aesthetics, which constitutes a different approach to identity.

In an aesthetic approach, the image is not primary. God has many faces. *The relational self can be imaged in many ways, but this self is no image.* It is not a position or an image, but a context and a relational process. The consciousness that feels and sees (and is felt and seen) through images and descriptions, to a deeper pattern that connects, is more basic. Thus, the identity question is answered not in terms of "I am the follower of orthodox images," but rather "I am (with you) the consciousness that experiences multiple truths." (In this way, the poetic is a more grounded, primary, direct language than the literal.)

As Bateson (1955/1972) pointed out, the simultaneous holding of multiple frames or truths underlies many distinctly human contexts, such as intimacy, play, hypnosis, mythology, and psychopathology. Stated simply, to generate a nonrational state of consciousness (love, intimacy, humor, pathology, trance, symptoms, play, etc.), one must activate two seemingly contradictory truths or experiences simultaneously. In intimacy, for example, once we get beyond the romantic ideal of 1 + 1 = 1 (where differences are obliterated), we see a more mature version of 1 + 1 = 3 (where the differences of "I" and "thou" held in a unified field of consciousness give birth to a third, shared "us"). Later in this chapter, I describe how shifts in identity engender the need to hold opposite or multiple frames simultaneously, and examine further how altered states of consciousness are inevitable at this time. I also describe how these altered states are symptomatic or therapeutic, depending on whether the opposites are regarded as complementary or as irreconcilable, and whether a common field is felt to underlie and imbue both simultaneously. For now, I would like to simply suggest that aesthetics is an approach to identity that seeks to see or feel through different images to what T. S. Eliot (1963) has called "a further union, a deeper communion" (p. 190). In holding multiple images or descriptions simultaneously, one is freed from the tyranny of what Bateson (1972) described as the pathology of operating from a single position.

## THE PREMISES OF SELF-RELATIONS

With these general distinctions in mind, we are now ready to examine how self-relations theory approaches the question of identity. There are three basic premises.

### 1. Self as Consciousness: The Principle of Beingness.

The first premise is meant as an alternative to the three major causal metaphors used in psychotherapy — namely, (1) you are your past (personal history); (2) you are your biology; or (3) you are your social context (ethnicity, gender, family, etc.). Self-relations acknowledges that these are immensely important factors in shaping your experience, and that you must come to terms with each of them. Like ignoring money in modern times, ignoring them is the kiss of death. But if you make any of them primary, you'll also go down. So, while respecting the importance of personal history, biology, and social place, self-relations says that you are something more: You are a one-of-a-kind being of consciousness.

This can be expressed as the principle of beingness:

1. The beingness of life is distinctively present in each person.

Its corollaries are:

2. When the direct experience of beingness is ignored, denied, or cursed in a person, symptoms are likely to develop.
3. To alleviate symptoms and relieve suffering, first connect with the basic goodness of beingness in a person.

The felt sense of distinct beingness is represented in Figure 13.1 by a simple circle, to indicate an existence ("ex" and "sisto," "stand" — to stand out). The point is that you really do exist as a human being. Your beingness is blessed. To forget or to ignore this leads to great suffering.

This may sound a bit esoteric, so let me give a few simple examples. If you were to meet my young daughter, Zoe, I could say to you, "Behold Zoe con-

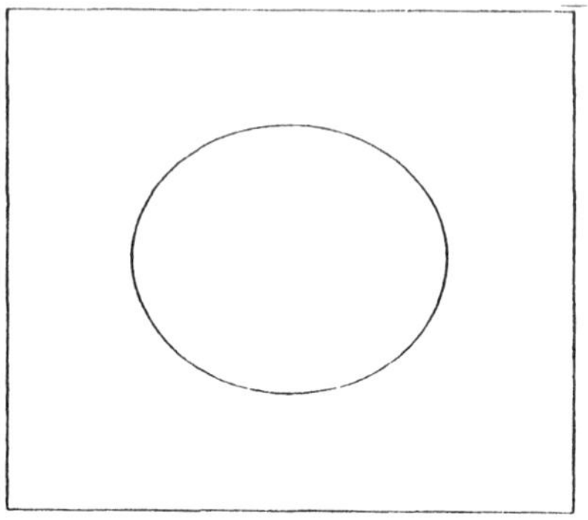

Figure 13.1.
A being is distinguished in consciousness.

sciousness!" and you would get it. You would understand that she's no story, she's no description — she's consciousness itself, she's the real thing! Or if you've ever had the privilege of sitting with a person dying, you probably felt a deep consciousness in his or her process of letting go. A client of mine recently spoke of her struggle to come to terms with her dying father. He had been a terribly abusive man all her life, violating her in many ways. She had had no contact with him for years, but visited him upon hearing that he was dying of cancer. When she saw him on his deathbed, she was shocked to see that his mask of hatred and violence had dissolved, and a gentle, lonely man was exposed. She described it like the scene at the end of *Return of the Jedi*, when Darth Vader ("Dark Father") is unmasked to reveal his atrophied human face. Her heart felt opened, but her behavior was still paralyzed by what had happened over the years. In the therapy session, she struggled to reconcile the lifelong image of her father and her last experiential sensing of the consciousness behind the image.

In a similar way, we all become caught in fixed images or static stories that obscure and deny the dynamic life force pulsating through everything. It is easy to become seduced to fixating on the image, and more difficult to feel through it to the self as consciousness. But I believe that this is one of our challenges as therapists — to sense and reconnect consciousness to itself.

The experience of beingness is first known via *blessings* from influential others. Most people can remember someone in their lives — a family member, teacher, or friend — who really saw them as special and unique. This is not a cognitive event; it is about seeing and calling forth the spirit of life that infuses each person. Blessings are crucial acts in the emergence of each person into the world. Without them, love and other skillful human acts are not possible.

The opposite of a blessing is a *curse*. Curses are prominent in most traumatic events that are the forerunners of many symptoms. A trauma typically involves not only a physical violation, but also a curse: The perpetrator invades and imprints life-denying ideas such as "You exist only to serve me," "You are stupid," "You deserve to be punished," "You are unlovable," and so forth. Self-relations refers to these events as "invasions by aliens," to emphasize that such ideas are not intrinsic to a person. They represent a sort of autoimmune disease in the "psychological immune system" — the part of a person that is needed to differentiate what's "me" from what's "alien to me." In other words, violence tears the "sheathing" that surrounds a being, and through the tear pour the aliens.[3] A person almost inevitably comes to misidentify these alienating ideas as his or her own and to act accordingly. Self-relations looks to discriminate alienating ideas from self-affirming ideas, and suggests methods by which a person may "externalize" these aliens and reconnect with internally resonant descriptions (cf. White & Epson, 1990).

Children rely exclusively on blessings at first to experience their beingness. But as they mature, they develop the possibility for knowing their beingness via self-generated means. Self-relations terms such methods *centering practices*, and is interested in identifying which ones might work for a given person. Such practices — such as walking, meditating, talking to a friend, or creating art — bring a person to a calming, nonintellectual center of being. Through

---

[3] The sheathing that surrounds each being can be seen graphically in the response of young children to strangers or unfamiliar situations. A three-year-old may be exuberant and completely outgoing while playing at home with friends or family, but may show great changes when a stranger arrives. Everyone has seen how such a child may grow shy and hide behind a parent's protective body while sizing up the stranger. Because a child's sheathing is so delicate, a parent is responsible for shielding it from events that might tear it. It is in this way that the idea of a "tear in the sheathing" is meant.

a combination of blessings and centering practices, a person may overcome the curses of alienation and recover the primacy of beingness.

**2. Self as Relational Field: The Principle of Belongingness.**

Self-relations suggests that the beingness of self is revealed in two complementary domains: (1) *a relational field* and (2) *a relational form*. The first is a felt sense of belonging to something bigger, to a field of consciousness; the second is a dynamic form of relationship playing through that field. To get a sense of the experience of self in a relational field, one might inquire along the following lines:

1. When do you feel most like yourself?
2. When you need to reconnect with yourself, what do you do?
3. When is life not a problem for you?

Typical responses might include playing or listening to music, going for a walk, being in nature, talking with good friends, reading, knitting, creating or performing art, dancing, and so forth. These activities constitute what I call "traditions of the aesthetic." They are traditions in that they are pulled from a large body of cultural practices that have been developed over many years, and aesthetic because of the nature of the experiences generated by such practices. If asked to describe what existential or phenomenological shifts occur during such events, most people will include responses such as decreased internal dialogue, timelessness, and an expansion of a felt sense of self. If you ask where the sense of self ends during such experiences, people will look at you quizzically, because no sharp boundary exists. *This expanded feeling of self beyond boundaries of skin and either-or ideology, while maintaining a center, is the experience of self as relational field.*

This relational field is described by the principle of belongingness:

1. The consciousness of self belongs to (or is part of) a larger relational field.

The corollaries are:

2. When a person experiences a sustained "break in belonging" to a relational field, symptoms are likely to develop.

3. To relieve suffering and reconcile symptomatic conflict, reconnect consciousness to its relational fields.

This relationship may be represented in the traditional figure/ground or figure-field diagram (see Figure 13.2). The relational field may be spiritual ("I belong to a higher power, and he or she or it moves through me"); organismic ("I belong to nature, and it moves through me"); social ("I belong to my marriage/family/culture, and it permeates my consciousness"); or psychological ("My experience/perspective is embedded within a larger field of experiences/ memories/archetypes, and they guide/inform me").

Self-relations makes the observation that this experience of the field is present when life is working for a person — when life is not defined or perceived as a problem. At the same time, a person struggling with a symptom has experienced a "break in belonging" to the field; such a person does not feel a connection or sense of connection to a power or place greater than himself or herself. The experience of self is contracted and split, and a unified field supporting self and other is not felt. This cutoff from context leads to identification with the intellect and its fear-driven strategies of control and domination (and experiences of being out of control and reactive), rather than to curiosity and connectedness. Again, this is the basis for fundamentalism.

The disconnection from field occurs in many ways, most of them involuntary. Some disconnections are the healthy first steps to individuation, as when an adolescent rebels against his or her family. Thus, breaks in belonging are not necessarily bad; they are inevitable steps of separation, and are ideally followed by a reunion with the field. But some experiences (such as traumas) don't allow such reconnection to occur. If the conditions or violence or trauma prevail, a sustained break occurs in which the person or experience is split off from its larger contexts of resources.

In this regard, symptoms are seen in part as unsuccessful attempts to reconnect with the field. For example, an addiction — whether to drugs or alcohol, food, sex, or cults — is initially an experience of losing one's self to a larger field. However, because the person attempts to get rid of part or all of his or her personal identity in this process, the results are emptiness and depression, followed by a downward spiral of further attempts to reconnect with the field by self-destructive activities. In this way, one part of the symptom is an attempt to return to the ground of being, while another is a reenactment of the violence that exiled one from the field in the first place.

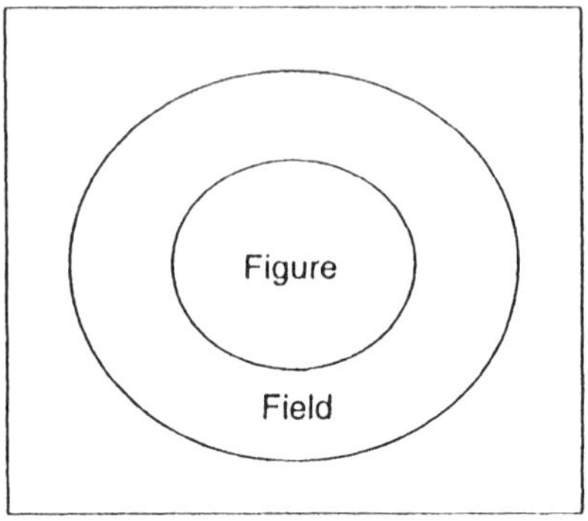


Figure 13.2.
Each distinction of consciousness belongs to a larger field.

Thus, a major focus of self-relations is on the nonviolent restoration of the felt sense of the field. It gently seeks to help a person unloose the grip of egoic control and rediscover the dynamic ground of natural being. In any performance art — dance, music, acting, aikido, sculpting, writing — one will hear from an artist the important of "relaxing" and feeling the rhythm. This is not the experience of a stuporous drool, but rather one of feeling centered and grounded in a way that allows the presence of the life force to move through one's being. In psychotherapy we help clients do this via many relational methods, including joining and validating experience, being in rhythm with the clients, encouraging centering and a felt sense of experience, and so forth. Disciplines such as prayer and meditation, service, and other mindfulness practices are explored and gently encouraged. In this regard, therapy is a process of reconnecting a person with his or her natural ground of being, so the sense of self as a relational field can be felt and used to gently ground and guide the person's activities.

**3. Self as Relational Differences: The Principle of Relatedness.**

In time ("successive moments of now"), the relational self comes to know itself by proceeding through conversations between relational differences: different positions, different truths, different people, different times or places, different values, and so on. As Bateson (1979) repeatedly emphasized, *mind is relationship,* and *difference is the basic unit of mind.* Self-relations suggests the self as the experience of a dynamic relatedness between differences. This is described as the principle of relatedness:

1. To learn (or become) who you are, relatedness between differences is required.

Its corollaries are as follows:

2. When a "break in relatedness" persists, the experience of self disappears, the fundamentalist ego-mind reigns, and symptoms are likely to arise.
3. To reduce suffering and to reconcile symptoms, reestablish dynamic relatedness between positions of identity.

Self as the conversation of differences is represented in Figure 13.3 by the simple figure of two interconnected circles. In terms of psychological identity, this may be described in terms of a subject-object relationship, in which the person is identified with one position (the subject, or what we might call the "me" position), while directing his or her attention to another position (the object, or what we might call the "not me" position). Thus, the relational self is a pattern of connections between "me" and "not me," experienced in a relational field.

Other pairs of relational differences relevant to psychotherapy include the following:

self (me, us, I)/other (you, them, it)
good/bad
power/love
inside/outside
masculine/feminine
healthy/sick
problem/solution
therapist/client
thinking/feeling
mind/body
conscious/unconscious

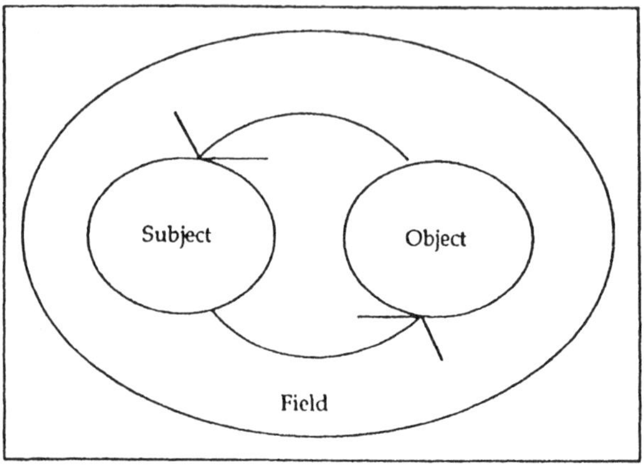


Figure 13.3.
The relational self as the pattern that connects differences.

In healthy situations, these relational differences operate in a conversational connectedness, the sort of "I-thou" relationship described by Martin Buber (1923/1958). In intimacy, there is an experience of a "me," a "you," and the relational self of "us" that is felt when both the "I" and "thou" are validated. The experience of therapeutic trance (Gilligan, 1987) reflects a similar "self-(other) self" relatedness. The fictional terms of "conscious-unconscious" are provided, the suggestions to do something while just letting it happen ("Your hand can lift involuntarily") are given, and the resulting experience of "It's happening but I'm not making it happen" (e.g., "My hand is lifting, but it's old Mr. or Ms. Not Me that's lifting it! ") is central to every hypnotic happening.

The examples above suggest that relatedness between differences is played out in different domains: Relational differences require a container, or a "temenos," as Jung (1916/1971) described it. The boundaries of "mind" may be intrapersonal or interpersonal; "mind" could be the individual, the couple, the family, the group, or the nation. For therapy purposes, self-relations generally emphasizes three types of relatedness required for conscious learning. The first is the *interpersonal,* involving the "I" and the "thou" described by Martin Buber. The second is the *embodied intrapersonal,* a felt sense of vertical relatedness between the cognitive/social self in the "head" and the emotional/archetypal consciousness in the "belly." The third is also intrapersonal — a horizontal *interhemispheric relatedness* required for experience to be processed and integrated (cf. Shapiro, 1995; Rossi, 1977). Self-relations posits that a sustained "break in relatedness" in any of these domains will result in an image of self that is "frozen in time," unable to learn, and thus likely to produce symptoms.

In problem situations, relatedness between different positions is denied or ignored. An interpersonal "thou" becomes an objectified "it," and the "beings in the belly" are reduced to an inhuman "other" to be removed by any means necessary. But as Jung (1957/1967) pointed out:

> We think we can congratulate ourselves on . . . having left the [archetypal] gods behind . . . but we are still as much possessed by autonomous psychic contents as if they were Olympians. Today they are called phobias, obsessions, and so forth; in a word, neurotic symptoms. The gods have become diseases; *Zeus no longer rules Olympus but rather the solar plexus.* (par. 54; emphasis added)

When things are working, life moves through us as we move through life, and is represented by the psyche in terms of different positions. The key is to find ways to respect and value each position as it moves through its ever-changing forms. This is a difficult process, as anyone involved in an intimate relationship soon realizes. It requires a centering within one's beingness, a grounding in one's field, and an openness to dialogue. Even under the best conditions, imperfection reigns. But as T. S. Eliot (1963) encouraged, humility is endless. Or as Bill Wilson (1967), the founder of Alcoholics Anonymous, noted: "This is no success story in the ordinary sense of the word. It is a story of suffering transmuted, under grace, into gradual spiritual progress" (p. 35).

As we come back to relatedness, our experience of the relational self as dialogue develops. Holding the tension between differences nurtures a deeper harmony and capacity to act with love and integrity. At some point in the cycle, what Jung (1916/1971) termed the "transcendent function" occurs: The opposites integrate into a united form, where a difficult contradiction moves into a beautiful paradox — a movement Jung described as the central means of individuation of Self. At that moment, we realize that the kingdom of God is within.

## A SELF-RELATIONS MODEL OF HOW SYMPTOMS DEVELOP

The three principles of beingness, belongingness, and relatedness suggest questions to hold for sensing a person and not getting trapped in a problem-defined self:

1. Can you feel the beingness?
2. Can you sense the belongingness?
3. Can you hold the tension of the opposites?

Conversely, the principles suggest that symptoms reflect three types of sustained breaks: a "break in beingness" (and the awareness of goodness or blessedness), a "break in belonging" to something bigger (spiritual, organismic, social, psychological), and a "break in relatedness" between differences.

From these premises we can build a working model for self-relations. Figure 13.4a represents a healthy learning situation involving three aspects of a relational self: (1) the *normal self*, (2) the *experiential/archetypal self* and (3) *influential others*.[4] The *normal self* refers to the basic, everyday egoic sense of self that a person is aware of when life is not a problem. It is the cognitive/social self, based on the person's present age, and centered in the head. It includes competencies, resources associations with present social others, skills, and multiple perspectives. It uses frames and models to plan, evaluate, and otherwise try to manage the world of experience. It is "normal" in the sense that it is what most people would think of as their typical sense of self. In a symptom, this sense of self disappears, contracts, dissociates, or is otherwise nullified. Some clients will talk about just wanting to get back to their "normal self."

The *experiential/archetypal self* lives in the belly. It is experiential in that it is a directly felt sense of self, and archetypal in that it is connected to many generations of psychological experiences. Some traditions call it the *center*, others call it *soul*. Self-relations asserts that life moves through a person (except when it doesn't), radiating out from this center. It assumes that this order of mind is, at its roots, collective and transpersonal. In healthy situations, there is

[4] Editor's note: In later writings (see Gilligan, 1987), the "normal self" was changed to "cognitive self," and the "experiential/archetypal self" was changed to "somatic self."

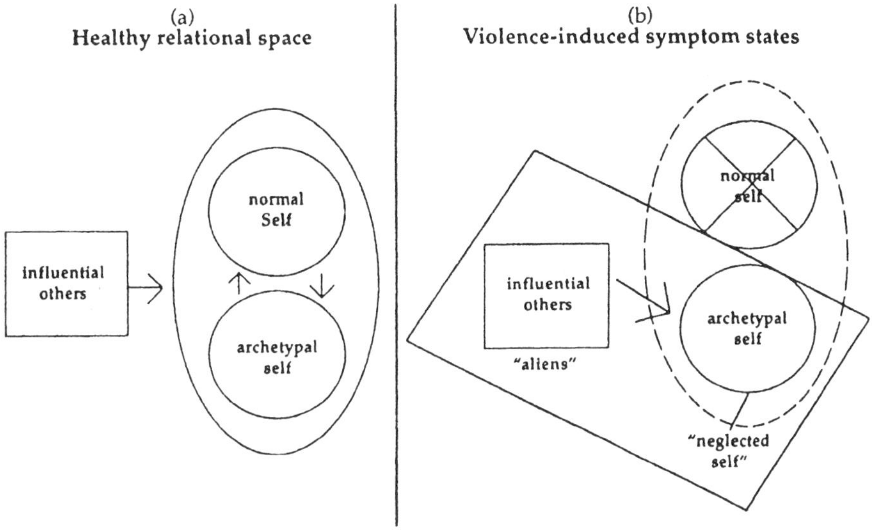


Figure 13.4.
Relational space of the normal self, archetypal self, and the influential others: a) healthy relational space and b) violence-induced symptom states.

no fixed text or single image tied to this center. It is not an inner child, although the inner child may at times be one of the "beings in the belly," as Isabel Allende (in Toms, 1994) described them. Just as children have multiple forms of expression moving through them, so does the archetypal self in the belly. Whenever a particular form becomes fixated in a person's expression — as the Mental Research Institute folks say, whenever "the same damn thing happens over and over again" (see Watzlawick, Weakland, & Fisch, 1974) — it can be said that the archetypal self is disconnected from the cognitive self. This becomes the main objective of self-relations work: to restore the spirit of relatedness that joins the two selves into a relational self.

The normal self and the archetypal self constitute a dual-processing model of the relational self. As Epstein (1994) has effectively argued, there is tremendous support for this type of model of human processing. He summarizes the many descriptions of this dual processing, including "holistic-analytical," "affective-logical," "receptive-active," "nonverbal-verbal," "experiential-rational," and "narrative-analytical."

A third aspect of the relational field can be described as *influential others*. One's sense of identity is always a function of the intrapersonal relatedness between the normal self and archetypal self, as well as the interpersonal and transpersonal relatedness between oneself and influential others. These others may include social individuals, such as parents, friends, enemies, children, spouses, and so forth; they may also include spiritual beings, such as one's sense of a higher power. The point is that one is always being influenced and influencing identity via these interpersonal or transpersonal connections. Self-relations is especially interested in identifying which influential others are in a person's current circuitry, and what types of conversations are taking place.

Of special interest is whether these influential others offer blessings or curses of one's beingness. In healthy situations, a person is seen and blessed by influential others; in unhealthy situations, curses reign, and self-denigration and other alienating practices are the order of the day.

Thus, as Figure 13.4a illustrates, a healthy relational process involves life-affirming processes at both interpersonal and intrapersonal levels. At early developmental stages these two levels are barely distinguishable, since the normal cognitive/social self is very undeveloped, such that the interpersonal others (e.g., parents) must fill in for and model the normal self. Maturity involves gradually developing one's own unique cognitive/social self that can both be "a part of" and "apart from" influential others, such that a person's intrapersonal relatedness becomes an increasingly important factor.

As Figure 13.4b illustrates, a symptomatic self occurs when one or more influential others invade the boundaries of self, leading to a break in relatedness between the cognitive and archetypal selves, as well as a break in belonging of the self to its larger field. These breaks are what allow alienating ideas ("curses") to be internalized. If processing of the traumatic event is inhibited, the alienating ideas are mistaken for one's own voice, and the traumatic relationship is mistaken for one's identity.

An identity based on traumatic experience leads to three types of symptoms (cf. Herman, 1992). First, the person's normal sense of self is constricted, dissociated, fragmented, or otherwise inaccessible. Second, the archetypal self is gripped in a state of "neuromuscular lock," a frozen state distinguished by out-of-control emotions, hyperarousal, hypervigilance, somatization, and regression. Third, the person cannot shut out intrusive, negative images and voices that define the self as bad, unlovable, deserving of violence. and so forth. Thus, in the language of self-relations, the normal self becomes disconnected; the archetypal self becomes neglected, literalized, and frozen into a fixed form; and the influential others lock into alien(ating) presences.

## A PROTOTYPE MODEL FOR SELF-RELATIONS WORK

Self-relations suggests some basic interventions that may be helpful in psychotherapy. The first is dissolving rigid attachment to a single text or description, so that other frames may be made equally available. The second is returning consciousness to a felt sense of the relational field, so that a person has a direct sense of belonging to the community, to the environment, and to an intelligence and power greater than the isolated ego. The third is reconciling or at least resolving the relational differences between the "me" and "not me" positions in a person's identity.

In the development of practices along these lines, a simple seven-step prototype has emerged. This is not a fixed prescription for how to do therapy with every person, but rather a pattern that suggests coherent principles that can be applied in various ways. In applying this model, it is important to reiterate the aesthetic base of self-relations: *The goal is to find a middle way between the alienation of intellectual discourse and the inflation of catharsis or regression processes.* The client should be helped to stay in the present, while also feeling a variety of experiences via the "other self." To allow for the emergence of this processing of the relational self, the relational connectedness between therapist and client must be developed and maintained throughout the application of the technique. This is not a model to be explored without a felt sense of ongoing collectedness; to put it bluntly, if you can't get it, don't use the model. This is difficult to convey in writing, but crucial to understand in practice. Based in part on the earlier legacy of Milton Erickson, a main focus of the method is on gently opening mind-body circuits, to move language from an "in-the-head" intellectual analysis to an "in-the-body" felt sense that evokes multiple levels. It should be used with a soft rather than a hard intensity, with relational grounding and nonverbal pacing. Many of the ideas, especially those of "aliens" and "neglected selves," will be unhelpful if they are not apprehended in the more primary felt sense.

With these considerations in mind, let us consider each step in turn.

### Step 1: Identify the Problem

In this first step, the therapist seeks to identify what the problem is, where and when it is occurring, and what specifically happens that moves an experience from mere unpleasantness (e.g., "I feel sad") to an identity-defining, self-disturbing symptom. The therapist's frame is something like this: "A funny thing happens on the way to this person's becoming more of his or her self. What is it?" Thus, after receiving the client's general description of the problem, the therapist may ask something like this: "If I were accompanying you on a day [or week, or month] in your life, where and when would I see this problem occur?" Clients often have difficulty getting specific, or may say something like "It happens all the time," so the therapist may need to be gently persistent — perhaps by asking, "When did it happen recently? Where was it really disturbing?" The movement into specific times and places helps to move the experience of the problem back into the body and other important realities, so this step is crucial.

As the person identifies a time when the problem occurred, the therapist slows down the processing to try to get a moment-by-moment, frame-by-frame description of the problem sequence. Clients will frequently rush through frames, so the therapist must try gently to get the details of both external behaviors ("And then he did that") and internal experiences ("And then I felt angry" or "Then I thought I was wrong"). The basic idea guiding the therapist is that circumstances at some point trigger the activation of the neglected self, which prompts the person to "leave time" (i.e., "successive moments of now"). This dissociation sticks the person in a loop; since he or she has left time, life moves from "one damn thing after the next" to "the same damn thing over and over." This is the "break in belongingness" as well as the "break in relatedness" that moves a difficult event to a symptom-producing clinical problem.

Here is an abbreviated example of this part of the interview:

CLIENT: Well, I guess the last time I got anxious was this morning when my friend came over.

THERAPIST: Your friend came over . . . May I ask your friend's name?

CLIENT: Bill.

THERAPIST: Bill. And before Bill came over, how were you doing?

CLIENT: Okay. I was feeling okay that morning, just making some phone calls and stuff.

THERAPIST: You were feeling pretty good, and then this event with Bill started happening. When exactly — if you can just take a moment to relax and remember back — when exactly did you feel the first moment of disturbance? Was it before Bill came, or was it when he actually was there, that you began to feel the first suggestion that the problem of anxiety was going to happen? [The therapist softens the tone to allow experiential accessing.]

CLIENT: [Pauses to think] Well, I began to feel a little weird as soon as he walked in.

THERAPIST: As soon as he walked in. And where were you?

CLIENT: I was sitting at my desk.

The therapist now asks a series of detail questions about the other furniture, what each person was wearing, what specifically was said, what was felt in the body at each point, and so forth. This procedure is an outgrowth of Ericksonian hypnotherapy procedures (see Gilligan, 1987), whereby associational questions are asked in a hypnotic-like focus to move attention to experiential revivification of the problem sequence, so that the emotional/imaginal/psychological components of the sequence can be heightened and utilized. (Remember, trance is the repoeticization of experience.)

**Step 2: Identify and Somatically Locate the Neglected Self**

At some point in the problem sequence, a felt sense of the problem will begin to develop in the client. This marks the appearance of the neglected self. An easy way to identify the neglected self is to ask the client to fill in the following statement: "If only I didn't experience/do [or could get rid of] X, then this really wouldn't be a problem." X marks the spot of the neglected self. For example:

- If only I didn't feel so inhibited, I would be successful.
- If only I didn't feel so angry, I could get on with my life.
- If only she wasn't so cold (and I didn't feel rejected as a result), our marriage wouldn't be such a problem.

The idea is that when this unacceptable experience or behavior arises, the person has to "leave town" or dissociate, because he or she cannot hold the tension between the opposites — between this experience and his or her egoic normal self. In other words, this is where the break in relatedness occurs, and where symptomatic behavior is likely to arise. Thus, self-relations seeks to bring the neglected self back into the field of the relational self in three subsidiary steps.

*Step A: Locate the Somatic Center.*

The therapist should ask the client: "When the problem is present, where in your body do you most feel its center of disturbance [or discomfort]?" Many people point immediately to their stomach, solar plexus, or heart area, even before conscious or verbal awareness has developed. If a person has difficulty understanding the question or feeling anything, a bit of relaxation helps to open awareness of somatic sensation. A major purpose of locating the neglected self is to form a relationship with it, so it may be both "apart from" the ego identity (to reduce what Jung (1928/1971, p. 88) called "psychic inflation") and "a part of" the relational self (to reduce "alienation" from the archetypal self). When the neglected self is brought into the body, experience is brought back into the reality of time ("successive moments"), where change is a constant process. Locating it in a specific center causes it to lose its amorphous quality and takes a specific "otherness" that allows relatedness.

*Step B: Identify an Age.*

The archetypal/experiential self has many identities and many ages. In fact, through its center in the body flows a progression of different psychological forms. A symptom represents a point where that flow of the psyche through the belly has been arrested, and its form fixed and "frozen in time." Reintroduction of trauma cues can reactivate the symptom, and it may be experienced without conscious understanding or meaning as an out-of-control feeling in the body that must be ignored, denied, repressed, or otherwise disconnected. In order to allow it to enter the change process of life, the self-relations therapist not only identifies its location but asks the person, "If you were to let a number come to mind that represents an age for that experience in your [identified somatic location], what number do you become aware of?" The language here is somewhat hypnotic, as should be the therapist's soft but focused attention. If a person tries intellectually to guess a number or has difficulty letting one develop, more relaxation is in order, so that the age can flow freely from the neglected self into conscious awareness.

Again, the point is not that the neglected self is always that age. It may help to point out to the client that a person's center carries every age and every emotion and every psychological form, but a particular one (such as the one the client keeps coming back to in the symptom) stays until it is accepted and loved. Acceptance allows release, and release allows new psychological ages and identities to emerge.

*Step C: Shift Pronoun from "It" to "He or She."*

A crucial question in psychological relationship, either internal or external, is whether the other is regarded as an "it" or a "thou." Self-relations looks to move the neglected self from an "it" that needs to be controlled or otherwise disregarded to a "thou" that can be accepted. For example, say the client responds to the question regarding age with the number "Three." The therapist may continue: "So ['seeing' and sensing the person at three] ... *she* is three." A number of clients will respond to such a comment, when it is delivered with appropriate empathic qualities and soft attentional focus, with gentle tears or other emotional softenings. Such a response will usually be experienced as coming from someplace other than one's intellectual "in control" normal self.

Other clients may feel something stirring inside when the neglected self is directly named, but may cognitively be confused and ask, "What do you mean, *she*?" The therapist may respond:

> Well, I mean that there appears to be something or someone other than yourself that gets active when the problem kicks in. If I'm hearing you correctly, you're saying that when the problem develops, one of the things that happens is you get an intense unpleasant feeling centered in your body that doesn't feel that it's coming from you or even belongs to you. Is that right? [Client usually agrees.] And it seems one of the most disturbing things is that when that feeling develops, somehow *you* feel like you disappear or disconnect or feel out of control. Is that right? [Client usually agrees.] So I guess an important question is this: If that response isn't coming from your normal self, who is it and where is it coming from? [Brief pause to let this sink in.]
>
> There's obviously a lot of ways of talking and thinking about it, and certainly the more traditional way is to think of that response as an "it" that has no meaning, that should be ignored or destroyed or gotten rid of. It seems, if I'm hearing you correctly, that you've tried that many times and have failed miserably. It keeps coming back over and over, more and more. ... It may be helpful to consider that the feeling belongs to *her*, to another aspect of you that is listening even right now.

> . . . She has her own feelings, her own thoughts and images, her own way of listening. . . . She's been ignored for a long time, but it doesn't seem like she can be denied any further.

Other comments may elaborate this theme of thinking of the neglected self as a separate, autonomous being. If this sounds too strange, it should be reminded that appreciation of, and relationship with this, "other self" is the basis for much of artistic expression. When the therapist delivers such comments in a relational, experiential, absorbing manner, the client has a hypnotic-like response of feeling that another part of his or her self is activated and listening.

**Step 3: Activate and Locate the Normal Self.**

One of the great dangers of attending to the neglected self is that one can become identified *as* it, rather than feeling a way to be *with* it. For example, a person may feel an emotion so strongly that his or her identity regresses to an earlier age. The goal in self-relations is to feel the presence of this neglected self in one's center, but to also stay present with one's normal cognitive/social self, thereby generating a felt field that holds and harmonizes both. Thus, it is important to activate and shift attention to the normal self periodically, especially when a client seems to be getting overwhelmed by and drawn into the neglected self. This method is akin to a form of systematic desensitization, in which the aversive stimulus (the neglected self) is progressively paired with a positive image (the competencies of the normal self).

The shift to addressing the normal self should generally be accompanied by a shift in nonverbal communication to a less hypnotic, more straightforward, but still engaging and gentle tone:

THERAPIST: So *she's* three . . . and, by the way, how old are you, in reality?
CLIENT: [Makes a nonverbal shift, coming out of light trance] I'm 43.
THERAPIST: Yes, I can see that you're 43. And can you tell me, what's the best thing about being this age compared to three?

A majority of people will say that the best thing about their present age is that they have more freedom, more ability to choose. Further questions to reconnect a person to his or her normal self include associations to work, present family and friends, interests, and so forth. It is important for the therapist to be connecting with the client relatively nonhypnotically during this time, or the client may slip back into the neglected self.

**Step 4: Identify and Externalize Aliens.**

A major obstacle to activating or maintaining the normal self is the presence of *alienating ideas*. This can be observed when clients appear unable to stay connected with themselves or the therapist; they withdraw, become critical, shut down, or the like. Such a "break in relatedness" signals that the alienating ideas have "taken over" the cognitive self.

I often approach the idea of "alien possession" with an "Irish twinkle" that conveys a gentle humor along with gentle, serious compassion. For example, with a person caught in negative internal dialogue, the therapist may say:

THERAPIST: As we're talking, I'm wondering if you're aware of *them*.

CLIENT: Them?

THERAPIST: Yes, it seems like you're coming under the influence of aliens.

CLIENT: Aliens? [Looking at therapist, not sure if therapist is kidding or serious, but intrigued.]

THERAPIST: [With mock somberness] I'm afraid so ... my professional opinion is that you're possessed by aliens. [Pauses, then smiles gently.] I'm only half kidding, but it seemed like when we were just talking all of sudden you weren't quite present. It seemed like some other presence came in and you had to leave, to withdraw, to go away. Did you feel that?

CLIENT: Yes ... I felt bad all of a sudden.

THERAPIST: Yes, I saw that. Are you aware of what those voices or ideas are saying about you then, or even right now?

CLIENT: They're saying it was my fault. [Other alienating ideas might be "You're unlovable," "You're stupid ... You're never going to be okay," etc.]

THERAPIST: That it's your fault ... Whose voices are those, anyway?

CLIENT: Well, mine, of course.

THERAPIST: [Gently, with serious focus] Where did you ever get the idea that those voices are yours?

CLIENT: Well, whose else could they be?

THERAPIST: I'm not sure, but they sure don't feel to me like *your* voices ... Because I notice that when they show up, you have to leave ... When they activate, you seem to feel smaller and less of a person. Is that right? [Client nods] So whoever they are, they sure as hell don't seem like they represent you ... I use the term "aliens" partly humorously, because you can't survive in these situations without at least a little bit of humor, but also with great seriousness, to suggest that whatever happened to you, you got invaded by something that led you to believe that the negative stuff that was conveyed to you was your voice. [With Irish twinkle] But you may be possessed by aliens . . . if so, there's a way out.

CLIENT: What's that?

THERAPIST: Reconnecting with that part of you that was wounded and had to be abandoned. Because when the relationship between you and her [the neglected self] is disconnected or abused, a break in relationship occurs — the elevators stop going up and down — and the aliens come. But there are other times when you feel that good connection between the cognitive stuff in the head and the feeling stuff in your belly — the elevators are going up and down. [The therapist might ask about times when the client doesn't feel alienated — i.e., the traditions of the aesthetic practices described above to point out that sometimes the aliens aren't around. The suggestion can then be made that such experiences reflect times when there is a connection between the egoic center and the archetypal self.]

Many clients find the idea of "aliens" exceptionally helpful. Like a meditation technique that teaches a person to detach from the thoughts in his or her mind, it helps to free a person from identifying with negative influences, thereby allowing reconnection to a calm "thinking center" in the belly. Again, the term is meant poetically and is designed to generate both lightness and seriousness, so the therapist needs to present it in such a context. The intent of naming aliens is not to give primary focus to them, but to differentiate them from a person's own voice and externalize them. The more primary relationship is the reconnection of the normal self and the archetypal self.

**Step 5: Connect Normal Self and Archetypal Self.**

When a person's consciousness is not subjugated by alienating influences, it is free to reestablish the circuitry of the relational self. The present model uses a scaling technique to identify the intensity levels of the normal self, the neglected self, and the spirit of connection between them. The therapist asks the client:

1. On a scale of 1 to 10, where 1 is the low end and 10 the high end, how much do you feel the presence of your neglected self in your solar plexus right now? Just let a number come to your mind.
2. On a scale of 1 to 10, where 1 is the low end and 10 the high end, how much do you feel the presence of your normal, everyday self in

your head (looking out from behind your eyes) right now? Just let a number come to your mind.

3. On a scale of 1 to 10, where 1 is the low end and 10 the high end, how much do you feel a sense of connection between the normal self in the head and the neglected self in the belly? Just let a number come to mind.

Again, the goal here is to foster a felt sense of each relational component. Once this has developed, the therapist can ask whether the client would like to experiment with lowering or raising an intensity value 1 or 2 points to see what happens. For example, if the normal self is at 5 and the neglected self is at 8, the client will often feel out of control. If the therapist helps the client to go inside and gently "shift knobs on the intensity controls," the normal self may be moved to 7 and the neglected self to 6. This small difference in relative values can often make a significant difference in the person's overall quality of experience.

When the therapist asks about the level of connectedness between the two selves, some clients will look blank, as if the idea of such a connection is entirely new. This is often the case; the normal self and the neglected self frequently have little or no history of coexistence. When a person feels normal, the archetypal self is ignored and forgotten; when the archetypal self is activated (i.e., whenever identity is at issue, via symptoms), the normal self disconnects (and is hence replaced by alienating influences). Thus, the goal of self-relations therapy is to examine what happens when a person feels a connectedness between the two selves. This is a structural description of wholeness, intimacy, love, and cooperation.

When the felt or "telepathic" sense of connection is made, the person will usually look different; a sense of beauty will often imbue his or her being. The person will feel aware of but not identified with each self. It is important to note that the connection is not the ego speaking (down) to the "inner child," but to a felt spirit that runs in full orbit.

**Step 6: Return to Original Problem Sequence.**

Since a problem degrades into a symptom when a sustained break in relatedness occurs, a reparation of the break will allow a person to move though a problem sequence without becoming symptomatic. The therapist may suggest that the client take a few minutes to close his or her eyes, feel the connection between the selves, and then imaginally go back through the problem sequence (as defined in the first step), this time keeping the telepathic inner connection.

**Step 7: Identify Further Tasks.**

An old saying laments, "We abandon our souls a hundred times, no, a thousand times each day." Thus, self-relations therapy is not a cure-all procedure, but the beginning of a tradition of being in relation with one's center regardless of circumstances. Much practice is needed, and the therapist should always be exploring with the client workable practices for continuing to nurture this tradition. We cannot hope never to disconnect, but we can grow stronger and more gentle in our commitment to keep coming to the relational self.

## CONCLUSION

This chapter began with a question of identity: "Who the hell do you think you are, anyway?" Now we can see that self-relations suggests that the answer to this perennial question is always dynamic and always relational. When beingness, belonging, or relatedness is broken, bad things happen. Psychotherapy can be seen as a devotional practice of restoring the sense of beingness of the relational self, in its field and dynamic form.

Walking this path, we are reminded of T. S. Eliot (1963, p. 207):

> Who then devised the torment? Love.
> Love is the unfamiliar Name
> Behind the hands that wove
> The intolerable shirt of flame
> Which human power cannot remove.
> We only live, only suspire
> Consumed by either fire or fire.

As we learn to hold the fire in the belly, we are guided further by Kahlil Gibran (1923, p. 51) in *The Prophet*:

> Among the hills, when you sit in the cool shade of the white poplars, sharing the peace and serenity of distant fields and meadows — then let your heart say in silence, "God rests in reason."
>
> And when the storm comes, and the mighty wind shakes the forest,

and thunder and lightning proclaim the majesty of the sky then let your heart say in awe, "God moves in passion."

And since you are a breath in God's sphere, and a leaf in God's forest, you too should rest in reason and move in passion.

May the force be with you.

# Chapter 14

# THE PROBLEM IS THE SOLUTION: THE PRINCIPLE OF SPONSORSHIP IN PSYCHOTHERAPY[1]

"Wake up to find out
that you are the eyes of the world."
— Robert Hunter

In the movie "Pleasantville," two adolescent siblings from the 1990s find themselves transported into a 1950s black-and-white TV sitcom landscape based on the old show "Father Knows Best." While on the surface everything seems perfect, there is no depth, mystery, color, or soul in this world. Everyone lives in an enclosed "pleasant trance" devoid of real liveliness, a sort of mindless "brave new world." The two "visitors" instigate a series of happenings that precipitate awakenings in each person, including themselves. Each awakening occurs when a person connects with a hidden or undeveloped part of his or her being. For a teenage athlete, it happens via love and romance; for the kids' "mother," it comes from discovering the sensuality of her body; for the father, it comes from recognizing his longings; for the girl, it comes from reading classics; for the boy, it comes from finding his fierceness. In each case, the experience and expression of undeveloped parts of the self transform the person into living "color." They and others around them have to deal with

[1] This essay appeared previously in Jeffrey K. Zeig and Brent B. Geary. 2001. *Handbook of Ericksonian psychotherapy*. Phoenix: Zeig, Tucker, & Theisen.

the myriad responses that arise in response to this awakening.

Pleasantville is all around us. It keeps us asleep through false smiles, violent threats, unspoken fears, disembodied thinking, numbness, consumerism, and other practices of the modern and postmodern world. A corporate woman in a poetry workshop (cited by Whyte, 1994, p. 31) wrote:

> "Ten years ago . . .
> I turned my face for a moment
> And it became my life."

We have all suffered those 10-year "gaps" in our lives, where we thought we were present but then, in hindsight, realized we weren't.

The damming of life cannot continue forever. Sooner or later, the river leaks through, bringing with it a myriad of memories, dreams, and reflections. This can be a frightening time, for the fear in exile is that we will be overwhelmed, perhaps even die, if we allow these currents to wash over and through us. New defenses arise — more dissociation, more compulsive behaviors, more "playing dead," more intellectualization, more violence against self and others — all desperate attempts to regain control and expel the "negative otherness" that presses upon us. At some point, it becomes clear that we're losing the battle — we're dealing with a presence stronger than our ego, and our vaunted defenses no longer can keep separate from it. In desperation, we may turn to a therapist in the hope of fortifying our ego and its defenses.

When clients visit us, how we regard the disturbances in their lives — the experiences and events that are throwing them into "organized chaos" — makes a great deal of difference. The traditional view is generally that we should help the client overcome these "pathological" forces that threaten well-being. This view regards the "problem" as an "enemy" that should be defeated, through any means possible. Milton Erickson (1980a, 1980d) pioneered an entirely different approach, one based on accepting and working with a person's "problems" as unique presences that could, under the proper conditions, be the basis for new learning and growth. For example, a young secretary was utterly convinced that a large gap in her teeth made her ugly and undesirable. Erickson had her learn to squirt water through the gap in her teeth until she was able to hit a distant target. He then got her to wait at the office water cooler to "ambush" a young man (to whom she was attracted) with a squirt of water. One thing led to another, and the couple lived happily ever after.

## The Legacy of Erickson

The legacy of Milton Erickson has been elaborated on and deepened in many ways in the last 20 years. My own work has moved from a more mainstream Ericksonian emphasis (see Gilligan, 1987) to the development of a neo-Ericksonian approach I call self-relations psychotherapy (see Gilligan, 1997). Like Erickson's work, self-relations emphasizes the positive aspects of problems and symptoms. It sees such disturbances of the "normal order" as evidence that "something is waking up" in the life of a person or community. Such disturbances are double-edged crises. On the one side, they are (often hidden) opportunities for major growth. Most of us, for example, can recall negative events — a death, divorce, illness, or addiction — that led to a significant positive change in our lives. On the other side, such disturbances can be very destructive; we *can* get lost in depression, acting out, or other problematic behaviors. Self-relations suggests that the difference lies in whether or not a disturbance can be "sponsored" by a skillful human presence.

The principle and processes of sponsorship are the cornerstone of self-relations. The word "sponsorship" comes from the Latin *spondere*, meaning "to pledge solemnly." So sponsorship is a vow to help a person (including one's self) to use each and every event and experience to awaken to the goodness and gifts of the self, the world, and the connections between the two. Self-relations suggests that experiences that come into a person's life are not yet fully human; they have no human value until the person is able to "sponsor them." Via sponsorship, experiences and behaviors that are problematic may be realized as resources and gifts. In this way, what had been framed and seen as a problem is recognized as a "solution."

The motto for therapeutic sponsorship may be found on the Statue of Liberty in New York Harbor:

> "Give me your tired, your poor,
> Your huddled masses yearning to breathe free,
> The wretched refuse of your teeming shore,
> Send these, the homeless, tempest-tost to me.
> I lift my lamp beside the golden door."
>
> — Emma Lazarus, 1849–1887

In self-relations, this motto refers not only to people, but to experiences and behaviors as well. For example, Fred was an academic who was seeing me for what he described as "low-grade, long-time depression." He arrived at one session complaining of being "a sexual pervert." Taking a sabbatical year off to write and to stay home with his baby son, Fred found himself downloading pornography from the Internet for up to three hours a day. He explained that it took him this long partly because his fear of being "caught" would not allow him to give his credit card number; instead, he would search for sites featuring free "teaser pictures," download them, and then meticulously organize them into a library that had to be constantly updated. I had been working with him for about three months on his presenting problems of feeling depressed and anxious in some work-related matters. He had let me know in general terms about the pornography interests when I previously inquired about his sexual and social life, but had strongly rebuffed my attempts to engage him around those topics.

In bringing it up now, he said it was draining his energy and he desperately wanted to do something about it. As I listened to him, I noticed that my early Catholic guilt had come back to visit me, suggesting I send Fred to Father McCarthy for confession, followed by a lifetime of very cold showers. I also noticed that this "suggestion" led to my feeling off-center and rigid, so I allowed it to pass. (A major benefit of both hypnosis and meditation is that they teach you a "just let it happen" attitude toward your mind, so you can compassionately observe each thought or feeling without identification, and then decide how you'd like to proceed.) I worked to develop a receptive state in which I felt connected, open, and curious as to the positive gift that was awakening in Fred. After several minutes, I became aware of what a beautiful man Fred was, something I had somehow overlooked previously. I found myself talking with him about how sexual energy is perhaps the most powerful, undefeatable energy in the world. I suggested that finding one's deep sexual identity is a lifelong challenge that takes everything one has. I complimented Fred on the amazing depth and intensity of his sexual presence, but said that I had little confidence in his repressing it.

The relational "field" seemed filled with a deep connection, probably the most connected I'd felt with Fred. He seemed touched and receptive to my compliments, and developed a light hypnotic state in response to them. I talked some more about how, for whatever reasons, his sexuality seemed to be calling him to a deeper awareness. He agreed, but said he was scared. I acknowledged that he was scared, noting with special emphasis, "Yes, Fred, as a sexual being, you are scared." Pausing to let this stand on its own, I then asked: "As a sexual being, who else are you?" He laughed a bit nervously before saying, "I'm also very horny!" I paused to sense this part of his sexual self before feeding back, "Yes, Fred, as a sexual being, you are also horny!" I then suggested that he continue with further answers to, "Who am I as a sexual being?" It took a little coaching for Fred to settle down so he could speak, feel, hold, and make visible one sexual identity at a time. For example, he might say, "As a sexual being, I am really ashamed," then be encouraged to let go, feel that identity in his bodymind as I fed it back and acknowledged the importance of that truth. The next one might be, "As a sexual being, I really get turned on by looking at beautiful naked female bodies." As he spoke it, I would see it, nonverbally connect with it, gently name it, encourage him to know it, and nonverbally witness it. After 10 seconds or so of silence, I would ask, "Who else are you as a sexual being?" This continued for about eight identities, including "I am . . . afraid, really turned on, interested in touch, numb, obsessed, paranoid, and intense." Each identity was individually sensed, felt, made visible, properly named, blessed, and allowed its special place.

Somewhere during the process, Fred looked so beautiful, the way people look in therapy when they're no longer dissociating. It was as though he somehow had found a way to begin to make room and to reveal the deepest parts of his sexual identity. We talked about how sexual identity had so many different emotional truths and other identities enfolded in it. I suggested that what really distinguished a "pervert" from a vital, healthy sexual being was the ability to sense the relational connections between these diverse identities, as well as to feel the "unitary field" of self that held all of them. (For example, many identities might be contradictory, but all can have a place in the field of self.) We talked about a few technical ways (extensions of the exercise) in which he could practice this sponsorship of sexual identity.

Two weeks later, at the next session, Fred shared his surprise that, for whatever reason, his preoccupation with Internet pornography had been virtually absent. At the same time, he began to focus on concerns regarding his wife and their relationship. Further sessions focused on couples work, especially in terms of the relation between intimacy and sexuality.

## IDEAS ABOUT SPONSORSHIP

This small example provides a few hints about a number of ideas of therapeutic sponsorship. We might note three basic ideas here.

1. *There are two modes of experience: the "fressen" of nature and the "essen" of culture.* In German, there are two words for eating: *fressen* and *essen.*

> *Fressen* means to eat like an animal, a pig; *essen* is to eat like a human being. As anybody who has raised a child can attest, the road from *fressen* to *essen* is a long one. It takes tremendous acts of sponsorship to help a child learn to eat like a person!

If we take this distinction and generalize it to other human activities, we can see that each aspect of being a person comes to us as "not ready for prime time" *fressen* energies. It is the "re-spons-ability" of the community to help a person develop social-cognitive relational skills to transform these energies into *essen* forms that have value to the person and the community. Thus, the fierceness that reveals itself as temper tantrums in a toddler can, if properly sponsored, developmentally progress into the admirable fierceness of the mature individual. If negatively sponsored, the same tantrums may later reveal themselves as rage, passive aggressiveness, violence, or other social forms that seem to have little or no value.

I discussed at length in *The Courage to Love* (Gilligan, 1997) what some of these sponsorship practices involve, including the following.

- Centering/opening attention
- Deep listening/proper naming
- Being touched by/touching
- Challenging/accepting
- Connecting with resources and traditions
- Developing multiple frames/practicing behavioral skills
- Cultivating fierceness, tenderness, and playfulness

These practices, some of which are elaborated below, are the ways and the social/cognitive/experiential means by which a *fressen* energy is awakened into consciousness and cultivated into the human value of an *essen* form.

2. *A Generative Self develops each time "essen" and "fressen" integrate.* In this view, the experience of a self arises at each moment that the *essen* mind — the *cognitive self* that performs acts of meaning and value — integrates with the *fressen* mind — the *somatic self* organized within the archetypal, experiential language of the body. The Generative Self is not a given, nor is it always present: it is a dynamic realization that awakens each time the cognitive and somatic selves are cooperating. A good example of this creative/created self can be found in artists. Most

> artists — writers, painters, poets, dancers — emphasize that their creative energies come from some place other than their cognitive (conscious) self. The task of the artist is to find ways in which to receive those energies and cultivate a relationship with them. This relationship is neither one of domination nor one of submission; the artist neither totally "controls" the creative energy nor has the luxury of just "passing out" and being overwhelmed. Rather, he or she must find a way to "sponsor" these energies, to midwife them into creative form.

In the same way, each person is a performance artist, and is visited regularly by creative but chaotic life energies that are calling the person to do something interesting. If he or she can develop sponsorship skills, these energies can take helpful forms in the social world. If not, they may become persistent, troubling feelings or behaviors — anxiety, depression, agitation, and the like.

3. *Symptoms and other acts of violence arise each time "essen" ignores, curses, or exploits "fressen" energies.* We can begin to see that while life flows through you, giving you everything you'll need to become a person, your presence also is deeply needed. If you do not "sponsor" the *fressen* gifts given in the moment, they will persist and repeat themselves with an even greater intensity. If you curse them, they will take on negative forms. If you exploit them, they will take on distorted forms. At some point, they seem to be a presence greater than the social/cognitive self, a repetitive experience or behavior beyond your control. The more you try to get rid of it, the deeper it becomes entrenched. This is what we call a "clinical symptom": a disturbing *fressen* energy that has not yet been therapeutically sponsored into a helpful *essen* form.

As therapists, we look for the unsponsored *fressen* energies. We become intensely curious about the disturbing experiences and behaviors by which a person feels overwhelmed, and welcome them as the basis for creative new developments. We realize that efforts to resist or overcome these "problems" not only are futile but typically have the effect of sustaining them. As Watzlawick, Weakland, and Fisch (1974) emphasized, the attempted solution is the problem. For example, a person who tried to overcome nagging doubts by obsessive "positive thinking" became even more agitated, self-absorbed, and ineffective. Self-relations posits that the opposite is equally true: the problem is the solution. That is, *what seems at first glance to be a terrible experience to be avoided at all costs is that which provides, under proper conditions and effective sponsorship, exactly what the person needs in order to grow and develop further.* For example, the client with "nagging doubts" was invited to welcome them while in a deeply relaxed state. While doing so, the client noticed a tender presence within the heart that had been ignored. Integration of this tender presence led to a calmer, more centered presence, one that was neither negative nor positive.

The presence of "proper conditions and effective sponsorship" is the key here. Without them, more ineffective suffering (Merton, 1964) and disturbing events will be the case. So our major challenge in psychotherapy is to define and effectively create the ways and means of transformational sponsorship.

## ASPECTS OF THERAPEUTIC SPONSORSHIP

### *Active Non-doing*

When clients enter therapy, they are often caught up in an obsessive mode of "What do I do? What do I do? What do I do?" Often therapists react to these anxious demands with the response, "What do *I* do? What do *I* do? What do *I* do?" The compulsive problem-solving that results is a major reason why therapy remains stuck. So one of the important things for a therapist (and client) to do is "nothing." The Chinese call this state *wu-wei*, or "active non-doing."

*Wu-wei* does not mean falling asleep, collapsing, resigning oneself, or withdrawing. On the contrary, it is an alert, yet relaxed, mode in which one feels centered and open to the entire field of activity. Erickson had this in mind when he said: "Too many psychotherapists try to plan what thinking they will do instead of waiting to see what the stimulus they receive is, and then letting their unconscious mind respond to that stimulus" (in Gordon & Meyers-Anderson, 1981, p. 17).

So *wu-wei* is a sort of a relational meditation process. It is what an artist does to invoke the creative spirit or an athlete does before a big event. The therapist practicing active non-doing feels connected to the self and client, deeply curious about whatever is "waking up" in the client's consciousness. The interest is in letting the client's spirit touch you, find you, and guide you. There are many ways to enter this process; most involve conscious breathing, somatic relaxing, attentional opening, and cognitive curiosity (see Gilligan,

1997). Sometimes I even say a little prayer to let whatever needs to be sponsored find me and teach me how to love it and support it.

A major skill being cultivated via *wu-wei* is attentional stability. In problem spaces, one of the first casualties is the destabilization of attention. When disturbing experiences arise, the result is often overrigidity, fragmenting, spaciness, constricting, and so on. A person loses his or her center, forgets about his or her embeddedness within larger fields, and becomes unhelpfully reactive (rather than responsive). *Wu-wei* is a relational meditation that allows one to reconnect with whatever is happening while regaining one's center. From there, helpful responses can arise.

Active non-doing is especially helpful for both client and therapist at the beginning of each session. It can be introduced through a meditation, light trance, or other simple mindfulness practices. It can be consciously returned to throughout the session, especially when it seems that the experience is stuck.

### *Therapeutic Focusing*

Eugene Gendlin (1996) found that one of the best predictors of the helpfulness of a therapy session is whether or not the client can develop, within the first part of the session, a "felt sense" of the problem. Gendlin (1996) points out that felt sense is distinct from simply emotions, physical sensations, or perceptions:

> A felt sense is the wholistic, implicit bodily sense of a complex situation. It includes many factors, some of which have never been separated before ... A felt sense contains a maze of meanings, a whole texture of facets, a Persian rug of patterning — more than could be said or thought ... One single thing, one statement, or next step can arise from the whole of it, if we allowed it to form. (p. 58)

In Gendlin's "focusing" approach, a client is asked to develop a "felt sense" by letting go of trying to figure things out and then sensing how the body is representing the problem. Further listening and dialoguing with the felt sense are the basis for therapeutic progress.

In the self-relations method of *therapeutic focusing*, both client *and* therapist are asked to connect with and track their respective felt senses. In the first step of this process, the therapist gives primary attention to the felt sense in his or her own body as the client talks about his or her problem. For example, the therapist may notice a sense of tightness, or emptiness, in the belly as he or she listens receptively to the client's presentation. The therapist allows his or her attention to drop into that place, making it a listening center. Mindfulness of this center continues throughout the method.

In the second step, the therapist also attends to the *client's* center of disturbance. The therapist might find the client's voice tonality leading to the center. Or he or she might look at the midline of the client's torso, noticing where the energy seems to be either intense (anxiety) or withdrawn (depression). Tuning into that place (while maintaining his or her own felt sense), the therapist gently asks the client to take a few moments of silence to sense where in his or her body he or she most feels the center of disturbances. The client is invited to gently place a hand on that center to bring more attention to it.

The simultaneous sensing and tracking of the two centers are then continued for the duration of the session. One value is that this centers and stabilizes the attention of both therapist and client. One of the major problems with problems is that they tend to destabilize attention; it can become fragmented, disconnected, too narrow, too intellectual, and so on. Therapeutic focusing can keep bringing both the therapist and client back to their felt senses.

Therapeutic focusing also helps the therapist to listen to the story without being involved with it. It is important to appreciate that the problem narrative typically leads one away from connection, not deeper into it. It is easy to get caught up in "talking about" the problem, or even forgetting it; therapeutic focusing teaches you a way to "be with it" without being affected by the explanations or "story line." In this sense, *self-relations sees problems in terms of a disconnection between the stories of the cognitive self and the felt sense of the somatic self.*

Therapeutic focusing also establishes a center-to-center relational connection between the therapist and client that can be used to track what's happening. For example, I was talking with a client about some difficult aspects of his marriage. We had established some form of therapeutic focusing, and the man seemed very connected. But after several minutes, I suddenly felt a disconnection to my own center. I noted this aloud to him, and wondered what he was feeling in his center. He started talking faster, but I gently asked him again. He said that he felt the same, that he had gone off somewhere. This awareness allowed us to reconnect with the felt center, so that what was being talked about was connected to felt sense.

### *Providing Sanctuary, Proper Naming, and Blessings*

As you connect with felt sense, you can begin to midwife new life into a person's being. Felt sense is a first stage of a new identity-related process that can be more fully developed through such sponsorship practices as providing sanctuary, proper naming, and blessings.

*Providing sanctuary* means offering a safe place, both in the bodymind and in the community, for a person or experience. This requires touching it with human presence, allowing it to be, listening deeply, and extending connection to it. It is what an artist does in welcoming creative impulses, or what a parent does when a child approaches with a skinned knee. If these felt senses are ignored, rejected, or cursed, they can turn nasty and unbearable. Their human value will go unrealized, and real suffering will result. So the stakes are enormously high.

Thinking in terms of sanctuaries suggests that we think of a person's center as having two levels: emotional context and emotional content. Virginia Satir pointed to this difference when she would ask a person two questions: (1) How do you feel about that? (2) How do you feel about feeling that way? The first regards emotional content; the second relates to the feeling context in which the content is held. The latter is especially important: The person who develops a bodymind sanctuary within which any experience can visit a feeling context has made it safe both for the experience and for the person(s) involved to "just let it happen."

A major value of creating a sanctuary is that it differentiates the experience from the person experiencing it. This is a central goal of many bodymind practices, including hypnosis, meditation, EMDR, and self-relations. For example, as the experience of rage arises, providing it with a place (say, in the belly) allows the person to bear witness to the rage without identifying with it. At the same time, providing sanctuary within a mindbody center (heart, solar plexus, or belly) gives it a specific container so that it doesn't spill out, project, or overwhelm the person or others.

As the person can bear witness to it, *proper naming* may develop. This does not mean an objective classification, but rather a touching of a felt sense with language. It is not an act of separation or dissection, but one of communion of subject with object. Naming adds an entirely human level to an archetypal experience, transforming it and extending it into the realm of human consciousness. (Without language, an experience is living but not human.) With most symptoms, a significant experience has not been properly named, held, and blessed; it is, therefore, dominant but seems to have no human value, for the simple reason that the sponsors involved have not properly welcomed and named it as "value-able."

For example, a man who had spent much of his adult life as a top-notch, hard-working lawyer began to slow down as he hit the age of 70. He was exhausted at night, his body wracked with anxiety, fear, and worries. His attempts to muscle the tiredness into submission just made matters worse. When he finally slowed down and listened to the felt sense in his heart, the presence of "death" was sensed and named. He broke out sobbing, continuing for some time. As the sobs subsided, he talked about how he had been running from death and that it was overtaking him. Further conversations with "death" clarified his interests in living and enjoying quality time as long as possible, which led to a significant change in his lifestyle, and the relationship of his "head" with his "heart."

There are many ways in which to name experiences properly that are felt but not sponsored. For example, a simple exercise that I often use with couples, and sometimes with individual clients, involves having the clients get comfortable, centered, open to the field, and tuned to each other. Partner A makes the following statements:

- Today my woundedness is about ______________ .
- Today my longing is for ______________ .
- Today my strength is about ______________ .

For each blank, the person lets a word or phrase come to mind, and then speaks it. It is important that it not be planned; the response should just come from listening to one's center and letting it happen. For example, the person might say: "Today my woundedness is about *missing my daughter* . . . Today my longing is *to be held* . . . Today my strength is about *reaching out to others*." In speaking each experience, the person seeks to let the energy lift from his or her center and extend into the relational field holding both partners. This is then released, a silent pause ensues, and the next sentence is undertaken. After Partner A finishes three statements, Partner B responds with his or her own three. This cycle can be repeated a number of times, five or six being typical.

Such an exercise, which can also be practiced alone or silently during a conversation, is a simple way to bring sponsorship to whatever is arising in one's center. Bringing mindfulness to an activated experience gives it place, and the connection between the cognitive self and the somatic center can allow each experience to be a valuable resource rather than a distracting or symptom-causing nuisance. This is the difference that sponsorship makes.

### *Cultivating Archetypal Energies: Fierceness, Tenderness, and Mischievousness*

Effective sponsorship, whether of one's self or of another person, requires the use of a number of complementary energies. For example, a helpful sponsor must be able to embody and extend *fierceness* in many ways: staying committed, seeing through "bullshit," remaining focused, taking a person seriously, respecting and defending boundaries, and so forth. A good sponsor must equally cultivate *tenderness* in the self and others via a soothing presence, an ability to touch and be touched emotionally, a gentle and kind presence, compassion, and so on. Effective sponsorship also requires a sense of playfulness or *mischievousness:* a twinkle in the eye, a sense of humor, a capacity to hold multiple perspectives and shift gracefully among them, and the like.

A sponsor lacking any of these energies might run into difficulty. Fierceness alone deteriorates into rigidity and crankiness. Tenderness by itself can sink into a sort of Barry Manilow–like sentimentality. Mischievousness in isolation makes everything a cynical game. Tender fierceness interspersed with timely humor has a much more powerful effect. Thus, effective sponsorship works to cultivate and blend these complementary energies within one centered approach.

At the beginning of a session, I typically check in with myself to ensure the presence of a felt sense of each of these energies. If there is not, I take a few moments to access each of them within me. I then look to sense the presence of each energy within the client. This may be challenging initially, as a client may seemingly present only one. For example, a new client recently presented primarily in a helpless, regressed, vulnerable mode. While accepting that mode as valid and genuine, I sought to sense her hidden fierceness and her "inner rascal" before proceeding any further. Once I could sense them, I felt a much deeper connection, respect, and calmness with her.

There are many ways in which to cultivate these archetypal energies. For example, one training exercise done in dyads is as follows:

1. Partners get comfortable, centered, open to field, tuned to each other.

2. Partner A says: See my tenderness . . .

See my fierceness . . .
See my mischievousness . . .
See me.

3. Partner B says: See my tenderness . . .
See my fierceness . . .
See my mischievousness . . .
See me.

4. Partner A says: I see your tenderness . . .
I see your fierceness . . .
I see your mischievousness . . .
I see you.

5. Partner B says: I see your tenderness . . .
I see your fierceness . . .
I see your mischievousness . . .
I see you.

6. Partner A says: May tenderness remain with us . . .
May fierceness remain with us . . .
May mischievousness remain with us . . .
May each of us remain with us.

7. Partner B says: May tenderness remain with us . . .
May fierceness remain with us . . .
May mischievousness remain with us . . .
May each of us remain with us.

As with the "today my woundedness" exercise, the major interest is in relaxing, dropping into center, connecting with the partner, using the mindfulness of speech to touch and awaken an emotional center, and then extending the energy into the interpersonal field. This is the purpose not only of hypnosis, but also of other performance arts: to develop and express an embodied experience within an energetic relational field. In this embodied relationality, old patterns may be reorganized into new meanings.

Each archetypal energy has many forms: integrated or unintegrated, undeveloped or mature, and so on. By recognizing this, the therapist can sense a "problem" as an undeveloped or unintegrated form of an essential human resource. Thus, an angry person can be deeply appreciated for his or her fierceness, and encouraged to "do it more, do it better," in ways that connect it with the other energies and allow new, more helpful forms to develop. Again, a basic principle of self-relations is that the problem is the solution: What seems to have no value may, under proper sponsorship conditions, be transformed into a deeply valuable expression.

### *Replacing Negative Sponsorship with Positive Sponsorship*

Each of us carries many sponsors within our head, some positive and some negative. A positive sponsor is one who (1) helps awaken awareness of the goodness and gifts of self, (2) helps awaken awareness of the goodness and gifts of the world, and (3) helps develop practices and understandings that connect the two domains. A negative sponsor is one who (1) turns awareness away from the goodness and gifts of the self, (2) turns awareness away from the goodness and gifts of the world, and (3) promotes practices and traditions of neglect or abuse against self, others, and the world. Using these definitions, it is easy for most people to identify examples of both positive and negative sponsors in their lives.

In exploring sensitive areas in therapy, it is common for negative sponsors to become activated. Self-relations suggests that a difficult experience becomes a clinical symptom when three things happen: (1) the somatic/archetypal self feels a disturbance (what we call the activation of a "neglected self"), (2) the normal cognitive self disconnects or dissociates, and (3) negative sponsors overtake the "neglected self." The therapist should be sensitive to when this happens, and work to replace negative sponsorship messages with positive ones.

One straightforward way to do this is by (1) identifying a repetitive problem sequence in a person's life, (2) tuning into where in the sequence the person accesses a felt sense of somatic disturbance (i.e., a neglected self), (3) identifying the negative sponsorship messages that are influencing the neglected self, and (4) replacing them with positive sponsors. For example, Jill was a 51-year-old woman building a successful business consulting practice. She complained about becoming anxious when talking to new clients. We explored an example of this, and she noticed herself beginning to feel "tension and fear" centered in her solar plexus about 30 minutes before an appointment. Self-relations emphasizes that such disturbing experiences are not the problem; the problem (or solution) arises in terms of how they are sponsored. To identify the negative sponsorship messages, Jill was requested:

1. As you experience those difficult experiences, just take a moment and sense the presence of your mother in the room. And as you do, just notice what she would say or do in response to witnessing the struggle you are voicing here right now.

Jill imagined her mother to be very silent and depressed, with an implicit message of, "You're asking too much of yourself, you're going to get hurt." When asked, she noted that her solar plexus responded to that message with a sinking feeling of fear. I commented, "That's good to know ... that when you hear that message, your inner self feels that way."

She was next requested:

2. As you return to sensing yourself struggling with that experience of anxiety, just take a moment and sense the presence of your father in the room. And as you do, just notice what he would say or do in response to witnessing your experience here.

Jill sensed her father getting tense, telling her just to focus on what needed to be done and to forget about her feelings. She felt her solar plexus respond to this message with a feeling of greater fear and confusion. I encouraged her simply to study and note each inner response to each sponsorship message.

I then suggested that this feeling of fear would probably revisit her many more times during her life. She was learning how her mother sponsored it and how her father sponsored it, and how her inner self responded to such sponsorship messages. While that was good to know, even better was that it was her turn now: She now had "first options" in terms of how to sponsor that feeling when it returned. We examined how positive sponsorship might involve creating a place for the feeling, touching it with kindness, deeply listening, properly naming it, and having a collaborative conversation with it. I pointed out that when the feeling came, her cognitive self could remain, with a resulting bodymind integration that would allow creative new responses.

As she developed this embodied relationality, a deep calm spread through her. She looked radiant and at peace. I suggested that she imagine herself going through the problem sequence while maintaining this positive sponsorship of herself. She successfully navigated the process, not only in the session, but also when facing actual challenges over the following several weeks.

This example suggests just one of many ways in which positive sponsorship can replace negative sponsorship (see Gilligan, 1997, for other examples). In encouraging this process, it is important to recognize that resistance sometimes occurs. A person might say, for example, that he or she doesn't deserve kindness or respect. In such instances, it can be helpful first to access that person's patterns of positive sponsorship toward significant others — for example, a child, pet, or best friend. (Most people know how to nurture others much better than they know how to nurture themselves.) For instance, Ray was a client who was feeling extremely insecure about losing his job. He flatly refused to provide positive sponsorship for his feelings of confusion and fear, claiming that they were undeserving of attention. I asked him if he had children, and he softened as he told me of his three young boys. Were one of his sons to experience confusion and fear, I asked, how would he respond? Would he scold him? Hit him? Electroshock him? Tell him to go to his room and not come out until he lost those feelings?

To each of my questions Ray responded "No," he would never do that. Each time, I acknowledged with a tender fierceness, "Yes, I see that you would not do that to your son." I then asked him how he would respond if it were a different son, or a friend, or anybody else? Would he hurt, punish, or ignore the person? To each question he again answered "No," which I continued to acknowledge. When asked what he would do in such situations, he replied earnestly that he would want to support and comfort the person in need. I said I believed deeply that he would provide tender support to anybody in that situation, so the real question remained: Wasn't he somebody too? Wasn't he a human being deserving of respect, love, and kindness? As tears fell from his eyes, I suggested he go inside himself, touch the place where he most felt the confusion, and provide positive sponsorship. Thus began a process of reconnecting with the center of his being, a process that continued in many positive ways over the next months.

## DISCUSSION

Each person is given a life to be lived and enjoyed. As this great gift opens across time, a multitude of primary experiences are brought through a person's center and into the field of awareness. Sponsorship is the relationship process that gives form, meaning, and value to each of these core experiences. Sponsorship can be positive — that is, it can awaken awareness of the goodness and gifts of the self and the world — or it can be negative, in the form of curses or inattentiveness that numbs or darkens awareness of the soul and the world. Sponsorship initially is held entirely by outsiders, but as psychological growth develops, the possibility of self-sponsorship is added. Positive sponsorship allows an experiential pattern to change and grow over time, while negative sponsorship freezes a pattern in form and meaning, forcing it to repeat itself over and over in a process that Thomas Merton called "ineffective suffering."

When the suffering from negative sponsorship becomes unbearable, disturbing behaviors may arise as unsuccessful attempts to resolve it. What seem like irrational or incomprehensible behaviors from the outside can be compassionately sensed as important efforts at healing. By demonstrating and encouraging positive sponsorship of these disturbing experiences, a wonderful transformation can occur. A life lived in fear and oppression can shift to one lived in courage, self-acceptance, and delight. Such is the difference that positive sponsorship can make.

## Chapter 15

# THE EXPERIENCE OF "NEGATIVE OTHERNESS": HOW SHALL WE TREAT OUR ENEMIES?[1]

Not too long ago, an American psychotherapist invited a Tibetan monk to his home for the weekend. During the visit, the therapist did what I guess one does when entertaining a Tibetan monk for the weekend — watch "The Exorcist," the movie in which the actress Linda Blair is possessed by the devil, who is then violently exorcised by a priest. Halfway through the movie, the therapist suddenly realized that Tibetans take their demons seriously — they have got a cartography of demonology more sophisticated than the psychiatrists' DSM-IV. He looked over at the monk, who was recoiling in horror at what he was seeing.

After the movie, the therapist expressed his apologies and hopes that the demon hadn't disturbed the monk too much. The monk replied that he wasn't disturbed by the demon, but rather liked him. The confused therapist pointed out that the monk had appeared to be upset, and that he was hiding his eyes. The monk again stated that he wasn't disturbed by the demon. "But why did you look upset?" asked the therapist.

"Oh, that," replied the monk. "I felt so bad for the priest because he so misunderstood the demon."

We all confront a lot of demons in the course of our lives. They may be the demons we call anger, depression, fear, or criticism. They may be the de-

[1] This essay appeared previously in Jeffrey K. Zeig. 2002. *Brief therapy: Lasting impressions*. Phoenix: Zeig, Tucker, & Theisen, Inc.

mons of addiction or compulsions, the demons of managed care or the patriarchal system, or the demons of social injustice. These demons may possess us, tell us we're worthless or no good, or induce us to sell our souls or prostitute ourselves.

Indeed, psychotherapy is, in large part, a conversation about our relationships to such enemies. These enemies embody what we might call "negative otherness." It is "otherness" in that it doesn't fit with our identity, ideals, values, hopes, or plans; it's negative in that it seems to want to negate our presence, our humanness, our integrity, our very lives. Without the presence of "negative others" — whether we think of them as internal states, behavioral patterns, external institutions, or other people or groups — we would have no basis for a psychotherapy conversation. So how we think about this negative otherness, how we understand our relationship to it, how we develop our responses to it, make a great deal of difference.

In long-ago times, the negative others were thought to be helpful. In *The Origin of Satan*, Elaine Pagels (1995) describes how the early Hebrew term for Satan meant "one who stands in the way of." It was thought that Satan was a great angel, a trusted servant of God who was sent down when God thought someone was on the wrong path. Satan was a bit of a trickster, a rascal who could engage you and get you out of your fixed ways so you could go back to where you belonged. This early Satan was not an enemy to be destroyed, but an honorable adversary who was there to help. It was only later that Satan was seen as outside the field of life, someone to be destroyed at any cost. I guess we should ask: Has this latter way of understanding Satan been helpful? Has it worked?

Also in earlier times, a struggle with a dragon appeared in many cultural myths. Again, the dragon was regarded as a presence that challenged you to grow up, to become a person, to learn how to negotiate crises skillfully. The dragon was not to be killed, but to be engaged in a way that would allow the transformation of both the person and the dragon. This was a dangerous undertaking, to be sure, for if one slipped, the results were catastrophic. But still, the relationship with the "negative other" of the dragon required not violence, but intelligence, courage, and self-transformation. It was only later, for example, in the Christian myth of St. George slaying the dragon, that the relationship shifted to violence and what Thomas Merton (1964) termed the "irreversibility of evil," — that is, the assumption that the enemy would never change, but would always stay in its state of "negative otherness" — an assumption that Merton described as the basis for the justification of violence.

Again I would ask, is the attitude of primarily opposing and destroying our enemies and their practices workable and helpful in the long run? This is not a moot question, for the modern myth of the "negative other" — whether our enemies, or a symptom, or an out-of-control experience — as an inhuman "it" that requires violence to be changed lives deeply within us. It is a core assumption of the modernist era, one that has led to much suffering and injustice. But does it really change in postmodernism? It doesn't seem so. I would like to suggest that, in many ways, this "us versus them" or "self versus it" frame continues unabated in many postmodernist myths and practices. I further suggest that this metaphor is both unnecessary and unhelpful in many ways. What Deborah Tannen (1999) has called the "argument culture" can only lead to greater violence, less community, more suffering, and deeper hopelessness. But until we develop more effective ways of transforming conflict nonviolently, we will perpetuate and exacerbate suffering in the name of ending it once and for all.

It is easy to talk about honoring differences and multiple possibilities, but the real test comes in our relationship to our "enemies" — the people, institutions, experiences, and practices that seem to threaten our survival. For example, take a moment to think of some person, experience, system that you really can't stand. Maybe it's someone who hurt you. Maybe it's an unjust system, perhaps managed care. Maybe it's the ideology and practice of, say, racism. Maybe it's a part of you, some lazy presence within you that's stopping you from being an important person, some fearful presence that just doesn't understand your repeated pronouncements that there's nothing of which to be afraid.

It's not too hard to come up with examples, is it?

As you bring that "negative other" into your awareness, just notice what your internal response is. It could be many things: fear, anger, disgust, numbness. What fantasies do you entertain about engaging with negative others? Would you like to hurt them? Scream at them? Run from them? Teach them lessons they'll never forget? What do you do with those feelings, those fantasies, those thoughts, those reactions?

In traditional terms, we generally respond to an enemy or threat in one of two ways: We fight it or flee from it. To fight it, we try to dominate it, repress it, destroy it, demonize it, analyze it, numb it, dissociate it. In trying to flee from it, we check out, drug out, give up, feel anxious, become paralyzed, get depressed.

Neither of these response styles is very helpful in the long run. The negative other keeps attacking, the conflict keeps recurring, and our human presence keeps diminishing. Such is the legacy of the fight-or-flight response.

Postmodernism is, in a significant way, about more options, more possibilities, more truths, more perspectives. For the promise of postmodernism to be realized, we need to develop more practices and understandings about how to deal with conflicts and "negative otherness," within ourselves and between ourselves. Gandhi (in Merton, 1964) used to say that if the only alternative to passive submission to injustice were violence, he would recommend violence in virtually every case, for no one should have to endure oppression and injustice. But he suggested a third path of what he called *satyagraha* (*satya*, "love" or "truth"; *graha*, "strength" or "force"), which involved neither submission to, nor violence against, one's enemies, as a more helpful alternative.

In the martial art of aikido, this third way, this alternative to fight or flight, dominance or submission, is sometimes referred to as "flow." This is not a flow whereby whatever the other wants, the other gets. It's a flow that allows one to stay relationally connected during conflict, both with our adversaries and with ourselves, so that the conflict itself is a creative, nonviolent event that leads to new understandings, new conversations, and new realities.

I'm suggesting that this is one of the great challenges of psychotherapy, and one of the great contributions that therapy can make to our culture today: offering creative ways to transform conflictual relationships. We need to accept that conflict is natural, inevitable, and helpful to human progress, both individual and collective. This is not to say that you look for conflict or seek to provoke. On the contrary, our hope is that we can advance peace however and wherever possible, but that when conflict arises, we can accept it and work with it as an opportunity for real growth. There are various paths to accomplishing this.

One path is the practice of aikido, which can be roughly translated as "the path of resolving conflict by blending with energy." In aikido, you try to open your heart, mind, and soul to your attacker in ways that protect you and the attacker. The interest is in how to join the attacker's energy to transform it. It's a beautiful and challenging practice. For example, one of the major learnings is letting go of taking things so personally. My aikido teacher, Coryl Crane, is a fifth-degree black belt, and an inspiring person from whom to learn. One day in class, we had about eight big guys who were dealing with each other's attacks in the traditional aggressive American way, slamming each other around to teach lessons that would never be forgotten. Coryl knelt on the side of the mat, watching the spectacle unfold. At the end of class, as we bowed in front of the altar, she said, "I just want to mention one thing: A lot of you are taking this very personally. When people attack, you think they're attacking you. So you're either backing up or trying to oppose them."

"If you look at me," she said, "you can see that I wouldn't last two minutes with such an approach. So you just might consider that the attackers are not attacking you, they're just trying to get somewhere. And so, if you can get out of their way, then you can join them and help them to get to where they want to go, maybe lessening a little bit of the violence and agitation as you walk with them."

Is such an approach workable? Is it possible to work with violence and injustice without punishing people, without hurting them, without your getting hurt or being destroyed? Is it possible to open your heart, mind, and soul to negative otherness as a way to help both yourself and others? Of course, it is. We see examples of it everywhere — not only in famous lives, such as those of Martin Luther King, Nelson Mandela, Gandhi, or Jesus, but in the lives of countless lesser-known people. As the poet W. H. Auden wrote, love is the only rational response.

Our challenge, then, is to articulate what love looks like as a skill, as a vibrant practice not only of protecting life, but also of transforming it. It's an enormous challenge, to be sure, one made all the more difficult by our deeply held assumptions. The roots of modernist thinking run deep within our consciousness. Of the many possible ways of describing, defining, or deconstructing modernism, I would like to offer a single phrase to describe its core: *disembodied, isolated intellect.* The great accomplishment of modernism, for better and worse, was to separate the intellect from the present moment of the body, nature, and life itself. Once this separation was done, it was never undone. The mind was elevated to a supreme position of will and solitary intelligence: its task was to monitor, control, and dominate all that to which it related.

The hope was that if we could just think clearly and rationally enough, we could overcome the major problems of life. If we could just get the right idea, the proper text, the accurate theory, the clearest diagnosis, then we could control things. And if we could control and predict things, happiness would follow. Did it? Well, advances certainly were made in technology, in rational thinking, in materialistic comfort, in medicine, in the production of food. And extremely important differentiations were articulated between the fields of science, art, and religion, such that thinking and artistic expression were liberated from the dictates of the state.

But with these advances came certain pathologies. Modernism bred urbanism, a strange lifestyle in which concrete is poured over everything, people live within walls and cars all day, and we communicate primarily through machines. The disembodied intellect dictates a mind/nature split in which the body is objectified, the intellect is seen as the only valid intelligence, human life is primarily viewed in terms of utilitarian values (what's in it for me?), spirit and soul and heart–mind are denied, interconnectedness is rejected, nature is exploited, death is feared above all, materialism becomes a cult, relationships are seen in dominance–submission terms, ritual is ignored, and everything outside the self-identity is seen and feared as an "it." In short, the disembodied intellect leads to a disconnection and denial of the precious life of the present moment.

See how that feels after 30 years. Or 40 years. Or 450 years.

If we allow these disconnections and denials to continue unabated, postmodernism can easily deteriorate into what Charlene Spretnak (1997) has called "hypermodernism," or what Bruce Springsteen had in mind when he wrote the song, "57 Channels and There's Nothing On." It can become a practice of advanced consumerism and its main tool, television. More shallowness, more cynicism, more channels, more wasteland, more splintering into ever-growing factions without any common base. Less soulfulness, less mystery, less healing, less deep listening, less sitting still, less wisdom, less hope for peace and understanding. Granted, we're not sure what these words mean anymore, and we've almost forgotten how to use them poetically. But what I'm trying to point here is a postmodern practice of what psychologist Marion Woodman (1993) calls "embodied consciousness," a consciousness that is full of living energy, connected to the world and the present moment, filled with vitality, sensitive to shifting differences, discerning of subtle patterns, expressive of wondrous mystery. Embodied consciousness allows one to deal with differences creatively, without demonizing one's adversary or getting locked into fixed understandings or rigid positions. I am suggesting that without some conscious practices of embodied consciousness, the hopes and dreams of postmodernism will go down the tubes.

Embodied consciousness can be discussed in various different ways. I'd like to address two complementary aspects of it, the experience of a mind/body center and the experience of a relational field. It should be emphasized that these distinctions don't make that much sense in academic, literary, or intellectual contexts, which are the bases for most of the thinking and practice of psychotherapy and social change. They are distinctions that come from performance-art contexts, such as music, dance, oratory, and the martial arts.

The experience of a mind/body center is the experience of a nonintellectual intelligence and presence within one's self. It is a felt sense of dropping down under the words into a balanced, calm, aware connection with self and others. The experience of centering is described beautifully by the artist M. C. Richards (1962) in *Centering in Pottery, Poetry, and the Person.* The Chilean novelist Isabelle Allende (in Toms, 1994) has talked about how she writes primarily from her belly mind. When you hear great singers or speakers, you can sense immediately their connections to their centers, how they are expressing themselves from a deep connection.

The idea of a center is central to many cultures. Malidoma Some (1994), a member of the African Dagara tribe, describes in his autobiography how he was kidnapped by the French Jesuits in Africa when he was four years old. They tried to raise him to be a priest, but he escaped his captors in late adolescence and returned to his people. Some finally underwent his initiation rituals; he described the initial instructions given by the ritual elder as follows:

> Somehow what he said did not sound strange to me or — I found out later — to anyone. It was as if he were putting into words something we all knew, something we had never questioned and could never verbalize.
>
> What he said was this: the place where he was standing was the center. Each one of us possessed a center that he had grown away from after birth. To be born was to lose contact with our center and to grow from childhood to adulthood was to walk away from it. The center is both within and without. But we must realize it exists, find it, and be with it, for without the center we cannot tell who we are, where we come from, and where we are going.
>
> He explained that the purpose of Baor (the initiation process) was to find our center. This school specialized in repairing the wear and tear incurred in the course of 13 rainy seasons of life. I was 20. Had I been home all that time, I would have gone through this process seven years ago. I wondered if I was catching up too late but then thought, better late than never.
>
> No one's center is like someone else's. Find your own center, not the center of your neighbor; not the center of your father or mother or family or ancestor but that center which is yours and yours alone. (pp. 198–199)

## "Negative Otherness"

The basic idea of a mind/body center is that there is a nonlinguistic presence within you that you can tune to, connect with, rest in, and receive from. It is not a linguistic distinction so much as a postlinguistic distinction, something that the poet Rilke (1981) perhaps had in mind when he said:

> It seems that things are more like me now,
> that I can see farther into paintings.
> I feel closer to what language cannot reach.

Dancers dance from their centers. Writers write from their centers. Political prisoners engage from their centers. I would hope that this skill would be available to the rest of us in our diverse situations.

In psychotherapy, this might be done in relation to the problem or complaint a client brings in. A complaint always involves a somatic component. That is, the problem always carries a disturbing feeling or lack of feeling somewhere in the body. Were this distress not there, I don't think most people would seek psychotherapy. They are not caught in a philosophical conundrum; they are experiencing suffering in their moment-to-moment life experience.

In our self-relations approach to therapy (Gilligan, 1997), we typically ask folks to notice, when they experience the problems, where they most feel the centers of disturbance in their bodies. Interestingly, most point to their hearts, solar plexus, or gut areas. Rather than regarding these as bad feelings that need to be removed, we become curious about listening to these felt centers of disturbances as ontological presences; that is, as the presence of another intelligence that is awakening in their lives. In other words, the onset of a symptom may be regarded as the awakening of a person's center. Therefore, we see problems and crises as positive events, as heralding the breakdown of the isolated intellect and the development of a more relational intelligence that is distributed throughout the mind/body.

For example, one of my clients was a man who said he was really depressed. He was 38 years old and had just gone through his second divorce. He was trying to start a new business, but wasn't into it. He was trying to date, but just wasn't into it. He was trying to connect with friends, but he just wasn't into it. He was very concerned because he couldn't get himself motivated to "get on with it." When I asked him what the problem was, he said "depression." When I asked where he felt the center of the depression feeling, he at first said that he felt nothing or had a big empty feeling. When I asked him to take some time to sense where he felt the center of the emptiness, he pointed to his solar plexus. When I asked him to listen to what that center of his experience was saying to him, he looked at me as though I were crazy. I asked him again, and he reported hearing a voice saying, "It's no use, nothing will ever work." I suggested that the voice that went with the felt sense in his belly perhaps spoke with a lot of integrity, and that it was worth listening to. The conversation continued to be organized around listening to the felt sense (Gendlin, 1978), and gradually its position of rejecting an old identity based on pleasing others emerged. In short, the depression in the belly transformed into a felt sense of acting with integrity, rather than following what his head "identity" had been conditioned to do.

In this view, the mind/body distress in a problem or complaint is indicative of the waking up of one's center. We welcome disturbances as signals of new life. But rather than trying to understand or interpret such disturbances from the head, we connect to and engage the language of the mind/body center. Through careful attentiveness, listening, and conversation, this center can be developed as a primary base for knowing and expressing identity.

Attending to a mind/body center has many other values as well. For example, it offers an important point for stabilizing attention, especially in stressful situations. In self-relations therapy, we ask the question: To whom or what or where do you give your first attention? First attention is like the cursor on the computer screen: you can move it around. For example, if a person is yelling at you, where do you focus: on the person yelling, on a memory from childhood that is activated by that yelling, on a theory or text that says that the person shouldn't yell? If it gets locked onto another person or an old memory, you become reactive rather than responsive; that other person or memory becomes the "higher power" that dictates your action. If it gets locked onto a text or theoretical model, you slip into ideology and fundamentalism, trying to force the world into your frame of reference. By letting your first attention gently drop and touch your center, whether it's in your heart or your belly, you can allow your attention to stabilize and still have the freedom to be flexible and responsive.

Mind/body centering is another way of talking about tuning into different types of intelligences. Centering in your heart yields a different type of thinking than does centering in your head. Centering in your belly tunes into a different brain, one that scientists are now calling the enteric nervous system, or brain in the stomach. The type of mental processing that comes from centering is quite different from just intellectual thinking. It tends to be more archetypal than personal, more intuitive than causal in its logic, more attuned to the present moment than to some grand theory about the ways things work.

Mind/body centering allows connection and responsiveness to other people, as well. It's what allows you to dance freely with a partner, not knowing what the next movement might be, but secure in knowing that you can find it in the moment. Centering allows you also to stay connected with yourself and a partner during conflict, so you can stay in tune with each moment. In aikido, we follow the relational principle of "heart to heart, mind to mind, center to center," which means that as you connect with your attacker in these ways, you can deal most effectively with protecting yourself and transforming the conflict. When you're just in your head, it's hard to stay connected to others, whoever they might be.

Mind/body centering also allows you to create a place or sanctuary for holding experiences. Without a place to go, experiences — like people — get a little agitated and crazy. The mind/body center can be used as a container in which any feeling, image, or presence can rest. It's sort of like when your six-year-old comes in with a skinned knee. She's crying as if there were no tomorrow. You allow her to climb into your lap, where your feeling is a container for hers. It allows her experience to play itself out.

In a similar way, we can ask, when you are visited by fear, anger, depression, or confusion, what you do with these visitors. One possibility is that you can give them place within your mind/body center. As you breathe, you can feel a sanctuary opening up in your belly, a safe place to which any experiential presence can come. Rather than having, say, a fear that permeates your body, you can let it rest in your sanctuary. You can then connect with it relationally, developing what Martin Buber (1923/1958) would call an "I–thou" relationship with it. This type of relationship is central to work in self-relations psychotherapy.

As you connect with your center, you also have a powerful place where you can move and extend your energies into the world. A center is a place in which to gather your strength, to focus your attention, to balance yourself. As you sink into it, your voice, your self, your presence are able to extend into the world. Again, this is obvious and inspiring in gifted performance artists: their energetic presence radiates into the world. We are all performance artists, of course. But when we lose connection with our centers, our expressions become less clear, less confident, less connected to life. By learning how to keep coming back and connecting with our centers, we can regain our power and keep it present in the land of the living.

This extension of the self into the world of the living leads us to the complement of the center, the relational field. The field is the larger space and context in which we live. When we feel connected to it and nurtured by it, we do all right. But when we lose connection to it, as when under stress, we tend to think and react in our isolated worlds with little effectiveness. The basic idea is that there is an intelligence greater than you. It's not about giving yourself, but about joining in an experience of communion with a wholeness deeper than your individual self. If you feel it and can listen to it, your capacity to act with effectiveness and integrity, especially in response to your enemies, is increased tremendously.

It's important to recognize that people know the experience of a relational field in different ways. You may know it through walking in the forest, and call it nature. You may know it by joining with others in social justice, and call it community. You may know it through athletic performance, and call it the zone. You may know it through prayer, and call it God. You may know it through an intimate relationship, and call it love.

There are many names for the field, but all involve an experience of being supported and guided by a deeper intelligence around you. If you want to find out how people know the field, ask them what they do to get back to themselves. For instance, you've worked all week and are really tired. What do you do to get back to yourself? Answers might include talking with friends, conscious breathing, going for a walk, meditating, playing or listening to music, knitting, reading, or gardening.

What happens when folks engage in such activities? For one thing, their intellectual self mellows out a bit. There's not so much chattering, controlling, agitating, conspiring, plotting. Second, people feel less of a need to control and more of a sense of relational connecting, curiosity, and quiet confidence. Third, if you ask people where their sense of self "ends" in such experiences — where their boundaries delineate self from non-self — most look puzzled by the questions, and then start moving their hands outward, saying, "It doesn't end. It is an expansive field that has no limit." The experience of this expansive, unitive feeling is what we call the field. Interestingly, as William James (1902/1982) and Aldous Huxley (1944) pointed out, this experience of unitive consciousness is a common element of so-called mystical experiences across many historical periods and many cultures.

It is one thing to know the field in positive circumstances, a place where you feel safe and accepted. Is it possible to stay connected and supported by the field under adversarial conditions? I think so. Although the general response to attack is to constrict your field, thus leaving you locked into a small space that is under the influence of negative otherness, you can train yourself to stay connected to both your center and the relational field even in difficult circumstances. When you stay connected to your center and the field, alienating, negative influences cannot take hold of you. What I'm saying is that connecting with a living field is about as good a technique for externalizing alien presences as you can find.

To me, a great example is Nelson Mandela. Reading his autobiography (Mandela, 1994) or watching him on television dancing at a political gathering, one cannot help but wonder what it is that he is connected to that allows him such grace and strength, such a lack of bitterness, throughout what he calls "the long walk to freedom." I would suggest that he is a beautiful example of somebody connected to the soulfulness of his center and to the depth and breadth of the larger field of life.

In aikido, we describe this connection with the maxim, "Drop into center, open into field." That is, when you're in a stressful situation, don't fixate on the stressor. Don't give first attention to the problem. Instead, drop down into your mind/body center as a base from which to listen, perceive, relax, and respond, and expand your awareness outward to connect with a field awareness that is bigger than the stressful event. Now your attention is not entrapped by the stressor; it's free to receive and give beyond the confines of the situation. This allows you to respond to conflict not in a dominant–submissive way, in which someone wins and someone loses, but in a relational way that protects both you and your attacker, and seeks to bring a resolution of whatever differences or agitation is present.

It's a simple but difficult challenge, something that T. S. Eliot called "a condition of complete simplicity costing not less than everything." Sometimes people say, "You're asking a lot." My response is: "What else are you doing? And what are the alternatives?"

What I've been suggesting so far is that throughout our lives, we will be confronted with "negative otherness," with what we perceive to be enemies. Negative otherness comes in all shapes and sizes, and has many names. It can be internal experiences, such as fear or anger, that grip us; addictive behaviors that overtake us; oppressive systems that try to dominate us; old memories that try to possess us; angry people who try to control us; or fixed ideas that try to seduce us. If you are alive, these experiences will continue to visit you. The question is: How will you respond to these negative others?

You can capitulate to them, you can try to oppose directly and eradicate them, or you can engage them relationally as opportunities for mutual growth. If we choose the third path, we need to overcome the modernist tradition of the disembodied intellect. We need to find ways to reconnect with a mind/body center and the relational field that surrounds us. By embodying consciousness and situating it in a larger relational field, we can become more attentive, more effective, more loving, and more skillful. We can find ways to work creatively and nonviolently with conflict, so that more connection to life and love may be made possible for all involved.

There are many examples of how this can be done. For example, Zen Roshi Bernie Glassman is one of the leading figures in what is called socially engaged Buddhism, an American movement that tries to integrate Buddhist mindfulness training with social change. Glassman, a self-described Zen entrepreneur, owns a number of businesses, including a large bakery, that are run and managed by homeless and ex-homeless people in New York. He has established a multifaceted social service agency in Yonkers, N.Y., called the Greyston Mandala.

Glassman (1999) has also developed a community called the Peacemaking Order, which has three basic tenets. The first is *not knowing* — being in the state of not knowing, letting go of fixed ideas. The second is *bearing witness* — totally immersing one's self in the situations in which one is involved. The third is *healing one's self and others* using the materials that result from bearing witness.

To apply these tenets, Glassman (1999) recommends entering into situations that you fear, situations in which you think it would be great if healing could happen. For example, Glassman and his students have sat for days at a time with homeless people on the streets of New York City, who then join the community, guided by the three tenets of opening up into not knowing, bearing witness, and healing one's self and others. On the basis of their experiences, they then initiate further action. For Glassman, starting businesses that employed the homeless came out of the sittings with them.

Another project involved sitting in the Auschwitz concentration camp for a week or so, a gathering in which numerous people participated: Jews, Germans, Poles, Catholics. The experiences and subsequent action that came from sitting in a not-knowing mindfulness state in the middle of the concentration camp were quite extraordinary.

We as therapists need to continue to cultivate a similar openness as we sit with our clients, bearing witness in a not-knowing state to their homelessness, their Auschwitzes, their unnamed, unwitnessed experiences. This cannot be done via the disembodied intellect. By "dropping into center, opening into field," our capacity not only to tolerate but to help heal ourselves and others is greatly increased.

In connecting to center and to field, perhaps one of the best outcomes is that our awareness returns to the value of stillness and silence. Modernism is in no small part an emphasis on a linguistic universe, where talking and thinking and action, the yang of the universe, are given total priority. The yin principle of empty space, listening, receiving, and silence is ignored and marginalized.

I know that in some quarters it is heresy to suggest that something beyond linguistic construction exists, but isn't it obvious when you hold a baby or a dying person, any time you connect in love or in wondrous amazement? Some deep presence, an extraordinary intelligence, lives in the gap between the words, the space between the notes, the silence in the conversation. We lost that connection in the language-dominated, yang-based world of modernism. In this regard, I hope that the postmodern world can become a postlinguistic one, where we use language to go beyond language, to what T. S. Eliot has called "a further union, a deeper communion" with ourselves and others. This is where the experiences of mind/body centering and relational field can help.

The Chilean poet Pablo Neruda (1969) said it this way in his poem entitled "Keeping Quiet":

> Now we will count to twelve
> and we will all keep still
> For once on the face of the
> earth, let's not speak in any language;
> let's stop for a second,
> and not move our arms so much.
>
> It would be an exotic moment
> without rush, without engines;
> we would all be together
> in a sudden strangeness.
>
> Fisherman in the cold sea

would not harm whales
and the man gathering salt
would not look at his hurt hands.

Those who prepare green wars,
wars with gas, wars with fire,
victories with no survivors,
would put on clean clothes
and walk about with their brothers
in the shade, doing nothing.

What I want should not be confused
with total inactivity.
Life is what it is about. . . .

If we were not so single-minded
about keeping our lives moving
and for once could do nothing,
perhaps a huge silence
might interrupt this sadness
of never understanding ourselves
and of threatening ourselves with
death.

Perhaps the earth can teach us
as when everything seems dead in winter
and later proves to be alive.

Now I'll count up to twelve
and you keep quiet and I will go.

# Chapter 16

# EMDR and Hypnosis: The Same or Different?[1]

Over the past decade, EMDR has emerged as a very promising therapeutic approach for treating trauma-related problems (Shapiro, 1995; Shapiro & Forrest, 1997). It appears to allow for the integrated processing of experiential learnings that have been "stuck" or "frozen" in the course of a person's experience. While its effectiveness seems clear, many questions still remain regarding how it works and its relationship to other therapeutic modalities. This chapter examines the question of whether EMDR is related to the experience of "hypnotic trance" and, relatedly, whether hypnotic forms of treatment may be used in conjunction with EMDR.

We will start by presenting a case description. Some general comments will be made regarding how direct hypnosis, Ericksonian hypnosis, and EMDR might approach the case. These three approaches will be compared at three levels: Level 1 involves a special "learning state" that is activated whenever identity is destabilized; Level 2 is a symbolic-procedural level which frames how this learning state is understood and formally developed; and Level 3 refers to the larger context (e.g., psychotherapy) in which the special state is utilized. We will see that while all three approaches share the special "learning state" of Level 1, EMDR and Ericksonian hypnosis differ markedly from

---

[1] This chapter originally appeared in F. Shapiro (Ed.). 2002. *EMDR as an integrative psychotherapy approach: Experts of diverse orientations explore the paradigm prism.* Washington, D.C.: APA Press.

direct hypnosis at Levels 2 and 3. These comparisons will allow us to propose a general model of how identity moves through cycles of stability and instability in its growth and development, and the role that trauma and trauma-related therapies may play in this growth process. We will then return to the original case to see how Ericksonian trance work and EMDR may be woven together in a clinical treatment.

## A CASE DESCRIPTION

Greg was a 27-year-old, college-educated man who called me for an appointment after reading an article I wrote for a local newspaper. His complaint was that he lacked confidence and felt depressed about his life in general. He had a dead-end secretarial job at a large corporate office, and few social connections. He was the youngest of four boys, growing up in an Irish-Catholic alcoholic family in the Midwest. Both parents were alcoholic and abusive to each other and their children, with a great deal of physical violence erupting on "bad nights." Communication was often bizarre and unpredictable. Part of Greg's response was to develop dissociative skills so he could "go away somewhere" while sitting in his room.

Greg was initially very anxious and fearful. He had only recently begun (two months previous) his first therapy experience with a psychiatrist, whose name he picked out of the yellow pages. The psychiatrist, described by Greg as aloof and judgmental, told Greg that he suffered from severe characterological disorders, and that long-term therapy would be needed. Over eight sessions with the psychiatrist, Greg found himself as increasingly confused, frustrated, and disoriented. He wondered whether he was "going crazy," and wondered if he could come in and talk with me about it. After suggesting that he notify his therapist he was doing this, I scheduled an appointment with him.

In early sessions, Greg was extremely self-critical. He described himself as "a loser," a "chickenshit," and a "fuck-up." It took him awhile to declare his goals for therapy, which included a better job, better social connections (especially regarding dating women), and an improved feeling of self-worth.

## THREE APPROACHES TO HEALING TRAUMAS

Before describing the actual details of the therapy, we might first examine how practitioners from the three distinct approaches of direct hypnosis, Ericksonian hypnosis, and EMDR might respond to this case. This will allow us to compare and contrast these approaches, and see if they are at all integratable.

## *Direct Hypnosis*

Hypnosis is the mother of all modern treatment modalities (Ellenberger, 1970). Starting in the late 18th century with Mesmer, and moving through the 19th century with Braid, Janet, Bernheim, and Freud, and into the 20th century with clinicians such as John Watkins and Milton Erickson, hypnosis has developed as an effective treatment modality for a variety of ailments.

The common understanding (and fear) about hypnosis is that it is a process whereby the practitioner "takes control over" the client's consciousness and "plants" suggestions or other (presumably therapeutic) ideas. This popular view is exaggerated, but not totally without merit. While there are many different theories about and approaches to traditional hypnosis, its clinical application usually involves a relationship where the client comes in with a problem and the therapist induces a "hypnotic trance," typically via repetitive suggestions for deep relaxation and concentration on the hypnotist's voice. The resulting state is one in which "subjects" have their eyes closed, do not move or talk, and are focused on the hypnotist's words. A general loss of connection to the outside world develops and this narrowed state of attention constitutes a "special learning state" wherein subjects are more open to new ideas and possibilities.

Thus, in the case of Greg, a practitioner of direct hypnosis might introduce trance work to induce relaxation, concentration, ego-strength building, symptom removal via direct suggestion, and controlled emotional abreaction. In all of this work, the "special learning state" of hypnotic trance would be seen as independent from the symptomatic experience, and the outcomes an effect of the hypnotist's suggestions and the client's susceptibility to those directives.

## *Ericksonian Hypnosis*

In contrast to this operator-controlled hypnosis, a more client-centered approach was developed by the late psychiatrist Milton Erickson (1980a, 1980d). Erickson (1948/1980a) rejected ideas of suggestibility, artificial trance, and operator-controlled effects:

> Direct suggestion is based primarily, if unwittingly, upon the assump-

> tion that whatever develops in hypnosis derives from the suggestions given. It implies that the therapist has the miraculous power of effecting therapeutic changes in the patient, and disregards the fact that therapy results from an inner re-synthesis of the patient's behavior achieved by the patient himself. It is true that direct suggestion can effect an alteration in the patient's behavior and result in a symptomatic cure, at least temporarily. However, such a "cure" is simply a response to the suggestion and does not entail that re-association and reorganization of ideas, understandings, and memories so essential for an actual cure. It is this experience of re-associating and reorganizing his own experiential life that eventuates in a cure, not the manifestation of responsive behavior which can, at best, satisfy only the observer. (p. 38)

Like his predecessors, Erickson (1948/1980a) emphasized hypnotic trance as a "special learning state" that could be very helpful to therapeutic goals:

> The induction and maintenance of a trance serve to provide a *special psychological state* in which patients can re-associate and reorganize their inner psychological complexities and utilize their own capacities in a manner in accord with their own experiential life. Hypnosis does not change people nor does it alter their past experiential life. It serves to permit them to learn more about themselves and to express themselves more adequately. (p. 38) (italics added)

This induction of a "special psychological state" in Ericksonian hypnosis is not done via some standardized technique. Instead, it is a naturalistic state developed by utilizing the client's unique behaviors, experiential states, and values. These client variables might be strengths as well as symptomatic aspects. For example, Greg experienced dissociation, self-criticism, and shyness. Based on the assumption that a problematic process may be utilized as the basis for developing a resource or solution, the Ericksonian practitioner would become curious about how those experiences might help Greg develop a therapeutic trance in which old experiences could be reorganized into new learnings. For example, Greg might be encouraged to go inside and discover the "proper distance" for a "critical bird's eye view" of himself, to discover a safe place for discovering his own healing abilities. To support his shyness, he might be encouraged to feel free to keep things to himself, to find a safe place where he might be alone comfortably with himself.

A major consequence of utilizing the client's experience as the basis for therapy is that the resulting experiences, including trance, are naturalistic and constructed from the person's emotional values. *This is a fundamentally different "special learning state" from the traditional trance constructed by standardized communications.* While traditional trance is based on the hypnotist's values, Ericksonian trances are developed from the client's values. As Rossi (1996) emphasized:

> Modern (hypnosis) appears to have lost all connection to the psychophysiological foundations of hypnosis that were emphasized by the fathers of hypnotherapy. Academic researchers who tended to standardize (hypnotic) scales on college students and normal populations lost touch with the emotional crises and phase transitions that made up the essence of therapy in historical hypnosis. Modern hypnosis became a student of normal psychology rather than the desperate transforming experiences between sickness and health, sanity and insanity, life and death itself in historical hypnosis. (pp. 28–29)

In other words, hypnotic trance came to be an artificial state constructed by the hypnotist, totally divorced from the identity values and emotional experiences of the client. As we will see, this Ericksonian emphasis on the client's experience aligns it more closely with EMDR work than with traditional hypnosis.

Another feature of Ericksonian hypnosis is its emphasis on the creative and healing potentials that each client carries. Trance is a special learning state where these resources may be accessed and actualized. With Greg, for example, the Ericksonian therapist would be curious as to how Greg's creative unconscious could accomplish effective work. The therapist would be primarily interested in setting up the proper contextual conditions for this to occur.

## *EMDR*

EMDR has been described by its founder, Francine Shapiro, as "an interactive, interactional, intrapsychic, cognitive, behavioral, body-oriented therapy" (1995, p. 53). It rests on the assumption that as the experiences of life flow through a person, an innate psychophysiological capacity exists for processing, transforming, and integrating each of these experiences. Some events, however, can be so extreme and traumatizing that this innate integrative system is disturbed or overwhelmed, resulting in a "freezing" of the event-in-processing into a state-dependent form that is "stuck" in the nervous system.

This creates an antagonistic state of affairs where (1) the event is trying to "process through" into a resolved or completed form while (2) the nervous system is shut down into a "neuromuscular lock" that inhibits all such integrative processing (cf. Gilligan, 1997). The result is akin to driving down the freeway with one foot on the accelerator and the other on the brake. In real terms, this is evidenced by PTSD and other symptoms that include intrusive phenomena, hyperarousal and hypervigilance, and a constriction of the normal sense of self (Herman, 1992).

The efficacy of EMDR is in its development of new techniques for resolving such experiences. At its most basic level, EMDR relies on a "special learning state" that it calls "accelerated information processing." According to Shapiro (1995), the "accelerated information processing model . . . opens up new territory by defining pathology as dysfunctionally stored information that can be properly assimilated through a dynamically activated processing system." (p. 52)

In the case of Greg, EMDR work might involve first identifying the experiences of depression or anxiety that are disturbing him. A visual image of a representative event from the past, present, or (anticipated) future would be selected. Somatic experience connected to the event (e.g., pain in the heart, headache) would be elucidated and rated in terms of its subjective level of distress. Then the core negative self-talk connected to the event (e.g., "I'm no good") would be identified, as well as a positive self-talk message (e.g., "I'm OK") that might be substituted. The brunt of the work would then involve asking him to (1) simultaneously hold the visual image, the somatic experience, and the cognitive statement while (2) tracking the movements of the therapist's fingers moving back and forth across his with his visual field. (While there are a number of alternative ways EMDR may be applied, we will limit ourselves to the most basic here.) During this time Greg would be asked to "just let happen whatever happens, trusting your inner healing principle to process whatever needs to be processed to a healing resolution." At the end of each 45-second cycle, Greg would be asked to take a moment of rest before verbally reporting what was happening. Generally, he would be encouraged to "go with that," and a new 45-second cycle of eye tracking would ensue.

The intent of such a procedure is twofold. The first goal is to desensitize the experience, freeing it up from its initial context, so that when the image comes up, it brings no corollary negative somatic disturbance or negative self-talk. If Greg was working on an event where his father was abusive, for example, this might mean that he could bring up the image without feeling lousy or believing it was his fault. Once this contextual clearing was achieved, the second part of the process would be to build a new context, so that Greg could view, understand, and relate to this originally traumatizing event from a centered, self-loving, and more mature context.

To get from the original experience to a full resolution would likely take numerous "sets," involving numerous different experiences. Thus, Greg might start with an abusive experience with his father, and require numerous 45-second sets to let it all process through to resolution. He might then move to a related experience with his mother, and move through another series of sets to resolve that. And so on. During this time, the EMDR therapist is creating a stable context where the client is given structured, safe ways to methodically allow their inner healing system to integrate and resolve an interconnected system of self-disturbing, self-immobilizing experiences.

## DIFFERENT FORMS OF THE "SPECIAL LEARNING STATE"

We have sketched how three different approaches to healing trauma might proceed. While these approaches seem quite different in many ways, there are some key similarities. Perhaps the most important is the premise that *there exists a "special learning state" where traumatic identity and disturbing experiences may be transformed into healthy, integrated states.* In direct hypnosis and Ericksonian hypnosis, the terms "hypnosis" and "trance" are used to describe this state; in EMDR, the new and somewhat unwieldy term of "accelerated information processing" is suggested. I propose that while the terms differ, the approaches are pointing beyond the terms to *the same basic state of accelerated learning that is intrinsic to human beings.*

This is not to say that the state is experienced and utilized the same across the approaches. In fact, the way one views and connects with this basic state makes a tremendous difference in its consequent form, meaning, and behavior. Indeed, the more authoritative and traditional direct hypnosis views the state as an extension of hypnotic suggestion, and thus primarily emphasizes the control of the hypnotist. This represents the old patriarchal style where power was invested in the hierarchical hands of the "father [who] knows best." Consequently, the subject was implicitly expected to experience the state as a passive one where they were "rewired" by a kind yet domineering parental figure.

Milton Erickson, in what I believe was for him a lifelong struggle to move from an authoritarian to a truly permissive helping mode, developed a new set of understandings, values, and techniques for how to access and work with this special learning state. In fundamentally emphasizing trance as arising from and reflecting the client's values and experiences, the resulting trance was qualitatively different from the old-style hypnotic trance. Individuals could move in and out of trance, could maintain their individuality, and could discover their own unique wisdom and healing capacities.

During the time I studied with Milton Erickson (1974–1980), I was a graduate student in psychology at Stanford University. My experimental research led me to have some connection with Ernest Hilgard and the Stanford Hypnosis Laboratory. Dr. Hilgard, one of the great figures of American psychology and a leading researcher in experimental hypnosis, was a kind and inspirational figure. He and Erickson were contemporaries. While both had grudging respect for the other, Hilgard once told me about Erickson, "He seems to see trance everywhere, even where it's not!" When I told this to Erickson, he responded, "Jack Hilgard wouldn't know a trance if he saw it!"

These respective positions speak volumes of the differences between traditional and Ericksonian hypnosis. Traditional hypnosis saw trance only as occurring when a situation was formally defined as such, and induced via proper measures. Erickson, on the other hand, saw trance as naturalistic and occurring under various conditions. It was the therapist's task to utilize trance when and how it actually occurred, rather than developing it artificially.

EMDR is a more recent arrival on this general scene. It seems to have made a deliberate decision to distance itself from hypnosis. Part of this seems to be wise "public relations," in that many people may be put off, scared, or misled if it were couched in hypnotic terms. A second reason is that by freeing itself from the tradition of hypnosis, it opens itself to new ways of understanding and working with the age-old phenomenon of traumatization and its sequelae. As Shapiro (1995) herself stated, ". . . if EMDR is defined simply as hypnosis, its usefulness will be limited to those effects already available to the therapist" (p. 52).

In other words, the traditions of hypnosis, direct or Ericksonian, have no exclusive hold on how healing works. To reduce EMDR to hypnosis, as some do, is inaccurate and unhelpful. To emphasize the common "special learning state" that both hypnosis and EMDR tap into is, I believe, a more helpful position. It suggests that this special state has multiple levels. Level 1 has to do with the intrinsic capacity of human beings to transform and heal their psychological identity. It is the "special learning state" that all the healing approaches tap into. It is not a property of the therapist's technique or theory, but an innate skill of human consciousness.

Level 2 regards the social-symbolic structures surrounding the special learning state. It refers to how this state is described, the procedures by which it is accessed and worked with, and the values underlying the work. Thus, traditional hypnosis reflects traditional Western medical understandings, which sees the patient's own consciousness and skills as irrelevant to the healing process. Accordingly, the "special learning state" is seen as one wherein the patient's consciousness is psychologically anesthetized so the doctor can surgically implant better ideas into the mind. Also, hypnosis generally reflects a Western orientation to the empirical world of the senses; hence, the "special learning state" of trance is one in which phenomenology ("the world of appearances") is amplified dramatically. (Contrast this to Zen meditation, which reflects Eastern values of seeing through the "veil of illusion.")

EMDR, perhaps reflecting Shapiro's personal process of discovering how it worked for her (see Shapiro & Forrest, 1997), strongly values the client's own innate healing potentials. It looks to activate and guide these potentials through safe, structured, repetitive processing cycles. It assumes a natural drive toward integration and growth. Hence, the techniques that evolved to express these values are client-centered and naturalistic, yet structured and rigorous. The experience of a "special learning state" in EMDR work is not the experience of "trance." While related to hypnotic experiences via a shared Level 1 state, the basic experience and values of the "accelerated information processing" state of EMDR are distinct. In this sense, EMDR has added a significantly new way to experience healing processes.

Level 3 refers to the larger context of the therapeutic work. As stated earlier, all approaches agree that the Level 2 experience is insufficient. The experience of trance or "accelerated information processing" must, in order to be effective, be grounded in a wider therapeutic context. The experiences that arise must be talked about, connected to other contexts in the person's life, combined with additional work such as behavioral assignments, relationship work, and so forth. Thus, to some extent both EMDR and Ericksonian hypnosis may be used within different therapeutic modalities and approaches. As we will see below, they may also be combined together in the same therapy.

## CYCLES OF IDENTITY: FROM UNCERTAINTY TO STABILITY TO CHAOS, AND BACK AGAIN

One of the major ideas proposed in this chapter is that the values and ideas of the practitioner/culture strongly influence how the innate "special learning state" of human consciousness is developed, experienced, used, and understood. This makes it crucial that practitioners have a clear understanding of how and why symptoms develop, and how one's approach relates to such symptomatic states. In the present view, clinical symptoms are seen as primarily related to shifts in a person's identity state; that is, they indicate that something has happened that makes the old identity obsolete, and that a new identity is struggling to emerge. The altered states of consciousness inherent in symptoms indicate the attempt to access the "special learning state" needed to progress from an old identity to a new one.

The key idea in this view is that the "special learning state" of trance or EMDR is a psychobiological process that is activated whenever a person's state of identity is significantly destabilized. It is not induced by the operator but initiated by life events outside of the clinical context. These events require the proper conditions to allow new integration and stability. This is what therapy seeks to provide.

Traditionally we have thought of identity as relatively fixed and stable over a person's life. Once you got to a certain age, the modernist myth said, the basic structure of your personality pretty much stayed the same. Of course, a closer examination of a given life would produce much evidence to the contrary. For example, the psychotherapist Bill O'Hanlon likes to tell the story of "the woman with five husbands." O'Hanlon was ready to marry his second wife and, to allay his insecurities about how to be successfully married, he tried talking with different people who had succeeded in marriage. In this process he happened upon a woman at a party who, his friends pointed out to him, had been happily married to the same gentleman for some forty years. He approached the woman, introduced himself, mentioned his situation, and wondered whether the woman could share any of her "secrets" for a happy marriage. The woman looked at Bill and exclaimed, "Young man, I don't know who told you that I was married to the same man for 40 years. I've actually had five husbands over the past 40 years!!"

Taken aback, O'Hanlon listened as the woman described her first husband. He was a romantic, thoughtful man who took her out to dinner, wrote love letters, went for long walks with her, and so on. When they had their first child, she said, that man left her. She was very angry and had to adapt to her second husband, who was hard-working, worried about money, didn't write love notes, and so on. But in time she grew to love this man, which made it upsetting when he was gone and she had a third husband. Somewhere between her descriptions of her third and fourth husbands, it finally dawned on O'Hanlon that this woman was talking about the same man! With the same man, she had experienced five distinct marriages, five distinct husbands. Each marriage had a beginning, a middle, and an end. Each was connected by a death and rebirth process.

In a similar way, each of us has multiple lives over the course of a lifetime. Many cycles of identity exist within a person's life. While the middle parts of each identity cycle have a somewhat predictable, orderly nature, the beginnings and ends do not. They are disorderly, chaotic, and unpredictable. This dynamic view has been described beautifully in chaos theory (Gleick, 1987), which originally developed as a way of modeling complex non-linear systems (e.g., weather patterns). In chaos theory, a system may be ordered in a fairly straightforward way. But when certain stimuli are introduced that cannot be straightforwardly processed by the system — for example, high degrees of stress that move the system beyond its equilibrium — its basic state changes, first to an oscillating system (going back and forth between opposite states) and then, if it still cannot integrate the stimulus, to what is called "ordered chaos." The surface pattern in ordered chaos seems to make no sense, not conforming to a normal logic or form; however, its underlying pattern has a deeper order. An example is a symptom: the feelings, images, and behaviors may seem chaotic and illogical, but on deeper inspection have their own meaning and order.

Under the proper conditions, ordered chaos will reorganize into a higher order system that can effectively respond to the initial disturbance. It includes all the information of the preceding system as well as new resources and information that combine with the old in a completely new form. The important phrase in all of this is "under the proper conditions." If the proper conditions are not met, this state of ordered chaos may remain indefinitely, wreaking havoc and overwhelming the conscious self.

This is when people end up in psychotherapy. Typically, their sense of self-identity has been disrupted and destabilized, and their efforts to remedy the problem have failed. This disruption may result from normal developmental events — leaving home, getting married, having children, retiring, etc. — or from unexpected events such as illness, financial troubles, or trauma.

The disturbance may be a single event or a pattern of events over time. Regardless, the person cannot effectively respond in their "normal" ways to the event(s), and the stability of their normal identity state gives way to an unstable, seemingly chaotic state — that is, the person's normal sense of self has been replaced by a seemingly disordered set of experiences and behaviors. The person feels overwhelmed, at the mercy of the disturbance, and increasingly desperate and hopeless.

In the present view, "ordered chaos" is another way of talking about the "special learning state" we have described. It is activated when an identity state is destabilized; it moves the person into primary process; it cannot be understood or controlled by "normal logic"; but it may be utilized as the basis for integration and growth of a new identity state. *The loss of cognitive control in such experiences, whether voluntary or involuntary, is what triggers the ordered chaos of the "special learning state", which in turn allows for new patterns of identity to develop.* In other words, "ordered chaos" is a prerequisite for evolution and growth. In this way, *all events that destabilize identity, including trauma, are potential bases for growth and reorganization of self-identity.*

The caveat, of course, is that such events may also lead to prolonged suffering and disintegration. The key difference is whether a safe context for reorganization is available to the person. The EMDR community implicitly understood this when it sent volunteers to immediately help the Oklahoma City bombing victims in 1995. Like the bomb that shattered the federal building, the multiple horrors of the event shattered the identity structures of the many victims. Nobody who experienced the event would ever quite be the same again. However, the EMDR response team recognized that with the proper healing conditions, the victims could be helped to integrate the experiences into a stronger sense of self.

If the proper conditions for such integration are not present — for example, the person continues to live under the traumatizing conditions, or no help is available — a regressive form of ordered chaos results. The old sense of self and its response patterns are lost, but the new identity and its deeper intelligence and skills are not yet developed. The symptom is the attempt to initiate this new identity, but without a therapeutic context the person cannot surrender to the "ordered chaos" of the "special learning state" to allow the transformation to occur. Thus, the person resorts to defending against the development of the special learning state through measures such as shutting down, dissociating, self-medicating, rigid control, and symptomatic behavior.

But when the proper conditions are present, the special learning state moves from a regressive to a progressive process. Out of the ordered chaos integration and new resources emerge. In this situation, the therapist is like a midwife, someone who recognizes that the intense non-rational processes of the symptoms are evidence of some attempt at healing and transformation. To allow this to happen, the therapist ensures the proper conditions of a healing context. These include general conditions such as safety and support, as well as more specific conditions that vary across approaches. Interestingly, EMDR and Ericksonian hypnosis share a number of specific conditions, including an emphasis on developing and maintaining (1) relaxation; (2) direct experiential accessing of the core experiences; (3) dual attention (i.e., simultaneously attending to the interior experiences and the outer environment); and (4) trust and guidance for the intelligence of the "ordered chaos" process to lead the way to integration (with a key suggestion to clients of "just let it happen"). Because of these similarities, EMDR and Ericksonian hypnosis can be used within the same therapy. Furthermore, their different forms make them complementary rather than redundant. To illustrate, we return to the case of Greg.

## CASE DESCRIPTION: GREG REVISITED

The work with Greg took place over a year period, with about 3 meetings a month. One of the first goals was to address his intense self-criticism. Continuing his father's tradition, he berated himself continually as "a stupid, worthless idiot." My initial efforts to be straightforwardly supportive and encouraging were rebuffed by hostile remarks to the effect that I didn't understand how worthless he was. Seeing this as a key identity, I decided to join with it, with a curiosity about how it might lead to an opening. Taking some time to just listen and gain an appreciation of Greg, I suddenly remarked that I agreed with him "fully and completely" regarding his stupidity. This comment shocked but absorbed him, so I continued by pointing out how stupid it was to not realize what incredible unconscious creativity he had. These comments were delivered seriously but with an "Irish twinkle." Greg was initially bewildered and confused, but as I continued with such remarks he grew increasingly intrigued until at some point we both broke out laughing. He commented that he didn't realize that therapy could be so playful, but really enjoyed it.

Once some rapport developed, I tried teaching him some general relaxation skills. Success seemed to be blocked by the internal criticism, so I introduced EMDR to clear out some of the anxiety. Several intense EMDR sessions oriented around childhood experiences of being screamed at and degraded. Greg's courage to reconnect with these difficult experiences and follow the process through to a "breakthrough" was admirable.

A second issue was his dissociation skills. He would "check out" at various times and not be able to easily "come back." I asked him if he ever allowed himself to "keep going" in dissociation to the "safe places" beyond the initial bumpiness and distress. He was intrigued by this statement, so I taught him to hypnotically dissociate as a way of gaining a safe place, as a way of connecting with deep inner resources, and as a way to learn to "trust not only the protective but the healing and wise aspects of his inner self." This proved to be very helpful, as he had always associated the dissociation as a weakness. Once we had claimed dissociation as a therapeutic resource, the complementary skill of staying "associated" (relationally connected) without going away was slowly developed.

Another area of therapeutic focus was his job situation. Anytime he imagined doing something he liked, he would feel overwhelmed. EMDR sessions were used to access and "process through" a network of childhood experiences, both at home and in school, where he concluded that he had nothing to contribute to the world. EMDR was also used to open a "future orientation" space where he felt hopeful and confident. Some hypnotic techniques, including future orientation in time, were also used.

This work, combined with various conversations about his vocational interests and how to pursue them, proved productive. Greg turned out to be amazingly creative and talented in advertising on the Internet. With a small loan from a relative, he started up a small business from scratch. Two years later, he was employing six people and doing moderately well. Most of all, he was extremely proud of himself and excited about continuing to develop his talents.

His sexuality and connection with women were another concern. We used some EMDR and hypnosis sessions to open the possibility of asking some women out on dates. Various initial attempts didn't pan out, but answering a computer ad proved positive. He corresponded via e-mail with the woman for awhile, and they then arranged to meet for coffee. Greg was very nervous, especially about his "excessive sweating." We did a trance session, involving multiple metaphorical stories and trance phenomena, around the issue of mind/body resources and mastery skills. It seemed to help, as the date went relatively well. The relationship continues several years later. Greg describes the woman as "not necessarily my dream mate," but someone whom he shares good times and a growing intimacy.

After about a year of therapy, sessions were scheduled periodically, according to Greg's sense of needing to talk about things or get some coaching. He is currently running his business, in relationship with his girlfriend, and taking night classes in art.

## SUMMARY

We started out asking whether EMDR and hypnosis were the same or different. We have seen that at a primary level, they both emphasize a "special learning state" that is activated whenever identity needs to be reorganized — e.g, in response to trauma, developmental transitions, extraordinary performances, or self-transcendent experiences. At a secondary level, the approaches differ in the symbolic-procedural approaches they use to activate and work within this "learning state." At a third level, both hypnosis and EMDR work within a larger therapeutic context that draws upon many additional therapeutic resources to achieve their clinical goals.

Because EMDR and Ericksonian hypnosis share similar theoretic assumptions yet complementary forms, they may go hand in hand in working with clients. They both emphasize the innate healing capacities of clients and seek to provide a space where clients can learn to trust these capacities on their path to greater wholeness and integrity. They both rely on the "special learning state" wherein old problematic ways of responding can be set aside, core experiences can be felt and listened to, and new identities can naturally develop. A major advantage of combining the approaches is that it opens the possibility that therapy can creatively adapt to the client rather than following a fixed protocol. In this way, combining the approaches is good for both clients and therapists alike.

# *References*


Achterberg, J. (1985). *Imagery in healing: Shamanism and modern medicine.* Boston: Shambhala.

Alexander, P. A. (1985). Systems theory conceptualization of incest. *Family Process. 24,* 79–88.

Bandler, R., & Grinder, J. (1975). *Patterns of the hypnotic techniques of Milton H. Erickson, M.D., Volume 1.* Cupertino, CA: Meta Publications.

Bateson, G. (1954). A theory of play and fantasy. Paper presented to the American Psychiatric Association Meeting on Cultural, Anthropological and Communication Approaches. March 1954, Mexico City. Reprinted in G. Bateson. (1972). *Steps to an ecology of mind.* New York: Ballantine.

Bateson, G., Jackson, D. D., Haley, J., & Weakland, J. (1956). Toward a theory of schizophrenia. *Behavioral Science, 1,* 251–264.

Bateson, G. (1972). *Steps to an ecology of mind.* New York: Ballantine Books.

Bateson, G. (1979). *Mind and nature: A necessary unity.* New York: Dutton.

Bateson, G., & Bateson, M. C. (1987). *Angels fear: Towards an epistemology of the sacred.* New York: Macmillan.

Bateson, M. C. (1988). Interview with Kevin Kelly. *Whole Earth Review, 61,* 136–137.

Beahrs, J. O. (1982). *Unity and multiplicity: Multilevel consciousness of self in hypnosis, psychiatric disorder, and mental health.* New York: Brunner/Mazel.

Bernheim, H. (1895). *Suggestive therapeutics: A treatise on the nature and uses of hypnotism.* New York: Putnam.

Bly, R. (1981). Four ways of knowledge. In *The man in the black coat turns: Poems by Robert Bly.* New York: Doubleday.

Bly, R. (1981). (Ed.). (Trans.). *Selected poems of Rainer Maria Rilke.* New York: Harper & Row.

Bly, R. (1986). The good silence. In R. Bly, *Selected poems.* New York: Harper & Row.

# REFERENCES

Bly, R. (1986). The watcher. In R. Bly, *Selected poems*. New York: Harper & Row.

Briere, J. (1984). The effects of childhood sexual abuse on later psychological functioning: Defining a "post-sexual-abuse syndrome." Paper presented to the Third National Conference on Sexual Victimization of Children. Washington D.C.

Brown, G. S. (1979). *Laws of form*. New York: E. P. Dutton.

Buber, M. (1923/1958). *I and thou* (R. G. Smith, Trans.). New York: Scribner & Sons.

Buber, M. (1947). *Tales of the Hassidim*. New York: Schocken Books.

Butler-Smith, S. (1985). *Children's story: Children in criminal court*. California District Attorney's Association.

Campbell, J. (1984). *The way of the animal powers*. London: Times Books.

Capra, F. (1975). *The Tao of physics*. Boulder: Shambhala Publishers.

Castenada, C. (1974). *Tales of power*. New York: Simon & Schuster.

Cooper, L., & Erickson, M. H. (1959). *Time distortion in hypnosis*, 2nd ed. Baltimore: Williams & Wilkins.

Davis, P. J., & Hersh, R. (1981). *The mathematical experience*. Boston: Houghton Mifflin.

de Shazer, S. (1982). *Patterns of brief family therapy: An ecosystem approach*. New York: Guilford.

de Shazer, S. (1984). The death of resistance. *Family Process, 23*, 79–93.

de Shazer, S. (1985). *Keys to solution in brief therapy*. New York: Norton.

de Shazer, S. (1988). *Clues: Investigating solutions in brief therapy*. New York: Norton.

de Shazer, S. (1991). *Putting difference to work*. New York: Norton.

de Shazer, S. (1994). *Words were originally magic*. New York: Norton.

Dolan, Y. M. (1991). *Resolving sexual abuse: Solution-focused therapy and Ericksonian hypnosis for adult survivors*. New York: Norton.

Edinger, E. G. (1990). *Goethe's Faust: Notes for a Jungian commentary*. Toronto: Inner City Books.

Eliot, T. S. (1963). Four quartets. In T. S. Eliot, *Collected poems: 1909–1962*. London: Faber & Faber.

Ellenberger, H. (1970). *The discovery of the unconscious: The history and evolution of dynamic psychiatry*. New York: Basic Books.

Epstein, S. (1994). Integration of the cognitive and the psychodynamic unconscious. *American Psychologist, 49*(8), 709–724.

# References


Erickson, M. H. (1943). Hypnotic investigation of psychosomatic phenomena: Psychosomatic interrelations studied by experimental hypnosis. *Psychosomatic Medicine, 5*, 51–58. Reprinted in Erickson (1980b).

Erickson, M. H. (1948). Hypnotic psychotherapy. *The Medical Clinics of North America* (pp. 571–584). New York: W. D. Saunders Co. Reprinted in Erickson (1980d).

Erickson, M. H. (1952). Deep hypnosis and its induction. In L. M. Lecron (Ed.). *Experimental hypnosis.* New York: Macmillan. Reprinted in Erickson (1980a).

Erickson, M. H. (1954). Pseudo orientation in time as a hypnotherapeutic procedure. *Journal of Clinical and Experimental Hypnosis, 2*, 261–283. Reprinted in Erickson (1980d).

Erickson, M. H. (1959). Further clinical techniques of hypnosis: Utilization techniques. *American Journal of Clinical Hypnosis, 2*, 3–21. Reprinted in Erickson (1980a).

Erickson, M. H. (1964). The "Surprise" and "My-Friend-John" techniques of hypnosis: Minimal cues and natural field experimentation. *American Journal of Clinical Hypnosis, 6*, 293–307. Reprinted in Erickson (1980a).

Erickson, M. H. (1965). The use of symptoms as an integral part of therapy. *American Journal of Clinical Hypnosis, 8*, 57–65. Reprinted in Erickson (1980d).

Erickson, M. H. (1967). An introduction to the study and application of hypnosis for pain control. In J. Lasner (Ed.). *Hypnosis and psychosomatic medicine.* Reprinted in Erickson (1980d).

Erickson, M. H. (1980a). *The nature of hypnosis and suggestion: The collected papers of Milton H. Erickson on hypnosis*, Volume 1. (Edited by E. L. Rossi.) New York: Irvington.

Erickson, M. H. (1980b). *Hypnotic alteration of sensory, perceptual, and psychosocial processes: The collected papers of Milton H. Erickson on hypnosis*, Volume 2. (Edited by E. L. Rossi.) New York: Irvington.

Erickson, M. H. (1980c). *Hypnotic investigation of psychodynamic processes: The collected papers of Milton Erickson on hypnosis*, Volume 3. (Edited by E. L. Rossi.) New York: Irvington.

Erickson, M. H. (1980d). *Innovative hypnotherapy: The collected papers of Milton Erickson on hypnosis*, Volume 4. (Edited by E. L. Rossi). New York: Irvington.

Erickson, M. H., & Rossi, E. L. (1975). Varieties of double bind. *American*

*Journal of Clinical Hypnosis, 17*, 143–157. Reprinted in Erickson (1980a).

Erickson, M. H. & Rossi, E. L. (1977). Autohypnotic experiences of Milton H. Erickson, M.D. *American Journal of Clinical Hypnosis, 20*, 36–54. Reprinted in Erickson (1980a).

Erickson, M. H. & Rossi, E. (1979). *Hypnotherapy: An exploratory casebook.* New York: Irvington.

Erickson, M. H., & Rossi, E. L. (1981). *Experiencing hypnosis.* New York: Irvington.

Erickson, M. H., & Rossi, E. L. (1989). *The February man: Evolving consciousness and identity in hypnotherapy.* New York: Brunner/Mazel.

Erickson, M. H., Rossi, E. L., & Rossi, S. I. (1976). *Hypnotic realities: The clinical hypnosis and forms of indirect suggestions.* New York: Irvington.

Evans, F. J., & Kihlstrom, J. F. (1973). Posthypnotic amnesia as disrupted retrieval. *Journal of Abnormal Psychology, 82*, 317–323.

Forward, S., & Buck, C. (1979). *Betrayal of innocence: Incest and its devastation.* New York: Penguin Books.

Fromm, E. (1956). *The art of loving.* New York: Harper & Row.

Gendlin, E. (1978). *Focusing.* New York: Bantam.

Gendlin, E. T. (1996). *Focusing-oriented psychotherapy: A manual of the experiential method.* New York: Guilford.

Gilligan, S. G. (1981). Ericksonian approaches to clinical hypnosis. In J. K. Zeig (Ed.). *Ericksonian approaches to hypnosis and psychotherapy.* New York: Brunner/Mazel.

Gilligan, S. G. (1982). *Effects of emotional intensity on learning.* Unpublished doctoral dissertation, Stanford University.

Gilligan, S. G., & Bower, G. H. (1984). Cognitive consequences of emotional arousal. In C. E. Izard, J. Kagan, & R. Zajon (Eds.). *Emotions, cognitions, and behavior.* Cambridge, MA: Cambridge Press.

Gilligan, S. G., & Kennedy, C. M. (1984). Solutions and resolutions: Ericksonian hypnotherapy with incest survivor groups. *Journal of Strategic and Systemic Therapy, 8*, 9–17.

Gilligan, S. G. (1985). Generative autonomy: Principles for an Ericksonian hypnotherapy. In J. K. Zeig (Ed.). *Ericksonian psychotherapy, Volume I: Structures.* New York: Brunner/Mazel.

Gilligan, S. G. (1987). *Therapeutic trances: The cooperation principle in Ericksonian hypnotherapy.* New York: Brunner/Mazel.

Gilligan, S. G. (1988a). Psychosomatic healing in Ericksonian hypnotherapy. *Hypnose und kognition, 5*, 25–33.

Gilligan, S. G. (1988b). Symptom phenomena as trance phenomena. In J. K. Zeig & S. Lankton (Eds.). *Developing Ericksonian therapy: State of the art*. New York: Brunner/Mazel.

Gilligan, S. G. (1994). The fight against fundamentalism: Searching for soul in Erickson's legacy. In J. K. Zeig (Ed.). *Ericksonian methods: The essence of the story*. New York: Brunner/Mazel.

Gilligan, S. G. (1996). The relational self: The expanding of love beyond desire. In M. Hoyt (Ed.). *Constructive therapies, Volume 2: Expanding and integrating effective practices*. New York: Guilford.

Gilligan, S. G. (1997). *The courage to love: Principles and practices of self-relations psychotherapy*. New York: Norton.

Glassman, B. (1999). *Bearing witness: A Zen master's lessons in making peace*. New York: Harmony Books.

Gleik, J. (1987). *Chaos: Making a new science*. New York: Penguin Books.

Gordon, D. (1978). *Therapeutic metaphors: Helping others through the looking glass*. Cupertino, CA: Meta Publications.

Gordon, D., & Meyers-Anderson, M. (1981). *Phoenix: Therapeutic patterns of Milton H. Erickson*. Cupertino, CA: Meta Publications.

Haley, J. (1955). Paradoxes in play, fantasy, and psychotherapy. *Psychiatric Res. Rep., 2*, 52–58.

Haley, J. (1963). *Strategies of psychotherapy*. New York: Grune & Stratton.

Haley, J. (1967). *Advanced techniques of hypnosis and therapy: Selected papers of Milton H. Erickson, M.D.* New York: Grune & Stratton.

Haley, J. (1973). *Uncommon therapy: The psychiatric techniques of Milton Erickson, M.D.* New York: Norton.

Haley, J. (1976). *Problem-solving therapy: New strategies for effective family therapy*. San Francisco: Jossey-Bass.

Haley, J. (1984). *Ordeal therapy*. San Francisco: Jossey-Bass.

Haley, J. (1985a). *Conversations with Milton H. Erickson, M.D., Volume 1: Changing individuals*. New York: Norton.

Haley, J. (1985b). *Conversations with Milton H. Erickson, M.D., Volume 2: Changing couples*. New York: Norton.

Haley, J. (1985c). *Conversations with Milton H. Erickson, M.D., Volume 3: Changing children and families*. New York: Norton.

Hall, E. T. (1983). *The dance of life.* New York: Anchor Press/Doubleday.

Hammond, D. C. (1988). Will the real Milton Erickson please stand up? *International Journal of Clinical and Experimental Hypnosis, 36,* 173–181.

Herman, J. (1992). *Trauma and recovery: The aftermath of violence from domestic abuse to political terror.* New York: Basic Books.

Hoffman, L. (1985). Beyond power and control. *Family Systems Medicine, 3,* 381–396.

Huxley, A. (1944). *The perennial philosophy.* New York: Harper & Row.

Imber-Black, E., Roberts, J., and Whiting, R. (1989). *Rituals in families and family therapy.* New York: Norton.

James, W. (1902/1982). *The varieties of religious experience.* London: Penguin Books.

Jeffares, A. N. (Ed.). (1974). *W. B. Yeats: Selected poetry.* London: Pan Books.

Jenkins, A. (1990) *Invitations to responsibility: The therapeutic engagement of men who are violent and abusive.* Adelaide, South Australia: Dulwich Centre Publications.

Jung, C. G. (1916/1971). *The Structure and dynamics of the psyche.* Section on the transcendent function reprinted in J. Campbell (Ed.). *The portable Jung.* New York: Penguin Books.

Jung, C. (1954). *Symbols of transformation.* Princeton, NJ: Princeton University Press.

Jung, C. G. (1964). *Man and his symbols.* New York: Doubleday.

Jung, C. G. (1967). Commentary on "The secret of the golden flower." In H. Read, M. Fordham, & G. Adler (Eds.) and R. F. C. Hull (Trans.). *The collected works of C. G. Jung* (Vol. 14). Princeton, NJ: Princeton University Press. (original work published in 1957).

Justice, B., & Justice, R. (1979). *The broken taboo.* New York: Human Sciences Press.

Keeney, B. (1977). On paradigmatic change: Conversations with Gregory Bateson. Unpublished manuscript.

Keeney, B. (1983). *Aesthetics of change.* New York: Guilford.

Korzybski, A. (1933). *Science and sanity: An introduction to non-Aristotelian systems and general semantics.* Lakeville, CT: The International Non-Aristotelian Library Publishing Company.

Laing, R. D. (1971). *Knots.* New York: Pantheon Books.

Lankton, S. R., & Lankton, C. (1983). *The answer within: A clinical framework for Ericksonian hypnotherapy.* New York: Brunner/Mazel.

Lazarus, R. (1965). *Psychological stress and the coping process.* New York: McGraw-Hill.

Leonard, G. (1978). *The silent pulse.* New York: E. P. Dutton.

Leonard, G. (1991). *Mastery: The keys to success and long-term fulfillment.* New York: Plume Books.

Lynn, S. J., & Rhue, J. W. (Eds.). (1991). *Theories of hypnosis: Current models and perspectives.* New York: Guilford.

Machado, A. (1983). *Times alone: Selected poems of Antonio Machado* (R. Bly, Trans.). Middletown, CT: Wesleyan University Press.

Madanes, C. (1990). *Sex, love, and violence: Strategies for transformation.* New York: Norton.

Mandela, N. (1994). *The long walk to freedom.* London: Little, Brown.

Masters, R., & Houston, J. (1972). *Mind Games.* New York: Dell Publishing.

Maturana, H. R., & Varela, F. J. (1980). *Autopoesis and cognition: The realization of the living.* Dordrecht, Holland: D. Reidel.

Melges, F. T. (1982). *Time and the inner future: A temporal approach to psychiatric disorders.* New York: Wiley.

Merton, T. (1964). *Gandhi on non-violence: A selection from the writings of Mahatma Gandhi.* New York: New Directions.

Moore, R., and Gillette, D. (1990). *King, warrior, magician, lover: Rediscovering the archetypes of the mature masculine.* New York: HarperCollins.

Neruda, P. (1969). Keeping quiet. In *Extravagaria,* A. Reid, translator. London: Farrar, Straus & Giroux.

Nhat Hanh, T. (1975). *The miracle of mindfulness.* Boston: Beacon.

O'Hanlon, B., & Wilk, J. (1987). *Shifting contexts: The generation of effective psychotherapy.* New York: Guilford.

O'Hanlon, W. H., & Weiner-Davis, M. (1988). *In search of solutions: A new direction in psychotherapy.* New York: Norton.

Orne, M. T. (1959). The nature of hypnosis: Artifact and essence. *Journal of Abnormal and Social Psychology, 58,* 277–299.

Orne, M. T. (1966). On the mechanisms of posthypnotic amnesia. *International Journal of Clinical and Experimental Hypnosis, 14,* 121–134.

Ornstein, R. (1969). *On the experience of time.* Baltimore, MD: Penguin Books.

Pagels, E. (1995). *The origin of Satan.* New York: Vintage.

Palmer, W. (1994). *The intuitive body: Aikido as a clairsentient practice.* Berkeley, CA: North Atlantic Books.

Pearce, J. C. (1981). *The bond of power*. New York: E. P. Dutton.

Pearson, C. S. (1989). *The hero within: Six archetypes we live by*. New York: Harper & Row.

Planned Parenthood of San Diego. *One out of 6*. Video presentation by Teen-Image Theater, 1985.

Pribram, K. H. (1971). *Languages of the brain: Experimental paradoxes and principles in neuropsychology*. Englewood Cliffs, NJ: Prentice-Hall.

Richards, M. C. (1962). *Centering: In pottery, poetry, and the person*. Middletown, CT: Wesleyan University Press.

Rilke, R. M. (1981). Moving forward. In R. Bly (Ed.). *Selected poems of Rainer Maria Rilke*. New York: Harper & Row.

Rosenhan, D. L. (1984). On being sane in insane places. In P. Watzlawick (Ed.). *The invented reality: How do we know what we believe we know?* New York: Norton.

Rossi, E. L. (1977). The cerebral hemispheres in analytical psychology. *Journal of Analytical Psychology, 22*, 32–51.

Rossi, E. L. (1986). *The psychobiology of mind-body healing*. New York: Norton.

Rossi, E. L. (1996). *The symptom path to enlightenment*. Pacific Palisades, CA: Palisades Gateway Publishing.

Rossi, E. L., & Cheek, D. B. (1988). *Mind-body therapy: Methods of ideodynamic healing in hypnosis*. New York: Norton.

Rossi, E. L., & Jichaku, P. (1984). Therapeutic and transpersonal double binds: Continuing the legacy of Gregory Bateson and Milton Erickson. Paper presented at the Annual Scientific Meeting of the American Society of Clinical Hypnosis. October, San Francisco.

Rossi, E. L., Ryan, M. O., & Sharp, F. A. (Eds.). (1983). *Healing in hypnosis: The seminars, workshops, and lectures of Milton H. Erickson*. New York: Irvington.

Sacerdote, P. (1982). Techniques for hypnotic intervention with pain patients. In J. Barber & C. Adrian (Eds.). *Psychological approaches to the management of pain*. New York: Brunner/Mazel.

Schwartz, W. (1978). Time and context during hypnotic involvement. *International Journal of Clinical and Experimental Hypnosis, 4*, 307–316.

Selvini Palazzoli, M., Boscolo, L., Cecchin, G. F., & Prata, G. (1978). *Paradox and counterparadox*. New York: Jason Aaronson.

Shapiro, F. (1995). *Eye movement desensitization and reprocessing: Basic principles, protocols, and procedures*. New York: Guilford.

Shapiro, F., & Forrest, M. S. (1997). *EMDR: The breakthrough therapy for overcoming anxiety, stress, and trauma.* New York: Basic Books.

Siddle, D. (1983). *Orienting and habituation: Perspectives in human research.* New York: Wiley.

Some, M. (1994). *Of water and spirit: Ritual, magic, and initiation in the life of an African shaman.* New York: Tarcher.

Spretnak, C. (1997). *The resurgence of the real: Body, nature, and place in a hypermodern world.* Reading, MA: Addison-Wesley.

Steele, B., & Alexander, H. (1981). Long-term effects of sexual abuse in childhood. In P. Mrazek & C. Kempe (Eds.). *Sexually abused children and their families.* Oxford: Pergamon Press.

Tannen, D. (1999). *The argument culture: Stopping America's war of words.* New York: Ballantine Books.

Terr, L. (1994). *Unchained memories: True stories of traumatic memories, lost and found.* New York: Basic Books.

Toms, M. (1994). Writing from the belly: An interview with Isabel Allende. *Common Boundary, 12*(3), 16–23.

Trungpa, C. (1984). *Shambhala: The sacred path of the warrior.* Boston: Shambhala.

Turner, V. (1969). *The ritual process: Structure and anti-structure.* Chicago: Aldine Publishing.

Van der Hart, O. (1983). *Rituals in psychotherapy: Transition and continuity.* New York: Irvington.

Varela, F. J. (1979). *Principles of biological autonomy.* New York: Elsevier North Holland.

von Forester, H. (1984). On constructing a reality. In P. Watzlawick (Ed.). *The invented reality: How do we know what we believe we know?* New York: Norton.

Watts, A. (1961). *Psychotherapy east and west.* New York: Random House.

Watzlawick, P., Beavin, J. H., & Jackson, D. D. (1967). *Pragmatics of human communication: A study of interactional patterns, pathologies and paradoxes.* New York: Norton.

Watzlawick, P., Weakland, J. H., & Fisch, R. (1974). *Change: Principles of problem formation and problem resolution.* New York: Norton.

Wechsler, J. (1979). *On aesthetics in science.* Cambridge, MA: MIT Press.

White, M., & Epston, D. (1990). *Narrative means to therapeutic ends.* New York: Norton.

Whyte, D. (1994). *The heart aroused: Poetry and the preservation of the soul in corporate America.* New York: Currency Doubleday.

Wilbur, K. (1983). *Eye to eye: The quest for the new paradigm.* Garden City, NY: Anchor Books.

Wilson, B. (1967). *As Bill sees it: The AA way of life.* New York: Alcoholics Anonymous World Services.

Woodman, M. (1993). *Conscious femininity: Interviews with Marion Woodman.* Toronto: Inner City Books.

Yapko, M. D. (1988). *When living hurts: Directives for treating depression.* New York: Brunner/Mazel.

Yeats, W. B. (Ed.). (1979). *The poems of William Blake.* London: Routledge & Kegan Paul. (original work published 1905)

Young, A. M. (1972). Consciousness and cosmology. In C. Muse & A. M. Young (Eds.). *Consciousness and reality: The human pivotal point.* New York: Avon Books.

Zeig, J. K. (1980). *A teaching seminar with Milton Erickson.* New York: Brunner/Mazel.

Zeig, J. K. (Ed.). (1982). *Ericksonian approaches to hypnosis and psychotherapy.* New York: Brunner/Mazel.

Zeig, J. K. (Ed.). (1985a). *Ericksonian psychotherapy, Volume 1: Structures.* New York: Brunner/Mazel.

Zeig, J. K. (Ed.). (1985b). *Ericksonian psychotherapy, Volume 2: Clinical applications.* New York: Brunner/Mazel.

Zeig, J. K. (1988). An Ericksonian phenomenological approach to therapeutic hypnotic induction and symptom utilization. In J. K. Zeig and S. R. Lankton (Eds.). *Developing Ericksonian therapy: State of the art.* New York: Brunner/Mazel.

Zeig, J. K. (Ed.). (1994). *Ericksonian methods: The essence of the story.* New York: Brunner/Mazel.

Zeig, J. K., & Lankton, S. R. (1988). *Developing Ericksonian therapy: State of the art.* New York: Brunner/Mazel.

Zimbardo, P. G., Maslach, C., & Marshall, G. (1972). Hypnosis and the psychology of cognitive and behavioral control. In E. Fromm and R. Shor (Eds.). *Hypnosis: Research developments and perspectives.* Chicago: Aldine.

Zukav, G. (1979). *The dancing Wu Li masters.* New York: Bantam Books.

# Index

# Index

# INDEX